Voice Rehabilitation

TESTING HYPOTHESES AND REFRAMING THERAPY

Celia F. Stewart, PhD
Associate Professor
Department of Communicative Sciences and Disorders
Steinhardt School of Culture, Education, and Human Development
New York University

Irene F. Kling, PhD
Assistant Professor
Mannes College
The New School for Music
Kling Voice & Speech-Language Therapy Services, PLLC

Elizabeth L. Allen, PhD
Associate Professor, Retired
Department of Communicative Sciences and Disorders
Steinhardt School of Culture, Education, and Human Development
New York University

JONES & BARTLETT LEARNING

World Headquarters
Jones & Bartlett Learning
5 Wall Street
Burlington, MA 01803
978-443-5000
info@jblearning.com
www.jblearning.com

Jones & Bartlett Learning books and products are available through most bookstores and online booksellers. To contact Jones & Bartlett Learning directly, call 800-832-0034, fax 978-443-8000, or visit our website, www.jblearning.com.

Substantial discounts on bulk quantities of Jones & Bartlett Learning publications are available to corporations, professional associations, and other qualified organizations. For details and specific discount information, contact the special sales department at Jones & Bartlett Learning via the above contact information or send an email to specialsales@jblearning.com.

Production Credits
VP, Executive Publisher: David D. Cella
Publisher: Cathy L. Esperti
Acquisitions Editor: Laura Pagluica
Associate Acquisitions Editor: Sean Fabery
Editorial Assistant: Danielle Bessette
Associate Director of Production: Julie C. Bolduc
Production Assistant: Brooke Appe
Marketing Manager: Grace Richards
VP, Manufacturing and Inventory Control: Therese Connell
Composition: Cenveo® Publisher Services
Cover Design: Michael O'Donnell
Rights and Media Manager: Joanna Lundeen
Rights and Media Research Coordinator: Amy Rathburn
Media Development Assistant: Shannon Sheehan
Cover Image: © Tina Rencelj/Shutterstock
Printing and Binding: Edwards Brothers Malloy
Cover Printing: Edwards Brothers Malloy

To order this product, use ISBN: 978-1-284-07746-9

Library of Congress Cataloging-in-Publication Data
Stewart, Celia F., author.
Voice rehabilitation : testing hypotheses and reframing therapy / by Celia F. Stewart, Irene F. Kling, and Elizabeth L. Allen.
p. ; cm.
ISBN 978-1-284-02225-4 (pbk. : alk. paper)
I. Kling, Irene F., author. II. Allen, Elizabeth L., active 2014, author. III. Title.
[DNLM: 1. Voice Disorders—rehabilitation. WV 500]
RF510
616.85'5606—dc23

2014041124

6048

Printed in the United States of America
19 18 17 16 15 10 9 8 7 6 5 4 3 2 1

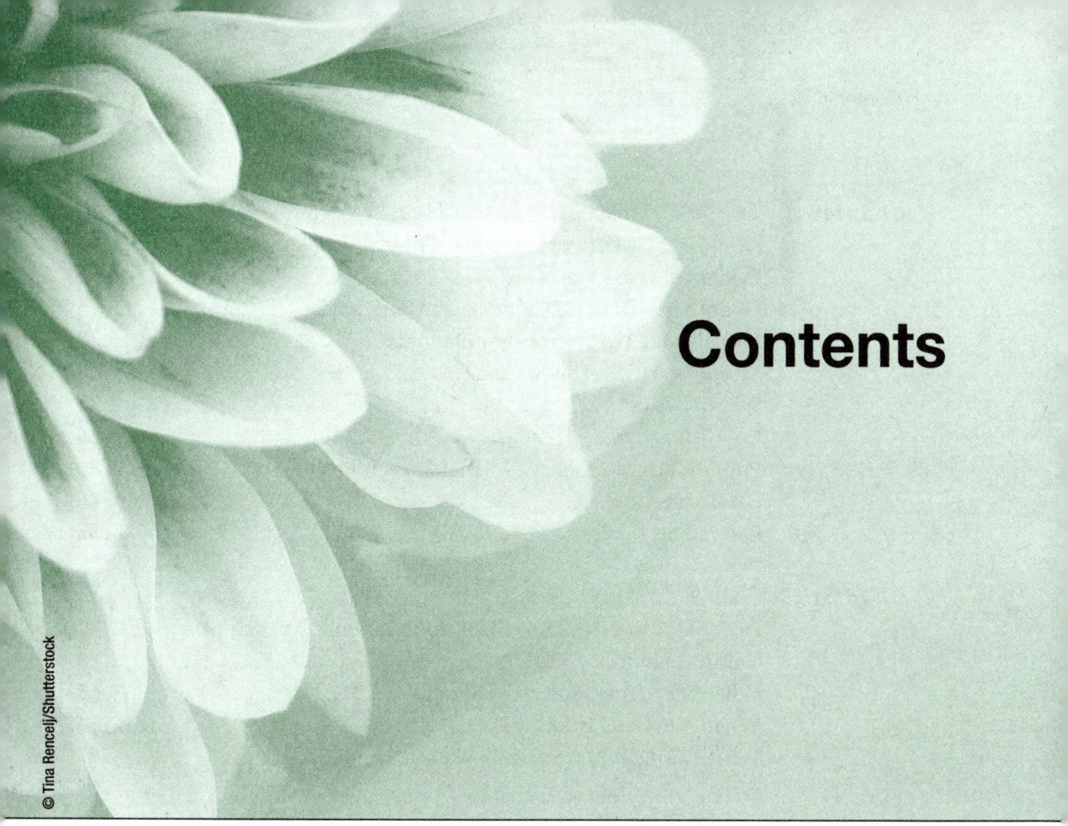

Contents

Preface

© Tina Rencelj/Shutterstock

Over the years, we have found that when we integrate hypothesis development and testing with the physiological underpinnings of voice production, motor learning patterns, and the principles of patient-centered care, our hierarchy of goals and procedures emerges as a logical and cohesive *gestalt*. The application of hypothesis development has made our thinking about the rehabilitation process more flexible and revealed logical connections that would not have been made otherwise. We believe that providing therapy without a theoretical basis is like walking through a room in the dark. Theory turns on the light.

Our goal as we wrote this book was to incorporate these principles into a hypothesis-driven framework that will support your development as a voice clinician. This text is suitable for an advanced graduate course dedicated to voice rehabilitation as well as the clinical practicum that typically follows that course. It is relevant to clinicians beginning to practice voice habilitation and rehabilitation as well as practicing clinicians who continue to develop their skills and reframe their treatment strategies to include the underlying physiological context for the presenting voice problem. Although it presupposes a working understanding of the normal anatomy and physiology of voice production and the laryngeal pathologies associated with voice disorders, we provide a review of the most frequently diagnosed laryngeal pathologies encountered by the voice clinician.

We have included the clinician's internal monologue within several treatment *Dialogues* to demonstrate and clarify the hypothesis-driven, clinical reasoning processes in action. The clinical application of the concepts of hypothesis development and testing, motor learning, physiology, and patient-centered therapy become apparent when the clinician's reasoning is made more explicit. It is also evident that clinical decision making is a logical process when practiced within the hypothesis-driven framework.

We are grateful to our patients and clients who participated in the video recordings and dialogues presented in this book. To protect their privacy and identity during the clinician–patient interactions, we have changed their names and personal details but not their symptoms and responses to treatment. Several of the dialogues are composites based on discussions over several sessions or across patients with similar symptoms.

The *Videos* of individual and group treatment that accompany this text can be accessed at http://go.jblearning.com/voicerehabilitation and have been selected to demonstrate the assessment, rehabilitation, and counseling procedures performed by the clinician and patient/client.

Finally, an Instructor's Manual featuring frameworks for class discussions, case studies, and key chapter terms and concepts is also available to qualified instructors. To gain access, contact your Health Professions Account Specialist at http://go.jblearning.com/findarep.

Acknowledgments

We are grateful to the many people who supported this work. First and foremost, we are indebted to Geoffrey Reid and Charlotte Stewart-Sloan for their ongoing love and unwavering support, insight, and analysis. Without them, this book would not have been possible.

We give special thanks to our students, whose questions have inspired us to deepen our understanding of the process of voice rehabilitation. We hope that this book will provide a direction and support as they develop their clinical skills.

A special thank you to our colleagues in the New York City Voice Study Group whose warmth and generous affirmation of this work gave us immense support.

We thank our patients, who have taught us so much about the treatment process, especially the relationship between patient and clinician.

We appreciate their generosity, allowing us to film their therapy sessions in order to make these video clips available with the text.

We are grateful to Jones & Bartlett Learning for the opportunity to develop this text and for their support, patience, and expertise.

Special thanks to Rick Mowat, Video Editor, Snackpack Productions, for our film clips and for his patience during numerous editing sessions.

© Tina Rencelj/Shutterstock

Reviewers

Karen Ball, MPA, MS, CCC-SLP, BRS-S
Lecturer
Department of Linguistics and Communication Disorders
Queens College, City University of New York
Queens, New York

Vicki L. Hammen, PhD, CCC-SLP
Associate Professor
Department of Communication Disorders and Counseling, School, and Educational Psychology
Indiana State University
Terre Haute, Indiana

Connie K. Keintz, PhD, CCC-SLP
Associate Professor
Department of Communication Sciences and Disorders
Florida Atlantic University
Boca Raton, Florida

Daniel Kempler, PhD
Professor
Department of Communication Sciences and Disorders
Emerson College
Boston, Massachusetts

Julia Rademacher, MM, MA, CCC-SLP
Clinical Assistant Professor
Department of Speech and Hearing Science
Indiana University
Bloomington, Indiana

Angela Bradford Wainwright, PhD, CCC-SLP
Assistant Professor
Center for Urban Education
The University of the District of Columbia
Washington, DC

Judith M. Wingate, PhD, CCC-SLP
Associate Professor
Department of Communication Sciences and Disorders
Jacksonville University
Jacksonville, Florida

Yihe Zu, MD, PhD
Department of Otolaryngology—Head and Neck Surgery
University of Southern California
Los Angeles, California

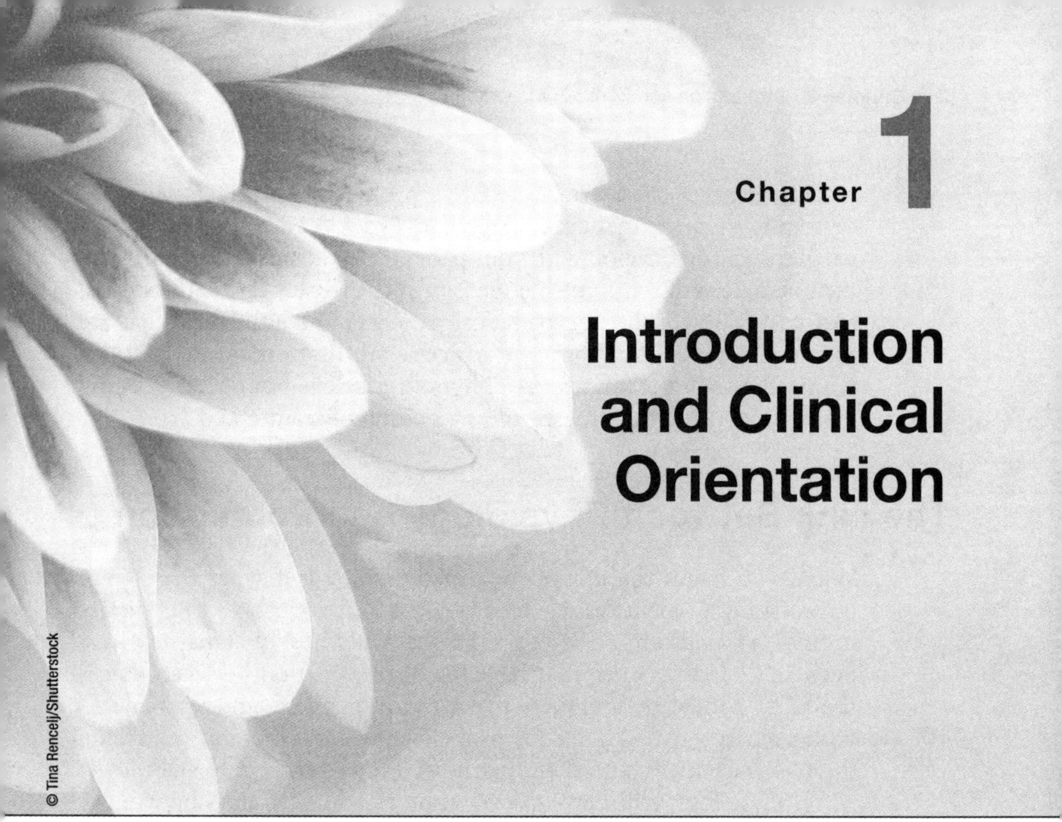

Chapter 1

Introduction and Clinical Orientation

"It is difficult to convince others how deeply voice disorders strike at the heart of the patient's total being and how special voice is in the average person's emotional and intellectual life."
(Aronson, 2009, p. 195)

The Voice

The importance of voice to communication, confidence, and one's identity often becomes evident only when a **voice problem** emerges. The patient experiencing the sudden or gradual onset of a voice disturbance may feel ashamed, embarrassed, isolated, angry, ineffective, helpless, and desperate to regain his normal voice use. The contribution you make to this patient's recovery will be a powerful one that rests on the application of your fund of knowledge as you develop hypotheses, consider the physiological underpinnings of the voice problem, and integrate principles of motor learning to solve problems and make decisions regarding a management plan (Freeman, Syder, & Nicolson, 1996). The partnership you develop with your patient and the **positive regard** you demonstrate will reinforce his sense of **self-efficacy** and **self-esteem**, and will facilitate the perseverance, patience, and adherence that are essential to a successful outcome. **Voice rehabilitation**, when practiced within the scientific framework of **hypothesis development** and testing and with compassion, is a seamless blending of science and art.

The Link Between Physiology and Perception

When you begin the practice of voice therapy it may, at first, seem intimidating to identify the characteristics that contribute to clinically normal or compromised voice production. Until now, you may not have been in a circumstance that requires discrimination between voices produced with effort and those that are **easy**, efficient, and resonant. As with all perceptual skills, your proficiency identifying and describing these characteristics and then linking the voice problem to the underlying physiology will develop over time as you have the opportunity to work with a broad spectrum of patients whose symptoms may not be immediately apparent or who do not follow an expected pattern of vocal behavior. The process of honing your **listening** and discrimination skills takes place as you listen to voices and critically evaluate the **efficiency** or inefficiency of production. These observations provide a starting point for the development of your treatment hypotheses, goals, and subsequent procedures. You then formulate hypotheses regarding the relative contribution of the subsystems of voice production to the manner of **phonation** and the individual's voice problem.

The Student Clinician's Voice

As a clinician, your voice is your most valuable credential. Your patient's first impression of you is, in part, based on his subliminal response to the sound of your voice. His confidence and trust in your skill to guide the treatment process begins when you introduce yourself, and he subconsciously responds to a voice that is produced effectively or one that is produced with effort. These first impressions are critical to the development of the patient's confidence in you, not only as a competent clinician but as someone whose voice exhibits the very qualities that he hopes to acquire.

Until this point, you may have taken your voice for granted. The normalcy of its pitch, loudness, and quality was assumed, but as a **professional voice user** you will now rely on your voice to demonstrate differences between ease and effort as well as consistently and reliably produce various levels of vocal intensity, pitch, and animation over prolonged periods. When you work with children, for instance, your voice will carry heightened enthusiasm and playfulness and will be used to modify the child's behavior. When you remediate an interdental lisp, you will **model** the standard production of the /s/ phoneme appropriately. Similarly, if you treat a patient who suffers from **expressive aphasia**, it is expected that you will produce models and utterances that meet the standard and complexity of the patient's primary language, and that you will modify your level of linguistic complexity to facilitate improvement in the patient's communication skills. Finally, your model of **effective voice** is essential to your patient's development of an appropriate **manner of phonation**. The flexibility required to achieve this goal as you use your voice in a variety of contexts and situations suggests an athletic and artistic coordination between respiration, phonation, resonation, and articulation.

If you habitually use an effortful, pressed manner of phonation, fade into vocal fry, or do not demonstrate vocal models easily and efficiently, how then can you provide an appropriate clinical model of your procedures? Although it may, at first, seem insurmountable to modify your manner of phonation before you begin to work with your patient, this challenge offers an opportunity for growth and clinical development as well as insight into the difficult job that lies ahead for your patient. Insight will contribute to **accurate empathy** (Rogers, 1951) with the patient and facilitate the development of a positive therapeutic relationship.

First Sessions: How Do You Prepare?

What are the options available to you as you develop and improve your model of voice production? Although little can be accomplished overnight, you can work to strengthen your **kinesthetic awareness**, your appropriate and effective models of voice procedures, and your physiologically-based rationales for procedures. A supervisor or colleague whose specialty is voice disorders may spend time with you modeling and shaping a more efficient production of techniques and/or suggest that you begin voice therapy while you are working with your patient. Certainly, your motivation to improve your manner of phonation and vocal flexibility will be high in order to meet the challenges presented by your patients. The work you do to develop these skills can only enhance your kinesthetic and physiological awareness as well as your insight into the process of change, thus facilitating your development as a competent clinician.

Your work with a supervisor or colleague to establish and habituate an appropriate clinical model of voice production can be further reinforced if you practice your chosen procedures independently. This practice may be remarkably similar to the therapy you provide for your patient. As you continue to practice, you will reflect on and rationalize the purpose of your chosen procedures in order to integrate your knowledge into the therapeutic process.

What is the most effective way to practice? Repetition, in and of itself, without attention to particular objectives will not only fall short of developing an appropriate clinical model for your patient, but may reinforce old, counterproductive habits. **Deliberate practice** (Ericsson, Krampe, & Tesch-Romer, 1993), on the other hand, is an entirely different experience. It is thoughtful and active. During deliberate practice you experiment with your manner of phonation, monitor and modify when necessary, and gradually improve the ease, consistency, and effectiveness of your model.

The time, patience, concentration, and attention required during deliberate practice can be fatiguing, especially given the coordination required to control and modify phonation as the phonemic contexts change. We ask our patients to practice for only two to three minutes at a time (but hourly) outside of therapy in order to maximize and maintain the high level of concentration and focus required during deliberate practice. Your practice sessions will be most effective if you follow a similar schedule with frequent, highly focused practice during the day in order to build the necessary **memory traces** that eventually construct a durable motor memory.

Memorization can be a useful way to acquire specific, concrete information quickly. It is very difficult, however, for most people to access that memorized information over time and then integrate and apply it. It is common, for instance, for a student clinician to memorize the directions for a procedure in preparation for its introduction, rather than integrating the kinesthetic, tactile, and motor patterns into a sensory-memory trace. In a face-to-face session, however, the memory of specific steps alone will not be enough to address the varied and individual responses that the patient may demonstrate, and these responses will require explanation, rationale, further description, and additional clinical modeling from you. To avoid this pitfall, take the time you need to practice the procedures you intend to use until you are confident that you know what sensations to expect and attend to during the procedure and can link that sensitivity to your knowledge of normal anatomy and physiology. It is necessary to practice a procedure until it becomes an appropriate clinical model even under pressure (i.e., when the patient is asking you to rationalize your procedures).

Motor learning theory provides a useful framework as you prepare to meet the challenges associated with introducing, describing, and then demonstrating new procedures to a patient. It suggests that attention to movement and behavior, deliberate practice (repetition), and use of a newly acquired motor skill (i.e., **motor program**) in a variety of contexts leads to integration and generalization. As you practice a procedure or new vocal behavior, you focus your awareness on what you feel in the larynx, neck, and respiratory subsystem. You will note variation among the trials of the specific procedures, and if you **attend to** those differences you can determine whether they are related to changes in your level of effort. Your mind continues to evaluate, analyze, and problem solve as you continue to practice the procedure on your own and, perhaps, with a peer clinician. As you practice and repeat procedures and attend to the motor differences between productions, you will attain consistency and reliability in the clinical model you eventually demonstrate to your patient. The next level brings an awareness of the smaller, fine motor adjustments that you make as you fine-tune your manner of phonation. Eventually, you will assimilate these new motor patterns and achieve a level of confidence that allows you to think on your feet during your interaction with the patient.

You may feel awkward when you begin to practice new procedures, but this feeling is a natural one as you work to develop and gain control of a new motor skill. Later on, when you introduce a new procedure and describe and demonstrate it to your patient, you will be under some pressure to perform. It would not be unusual under this circumstance for the motor skill that you have acquired only recently to be affected by the performance anxiety you experience as you attempt to provide education and integrate clinical modeling, **modification**, and feedback in these early sessions.

Therapeutic Procedures for the Beginning Clinician

As you prepare to work with your patient it may be useful to begin the process with procedures that address the symptoms most commonly observed in patients with voice problems. Exercises that facilitate the optimum coordination among the vocal subsystems (respiration, phonation, resonation, and articulation) will always be useful as you expand your therapeutic repertoire. These procedures are deceptively simple and your early attempts should be monitored by a specialist in voice before you practice them on your own. Nevertheless, we believe that one of the best ways to become confident and comfortable with voice exercises is to practice and perform them in a turn-taking format with a colleague. Given that so many voice problems are associated with excessive medial compression of the vocal folds we have provided several **back pressure** exercises that you can practice to build your kinesthetic awareness.

Although some voice patients will not demonstrate stiffness in the jaw, it is not unusual for jaw stiffness to co-occur with a voice problem. Given the frequency with which we have observed this common **counterproductive compensation**, we have included two jaw release exercises that are useful when you observe this behavior or when your patient reports discomfort or restriction in range of motion. The following procedures reduce **extraneous muscle activity** in the head, neck, and thorax (e.g., jaw release procedures) (Angsuwarangsee & Morrison, 2002) and increase **supraglottal pressure** by creating a semi-occlusion in the anterior portion of the **vocal tract** (Titze, 2006).

The jaw release exercises demonstrated on the film clips set the larynx up for easy and effective voice use. They work well, not only as a warm-up at the beginning of a session, but if you observe re-emergence of inefficient vocal behaviors during your patient's connected speech production. These procedures are useful early in the therapeutic process because they require little voluntary control from the patient, almost "tricking the larynx" to decrease **subglottal pressure**, medial compression, and stiffness of the vocal folds.

Jaw Release Exercises

Tightening or clenching the jaw can indirectly stiffen the muscles that support the larynx. When you release the jaw (including the masseters, pterygoid, and orbicularis oris muscles), the larynx has an opportunity to lower in the neck to its resting position (Sundberg, 1977) and, when appropriate, to rise and fall during phonation and swallowing. This released posture supports a more flexible and dynamic production of voice. When the jaw is released it drops "slightly downward and backward" (Chapman, 2012, p. 123), releasing the muscles surrounding the temporomandibular joint (TMJ).

Below are two procedures that effectively release the jaw. Certainly, there are numerous methods that achieve the same goal (the **Alexander Technique** [Leibowitz & Connington, 1990], the **Feldenkrais Method** [Nelson & Blades-Zeller, 2002], etc.). The following techniques facilitate awareness of stiffness in the jaw, decrease that stiffness, and, with deliberate practice, promote a new (released) customary mandibular carriage. You can adapt these exercises or develop new ones to meet your patient's specific needs.

The jaw release exercises should be integrated into a daily practice routine. If you draw your patient's attention to the jaw, he may notice that he maintains an appropriate **freeway space** (~2–4 mm between the upper and lower teeth) (Fenn, Liddelow, & Gimson, 1961; Johnson, Wildgoose, & Wood, 2002) following the exercise and finds that the posture of the jaw (at rest) remains released. He can check the status of the jaw periodically to see if the upper and lower teeth remain separated, or if the clenching returns as the session progresses or when he is under stress. Over time and with deliberate practice, the muscles will develop a new sensory memory, as the stiffness originally felt in the cheeks and temporomandibular joint areas diminishes. This released position is the normal rest position for the jaw for all activities except chewing and producing sounds that require close approximation of the upper and lower teeth (e.g., /s/).

Although the following jaw release exercises (**Boxes 1-1** and **1-2**) lead to similar results, the time required for each one varies. The first exercise is a good choice when you have the time to allow *gravity* to work and your patient needs a deep release in the musculature. The Modified Jaw Release Exercise (Box 1-2) can be easily integrated into daily life because it takes only a few moments and can be done often and in any setting. The following procedures are presented as though you are speaking directly to the patient.

The *Jaw Release Exercise* video provides a model of the clinician's facilitation of the procedure and the patient's response to it. The directions should be modified to meet your patient's needs.

Box 1-1

Jaw Release Exercise

This exercise uses time and gravity to release the jaw. No active (muscular) work is required.

1. Sit comfortably in a chair with your eyes closed, shoulders released, and thighs settling heavily into the chair. Breathe easily and naturally.
2. Clench your teeth and hold for a moment; feel the tightness inside your mouth.
3. Release the jaw (allow the jaw to be limp). Allow time and gravity to lower the jaw for you. Your jaw feels heavier and heavier. Even the lower lip and chin begin to feel heavy. As you let time pass and gravity work, the muscles in the cheeks begin to let go, and the jaw releases more and more. The muscles simply cannot hold the jaw up (and you are not going to try).
4. Feel the heaviness in the tongue as it rests on the floor of your mouth.
5. Allow the jaw to descend as far as it can comfortably go. Tilt the head back slightly (only as far as you are comfortable). Remember to allow the jaw to release as the head tilts back. Feel the stretch in your jaw while the head is tilted back.
6. After a few moments, slowly bring the head back to the rest position (the jaw is now parallel with the floor). Pay attention to the sensations in your lower face. Following your first attempt, you may notice that your jaw feels somewhat freer.

Nota bene: For optimum benefit the jaw release exercise should be performed at least twice daily in order to habituate the new released posture.

Box 1-2

Modified Jaw Release Exercise

This exercise is used to release the jaw to the neutral, rest position.

1. Sit comfortably with your feet flat on the floor. Rub your hands together rapidly to warm them.
2. Close your eyes and gently cup your jaw so that it rests in the warm palms of your hands.
3. Ask your jaw to release and allow the teeth to part slightly. You can now feel the freeway space of ~2–4 mm between the teeth.
4. Gently remove your hands without adjusting your jaw and note what you feel in your jaw.

Nota bene: The exercise can be used during a session to set the larynx up for an easy manner of phonation prior to voicing exercises. Hourly practice during the day will reinforce a more released posture. Over time and with deliberate practice, your jaw will maintain this released position with only the mental suggestion of release.

As you view the *Modified Jaw Release Exercise* video, note the small adjustments in the jaw and the change in facial expression following release of the jaw.

Back Pressure (Supraglottal Pressure/Semi-occluded Vocal Tract) Exercises

The term *back pressure* is derived from fluid mechanics to describe any **resistance** that opposes the flow of a fluid or gas through a tube, such as coolant in an air-conditioning unit, exhaust through a muffler, arterial blood flow (Archie, 1977), or air particles through the vocal tract. When a tube lengthens, bends, twists, narrows, or closes, resistance to the movement of the fluid or gas increases. When applied to voice production, this phenomenon releases stiffness in the vocal tract.

If voice is produced with excessive stiffness and **medial compression of the vocal folds**, and if the vocal tract is stiff (i.e., excessive constriction of the **epilarynx**, hypercontraction of the pharyngeal muscles), the manner of phonation will be compromised. An increase in back pressure (resistance that occurs when the flow of air from the lungs is slowed due to constriction in the vocal tract) will release the laryngeal and pharyngeal musculature without any direct voluntary control (Chapman, 2012; Laukkanen, Titze, Hoffman, & Finnegan, 2008; Titze, 2006).

The following back pressure exercises in **Boxes 1-3** to **1-6** lead to similar results and are interchangeable. Your choice of procedure will depend on the amount of physical space you have to perform the exercise (airway reflex), or if you are sitting at a desk with

Box 1-3

Airway Reflex Exercise

1. Stand in a relaxed manner with your arms at your sides.
2. Slowly raise your arms above your head like a bird gently flapping its wings as you inhale through your nose. The elevation of your arms reinforces the expansion of the chest wall as you inhale.
3. Using a strong expiratory drive, sustain the /tʃ/ (church) sound (like air escaping from the brakes of a bus or train, which creates a strong resistance at the level of the teeth and velopharyngeal port), as you simultaneously lower your arms to your sides. As you lower your arms, maintain the expanded, lifted posture (Franco et al., 2014) that you achieved when you raised your arms.

Nota bene: Repeat this procedure no more than *three times per hour*, in order to avoid dizziness (hyperventilation). The procedure should be performed at several intervals throughout the day in order to maximize its effectiveness by creating a new muscle memory.

Box 1-4

Back Pressure Exercise

This exercise uses a small diameter hollow, stir-straw cut to a length of 2.5 inches.

1. Place the small diameter stir-straw between your lips.
2. Inhale deeply through your nose.
3. Blow steadily through the stir-straw (without voicing).
4. Notice the changes in your throat.

Nota bene: This exercise should be performed *only once per hour* because the stir-straw creates a high level of back pressure, which may lead to dizziness if repeated. It can be performed several times throughout the day.

Laukkanen, A.M., Titze, I.R., Hoffman, H., and Finnegan, E., 2008.

others present (straw phonation, puffy cheeks). It is useful to alternate between these exercises to add variety and develop several ways to increase back pressure. In addition, some patients respond better to one procedure than another.

The patient's demonstration in the *Airway Reflex Exercise* video is produced with a fluid movement of the arms and a **semi-occluded vocal tract**. Note the strong expiratory drive during production of the /tʃ/ phoneme and the continuation of the released, open posture as the arms lower to the sides (Franco et al., 2014). If you practice with the video you may note the high back pressure and expansion through your upper torso.

Box 1-5

Straw Phonation

1. Place a drinking straw (that is 2.5 mm wide) between the lips.
2. Sustain a quiet phonation through the straw on a comfortable pitch. (This procedure can be varied with ascending and descending glides, crescendo and decrescendo [*messa di voce* and singing a simple tune).

Nota bene: This exercise creates high back pressure to facilitate easy, efficient phonation. It can be repeated several times throughout a session and the day.

Laukkanen, A.M., Titze, I.R., Hoffman, H., and Finnegan, E., 2008; Titze, I.R., 2006.

Box 1-6

Puffy Cheeks Exercise

The Puffy Cheeks Exercise creates a high back pressure (supraglottal pressure) with little need for voluntary control or skill on the part of the participant. An aspirated /hw/ (as in the words *what* and *where* as produced in England or Scotland) creates a tight constriction of the lips, a reflexive release of the pharyngeal and oral musculature, and contributes to efficient self-oscillation of the vocal folds.

1. As you form a tight constriction at the lips, puff the cheeks and begin phonation of the /hw/.
2. The cheeks remain inflated while you sustain the /hw/, but slowly deflate with continued phonation.
3. You will be aware of a release in the facial musculature as the buccal area and the space between the teeth and the lips expands.
4. If you place your finger in front of the lips you will feel the release of air as you phonate.

Nota bene: This exercise not only establishes a high back pressure, but it primes the larynx for an easy manner of phonation. For maximum benefit, it should be performed several times throughout the day.

Chapman, J., 2012.

The patient in the *Puffy Cheeks Exercise* video experiences a decrease in extraneous muscle activity in the head, neck, and thorax. Note the high back pressure as you imitate her model and sustain the /hw/ through a very small lip opening.

Summary

During your development as a voice clinician, you will strengthen your knowledge base, enhance your perceptual observations, fine-tune your clinical models (kinesthetic sensitivity), and build the confidence and experience you need to provide effective and insightful feedback. You will use several theoretical constructs and approaches to critical reasoning in order to support the decisions you make when you create a hierarchy of goals and procedures. When you use a theoretical model to rationalize the choices you make, you will understand the "why" and "how" of your choices.

References

Angsuwarangsee, T., and Morrison, M. (2002). Extrinsic laryngeal muscular tension in patients with voice disorders. *Journal of Voice, 16*, 333–343.

Archie, J.P. (1977). Hemodynamics of carotid back pressure and cerebral flow during endarterectomy. *Journal of Surgical Research*, 23, 223–232.

Aronson, A.E., and Bless, D. (2009). *Clinical Voice Disorders: An Interdisciplinary Approach*. New York, NY: Thieme.

Chapman, J. (2012). *Singing and teaching singing: A holistic approach to classical voice* (2nd ed.). San Diego, CA: Plural.

Ericsson, K.A., Krampe, R.T., and Tesch-Romer, C. (1993). The role of deliberate practice in the acquisition of expert performance. *Psychological Review*, 100(3), 363–406.

Fenn, H.R., Liddelow, K.P., and Gimson, A.P. (1961). *Clinical dental prosthetics* (2nd ed.). London, England: Staples Press.

Franco, D., Martins, F., Andrea, M., Fragoso, I., Carrao, L., and Teles, J. (2014). Is the sagittal postural alignment different in normal and dysphonic adult speakers? *Journal of Voice*, 28(4), 523.e1–523.e8.

Freeman, M., Syder, D., and Nicolson, R. (1996). Bridging the gap between theory and practice: A multimedia tutorial for students of voice therapy. *Journal of Voice*, 10(3), 292–298.

Johnson, A., Wildgoose, D.G., and Wood, D.J. (2002). The determination of freeway space using two different methods. *Journal of Oral Rehabilitation*, 29, 1010–1013.

Laukkanen, A.M., Titze, I.R., Hoffman, H., and Finnegan, E. (2008). Effects of a semi-occluded vocal tract on laryngeal muscle activity and glottal adduction in a single female subject. *Folia Phoniatrica et Logopedica*, 60, 298–311.

Leibowitz, J., and Connington, B. (1990). *The Alexander technique*. New York, NY: Harper Perennial.

Nelson, S.H., and Blades-Zeller, E. (2002). *Singing with your whole self: The Feldenkrais method and voice*. Lanham, MD: Scarecrow Press.

Rogers, C.R. (1951). *Client-centered therapy: Its current practice, implications, and theory*. Boston, MA: Houghton Mifflin.

Sundberg, J. (1977). Studies of the soprano voice. *Journal of Research in Singing*, 25–35.

Titze, I.R. (2006). Theoretical analysis of maximum flow declination rate versus maximum area declination rate in phonation. *Journal of Speech, Language, and Hearing Research*, 49, 439–447.

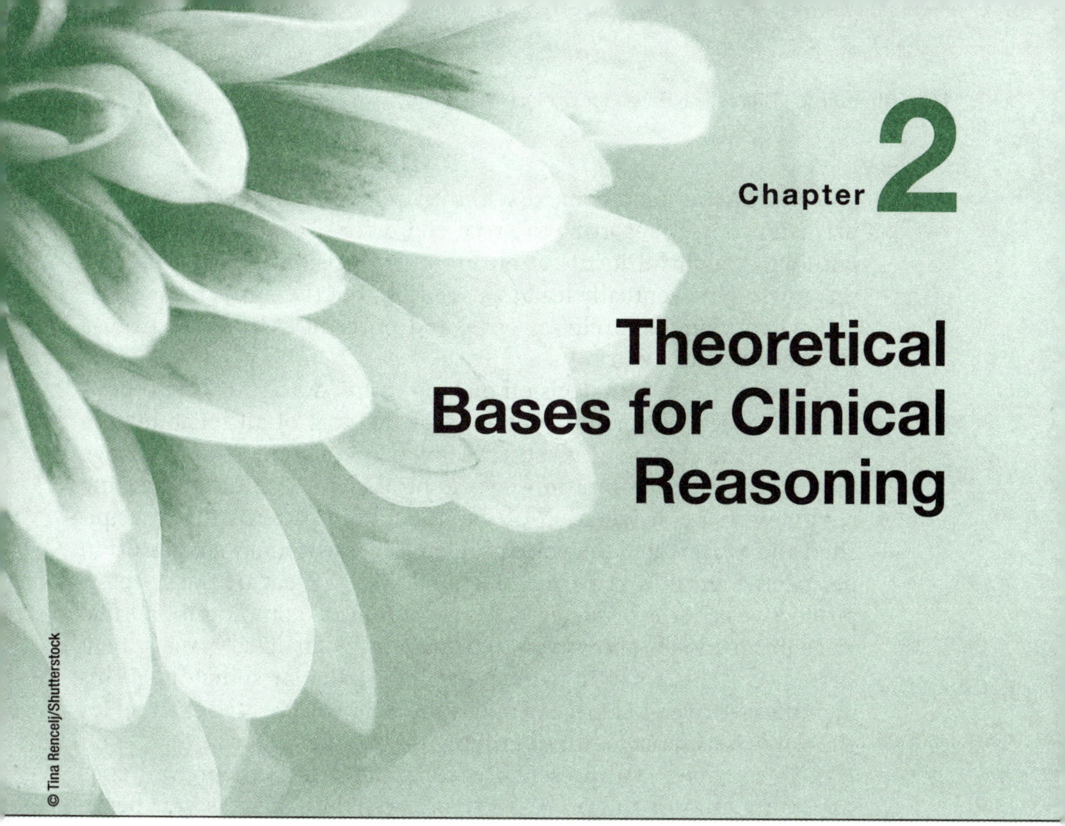

Chapter 2

Theoretical Bases for Clinical Reasoning

"Only as experiment and tentative theory are together articulated
to a match does the discovery emerge and the theory become a paradigm."
(Kuhn, 1970, p. 61)

How Do I Use Theory to Solve Clinical Problems?

At this point in your training, you have developed a good theoretical background in the anatomy and physiology of normal and disordered voice production, but you have little practical experience in the management of voice disorders. How, then, do you develop a hierarchy of goals and procedures if you have not yet had this experience? How do you answer your patient's questions competently? If your first question to yourself is, "What am I going to do?" you are focusing on procedures without a context within which to frame them, and you may find yourself resorting to a trial-and-error selection of techniques without thoughtful justification for your decisions. Trial-and-error therapy might eventually lead to a solution, but therapy is most effective when your hierarchy of goals and procedures emerges from a **theoretical framework.**

The subtle shift in decision making from "doing" to "hypothesis testing" reflects the critical notion that the goal of all rehabilitation is to facilitate change. If you ask, "How can I help my patient change the behaviors that compromise voice production?" critical reasoning begins with a consideration of the underlying patterns that precipitated and exacerbated the voice problem. This seemingly small shift in perspective from "What am I going to do?" to "What are the counterproductive patterns that triggered and continue to compromise normal voice production?" allows you to plan an individualized management strategy for this specific patient and his particular symptoms. This hypothesis-driven perspective opens the door to a creative channel for choosing, developing, and modifying therapeutic procedures.

This chapter will present and integrate several theoretical constructs to support the process of voice rehabilitation as you begin to plan a management strategy: evidence-based practice, hypothesis development, **motor learning theory**, and the **physiology of voice production**. These models are meant to facilitate the decision-making process by providing a foundation from which your goals, procedures, and rationalizations will emerge. As you become comfortable using theory to support the treatment process you will, no doubt, incorporate additional theoretical constructs.

You may not realize that you are already using theory to support you as you prepare your treatment plan. If, for instance, you describe the rationale for the Airway Reflex Exercise to your patient, you are incorporating a physiological model and using your expertise. When you ask the patient to attend to how an exercise feels, you are incorporating motor learning and kinesthetic sensitivity. That is to say, you are using an organizing principle to develop, explain, and support the procedures you have chosen. As you gain confidence and experience, these conscious and deliberate choices will flow from one to another and become subconscious as you respond to the patient in the here and now.

Evidence-Based Practice

As Kent (2006) suggests, "theory is important to connect facts and to formulate testable hypotheses" (p. 269). **Evidence-based practice (EBP)** encourages the clinician to read and interpret research and to link theory and data from the literature with clinical expertise in order to determine the most appropriate course of therapy. The concept of EBP emerged in the medical profession, providing a context within which to identify and measure progress as well as effectiveness of treatment. Based on a **disease-oriented approach**, EBP relied on scientific evidence and clinical experience to establish the most appropriate treatment.

In the past several years, practitioners have begun to include the patient not only as a *partner* in the treatment process, but as an *expert* whose perspective is critical to the resolution of the problem. When you incorporate the patient-centered model into EBP, you filter information through the eyes of the patient and tailor the treatment to his specific needs—his preferences, life experience, perceptions, and expectations (Ratner, 2006). As clinical expertise, appropriate research evidence, and the client/patient perspective of the problem merged with EBP, it became a more humane approach and spread to other disciplines including psychology, physical therapy, and speech-language pathology.

If you consider that theoretical constructs govern treatment across professions, you have the option to connect theoretical constructs across professional disciplines to enrich and guide your voice treatment. When you integrate theory and research from related areas into your practice of voice therapy, they will inform and shape your practice. This inclusive perspective fosters a broader, more inclusive view of the voice patient and his voice problem from several vantage points. Fortunately, a wide variety of approaches and procedures are available to address voice problems. Most voice clinicians use EBP as they develop a multidimensional, eclectic approach that links personal, clinical experience with scientific evidence and patient concerns to make decisions regarding clinical practice (Chan, McCabe, & Madill, 2013).

Hypothesis-Driven Diagnosis and Therapy

The scientific method provides a sound framework for voice treatment and can be adapted to plan, execute, and evaluate the accuracy of your **assessment** and the success of your treatment (Maxwell & Satake, 2006). Simply stated, the scientific method (**hypothesis-driven therapy**) encourages a clinician to identify and describe clinical problems, to develop hypotheses regarding the origins of the voice problem, to devise appropriate hierarchies and methods of treatment, and to collect data and assess the effectiveness of the treatment based on the outcomes.

What Is a Hypothesis and How Is It Conceived?

A hypothesis is a simple declarative statement that incorporates cause and effect and can be tested (Bowen, 2006). The statement is based on behavior, not judgment or assumption. Hypothesis-driven therapy sets the stage for the critical reasoning process as you observe behavior, listen to the voice, take the history, and incorporate the patient's perspective in your management plan.

At first, it may be difficult to distinguish between judgments based on assumption and behavioral observations that can be tested. Nevertheless, it is necessary to distinguish between them in order to formulate a hypothesis-driven treatment plan that is guided by problem solving. For example, when you choose a procedure, you hypothesize that it will yield a change in the patient's vocal behavior. You then observe the patient's response to the procedure (data collection), and based on his response you accept or reject your hypothesis.

If your cat is yowling, you might make the following hypothesis. *The cat is yowling because it has not been fed today.* (Not: *the cat likes to eat, the cat is unhappy,* or *something is wrong with the cat.* None of these hypotheses is testable.) When testing the hypothesis that *the cat is yowling because it has not been fed today,* you use behavioral observations to discover whether the cat has, in fact, been fed today. If you observe that it has fresh food in the dish, you will reject your hypothesis, especially if you know from many past observations that your cat eats its food as soon as it sees it. Similarly, if you find the cat's dish empty, you cannot accept the hypothesis—you must feed your cat—because you know that it eats the food when the bowl touches the floor. After you feed your cat, if it stops yowling you can accept your hypothesis. But, if it does not stop yowling, you must reject your hypothesis and modify or develop a new one, such as *the cat is yowling because the food is spoiled, the cat is yowling because it has a thorn in its paw,* and so on. Each of these hypotheses is testable through observation of a behavioral change. **Table 2-1** illustrates two methods of describing behavior: judgment/assumption or cause and effect.

Table 2-1 Assumption Versus Hypothesis

Judgment or Assumption (Not Testable)	Observable Cause-and-Effect Hypothesis (Testable)
The server is clumsy.	The server dropped the tray because it was wet.
The baby is hungry.	The baby is crying because he has not been fed today.
The girl is cold.	The girl is shivering because the temperature is 40 degrees.
The dog is thirsty.	The dog is barking because he has no water.
The patient is aggressive.	The patient exhibits stridency due to laryngeal and supralaryngeal constriction.
The patient is anxious.	The patient uses **abrupt onset of phonation** because of high **subglottal pressure** and excessive medial compression of the vocal folds.

You can develop hypotheses related to voice disturbances based on your knowledge of the normal system, manner of phonation, anatomical changes, and the characteristics of the dysphonia/**aphonia**. You can test those hypotheses in many ways—you can ask the patient to engage in specific behaviors, observe the results of those activities, or ask for feedback from the patient regarding how his throat feels during those procedures. If the results support your hypothesis, you accept it, and if the results do not support your hypothesis, you modify or reject it in favor of a new one. *This process is known as voice rehabilitation.*

When testing a hypothesis related to a voice problem, one applies **empirical observations** that are based on behavior and that can be evaluated according to its severity (e.g., mild, moderate, severe) and characteristics. For instance, when assessing a patient's manner of phonation you might observe extraneous muscle activity in the head and neck (clenching of the jaw and tightening of the strap muscles) (Angsuwarangsee & Morrison, 2002). Your understanding of phonatory control informs you that stiffness of the jaw can have a negative impact on both the singing and speaking voice—elevating the hyoid bone and larynx, increasing stiffness in the **tongue base**, and leading to undifferentiated movement of these structures (Chapman, 2012; Dimon, 2011). Such stiffness involves the jaw in the pitch raising mechanism, and negatively affects articulatory precision (Chapman, 2012). Based on these observations, you hypothesize that a decrease in jaw stiffness will facilitate independent movement of the jaw, tongue, and larynx. You test your hypothesis by asking your patient to perform the Jaw Release Exercise or the Modified Jaw Exercise. Immediately following several demonstrations of the procedure, you observe a decrease in the stiffness and fixed posture of the jaw, tongue, and larynx accompanied by reduced effort in the manner of phonation. Based on this observable, behavioral change, you accept your hypothesis. Conversely, if the patient performed the Modified Jaw Exercise several times and the stiffness in the jaw and larynx did not abate, you would reject or modify your hypothesis and choose an alternate hypothesis to address the problem.

Vocal symptoms can be similar across pathologies. Without hypotheses and a grasp of the underlying physiology, you may overlook individual differences among patients, fail to notice detrimental vocal behaviors, and possibly misunderstand or misinterpret the rationale for a given procedure's success or failure with a specific patient. The flowchart in **Figure 2-1** illustrates an example of hypothesis-driven decision making for continuing or rejecting a treatment hypothesis.

With the accumulation of practical experience, the current research evidence, and the conscious application of a hypothesis-driven approach, you will begin to retrieve information from memory of previous patients to assist in the identification and treatment of the

Figure 2-1

Flow Chart of Hypothesis Development and Testing

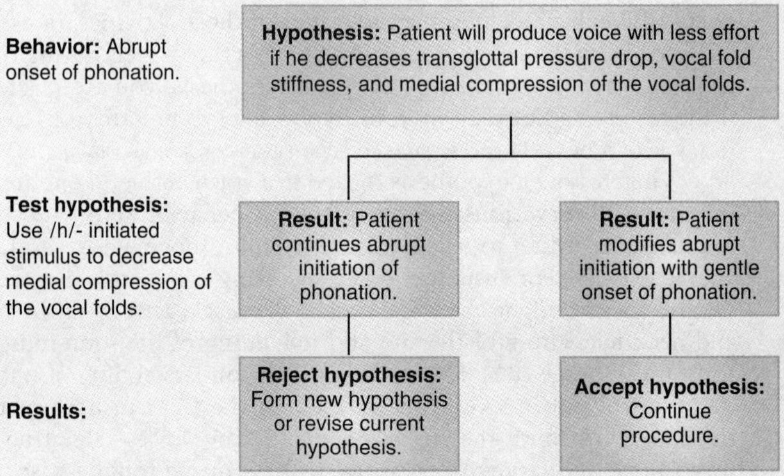
Behavior: Abrupt onset of phonation.
Hypothesis: Patient will produce voice with less effort if he decreases transglottal pressure drop, vocal fold stiffness, and medial compression of the vocal folds.
Test hypothesis: Use /h/- initiated stimulus to decrease medial compression of the vocal folds.
Result: Patient continues abrupt initiation of phonation.
Result: Patient modifies abrupt initiation with gentle onset of phonation.
Results:
Reject hypothesis: Form new hypothesis or revise current hypothesis.
Accept hypothesis: Continue procedure.

source of effort. Hypothesis development will become second nature, and your hypotheses will be richer and more complex, allowing you to discern patterns in symptomology and behavior that enhance the clinical reasoning process (Mandin, Jones, Woloschuk, & Harasym, 1997).

Models and Theoretical Frameworks

Motor learning theory, cognition, self-regulation, and vocal physiology provide a context from which you and your patient will develop the goals that inform your treatment plan. These models account for the process of skill acquisition, stabilization, and the expected, temporary fluctuations in performance that we observe as the patient works to achieve automaticity. In the following sections we will examine these theories and their application to voice habilitation and rehabilitation.

Motor Learning Theory

As you begin to implement procedures and test hypotheses that directly address vocal fold vibration, it will be useful to think about how individuals learn and incorporate new motor patterns of behavior into daily life. Your patient has spent a lifetime acquiring and perfecting a variety of common motor skills such as riding a bike, rollerblading, typing, drawing, standing in the shower with eyes closed, finding keys in a bag without looking, or knowing where the light switch is in the dark. He may be a singer, functioning at an elite level of performance with a specialized knowledge of how he produces his singing voice (but not his speaking voice), or he may be a customary voice user with little conscious awareness of how he uses his speaking voice. During your initial meeting, he may tell you that he learns best with tactile feedback, with observation, by doing, by listening, or that he learns cognitively and benefits from verbal rationales and analogies in order to process and integrate new motor patterns. He may even say that he is completely unaware of how he learns. Regardless of his preferred learning style or level of awareness, *your* continued observation and consideration of his learning style will facilitate a clinical integration of motor learning theory and motor control as you make treatment decisions. The choice of the appropriate sensory mode to match the procedure (e.g., **tactile-kinesthetic**, visual), the patient's learning style, and level of awareness takes vigilance and a conscious intention that becomes an implicit, subconscious part of your thinking as you gain clinical experience.

Motor Learning Theory: Historical Context

Schmidt and Lee (2011), define motor learning as a process that takes place as a result of deliberate practice and repetition of a specific sequence of motor patterns, eventuating in the "relatively permanent" (p. 327) capacity to execute a skilled movement. The integration of the countless individual components of motor learning rests on a foundation of cognitive processes, including attention, concentration, focus, working memory, task perseverance, executive function, and self-regulation (Adams, 1971; Vinney & Turkstra, 2013). The study and application of motor learning concepts crosses many disciplines and involves the acquisition, modification, consolidation, and habituation of skilled movements such as walking, typing, dancing, drawing, writing one's signature, playing the violin, and voice production. This process ultimately leads to the acquisition of a skilled movement via shaping the movement (reinforcing or modifying), stabilizing the movement (accounting for temporary variability in performance of the movement), reinforcing the accuracy of the movement (identifying the range of accepted performance), realizing the automaticity of the movement, and generalizing the movement within more and more challenging situations (Schmidt & Lee, 2011). Of course, some individuals develop greater motor control than others and evolve into highly trained athletes who can not only walk but walk on a tightrope, not only drive a car but race cars, or those who not only learn to speak effortlessly but are vocal professionals who are sought after as singers, actors, and voiceover artists.

Closed- and Open-Loop Theories of Motor Learning

Our discussion of motor learning begins with a description of closed- and **open-loop theories** of the acquisition of skilled movement. Adams (1971) hypothesized that motor control develops with the practice of a specific movement. Each time the movement is performed, a memory trace remains so that with repetition the memory trace strengthens and a motor template is developed. A closed-loop system uses proprioceptive and sensorimotor feedback to monitor and shape a new behavior during its acquisition. According to the closed-loop theory, when an individual moves he judges the accuracy of the movement against a template of the intended action, and when the action matches the template, the action continues (Adams, 1971). If a difference is perceived between the template and the movement, a correction is made. Adams suggested that the strength of these memory traces and templates diminishes with disuse.

Adams' theory reflects life experiences: a baby taking his first steps, falling and coming to his feet until walking becomes consistent and automatic, or a musician strengthening his skill by practicing a musical piece until it is perfect. The practice required to master a piece of music builds a strong motor memory trace that is then applied to repeated performances.

Closed-Loop Systems

In the closed-loop model, sensorimotor feedback comes from hearing, vision, touch, taste, smell, and proprioception (Adams, 1971; Fairbanks, 1954). If we apply this model to the process of voice therapy, we can identify several sensory contributors that are commonly used to heighten awareness of the manner of phonation and to enhance motor control of the voice. When your patient feels and then reduces an effortful manner of phonation (kinesthetic), when he modifies his posture to increase flexibility (Franco et al., 2014) in response to hands-on adjustment (tactile), when he watches his stance in a mirror and adjusts alignment to reduce stiffness (visual), or when he counterproductively *listens* to the sound of his voice (audition) and either increases effort or effectively decreases effort, we can say he is using sensory information to modify motor output. **Auditory feedback** provides unreliable information for voice modification because of the many counterproductive strategies patients often use to improve their voice quality. We encourage our patients to focus on sensory feedback to more accurately self-monitor their manner of phonation.

Open-Loop Systems

As opposed to a closed-loop system, in an open-loop system movement takes place without attention to its effect on the environment (Schmidt

& Lee, 2011). These authors give us a striking example of an open-loop system using a traffic light at a major intersection. The changes from red to green lights take place via a program that does not interact with the actual traffic pattern, thereby offering no feedback from the ongoing traffic. Is there an accident? Is the traffic suddenly heavy?

In humans, it is possible for a closed-loop system to become a partial open-loop system, as in the case of an individual with normal hearing acuity who develops a severe hearing loss or deafness. Here, the flow of sensory information is interrupted, blocking the flow of sound and interfering with comprehension and, ultimately, the regulation of speech production. Over time, articulatory precision may deteriorate and vocal intensity may increase or decrease. Auditory comprehension and articulatory precision may be restored when the individual closes the sensory loop with consistent use of amplification or focuses on other forms of feedback (e.g., tactile, visual) (Silman, Silverman, Emmer, & Gelfand, 1993).

Schema Theory

Although the closed- and open-loop models explain the acquisition and coordination of motor patterns to some degree, they fail to account for the novelty and possible storage problems that are a result of accumulating more and more memory traces and motor skills (Schmidt & Lee, 2011). Bernstein (1967) asks us to consider that any discrete action (e.g., hitting a baseball) requires coordination of a large number of independent, sequential movements, and if the context of the movement is changed (e.g., a curve ball; a low, slow, or fast ball) the batter must make adaptations to the swing. Bernstein calls these independent adaptations **degrees of freedom**. He suggests that if we consider each individual variation (degree of freedom) consciously and independently when executing a motor act, it would overwhelm the central nervous system and it would be impossible to perform the movement (Bernstein, 1967; Greene, 1972; Whiting, 1984). There would literally be no room to store all of the necessary motor traces in our memory or to store anything else.

Schmidt (1975) developed **schema theory** in an effort to account for these novelty and storage problems, as well as the adaptations made to cope with variability during acquisition, performance, and integration of a newly acquired motor pattern. Schmidt expanded Adams' (1971) open- and **closed-loop theory**, suggesting that with each repetition of a movement a memory trace remains, and as we accumulate these memory traces with repetition these perceptual traces become stronger and are distilled into a general trace that is adaptable to new situations. Schmidt's (1976) schema theory proposes that when a person sets a goal, he uses his knowledge from a related procedure to select and fine-tune the schema that will help him achieve the desired movement.

Schmidt theorized that a common conceptual representation or **prototype** for related movements would require less storage space in memory than the Adams' (1971) model and would explain the process of mastery and continuing control of skilled movement. Schmidt (1975) further postulated that the abstracted memory is distilled from four types of memory trace information, all of which are necessary to build a memory trace. The following categories of information are stored following a skilled movement: (1) proprioceptive/sensory information from the body *prior* to the initiation of the movement; (2) the sequence of the actions and the speed, duration, and strength of the movements; (3) the proprioceptive/sensory feedback *during* the movement (how it feels); and (4) the outcome of the movement. He proposed that the shared rules for a **motor archetype** are built in memory by the accumulation and refinement of these memory traces to identify the essential invariant features concerning the relative order of the actions, the timing of events, and the corresponding strength with which movements are executed. Schmidt called this motor prototype a generalized motor program.

Schmidt (1975) used the concept of a generalized motor program to explain how movement is acquired, repeated, varied, modified to meet new requirements of the environment, or adapted to produce similar movements without overtaxing our memory storage space. According to Schmidt's theory, by using a generalized motor program that predetermines the order, strength, and duration of the contraction of the muscles involved in the movement and then verifying that the movement occurred as planned, a new movement could be learned by either developing a new generalized motor program or by adapting an existing one. He hypothesized that the choice was made based on the strength of the individual's prior experience using the **generalized motor program** for similar tasks.

According to Schmidt's theory (1975), the schema is a motor rule or abstracted memory built by repeated practice of a motor action and the storage of the extracted memory trace. Schmidt's theory makes a distinction between two closely related components of memory—**recall schema** and **recognition schema**, which are relevant when you are assisting your patient through the bumpy process of generalization. An individual uses recall schema to identify and use the memory trace that is developed by the repeated enactment of a movement and to select and implement the specific, desired motor pattern that governs the desired movement. The implementation of schema theory to the treatment of voice disorders is explored in **Box 2-1**.

The individual uses the recognition schema to attend to sensory feedback from the ongoing movement in order to evaluate and monitor its effectiveness and accuracy. Throughout a movement, the recognition schema compares the expected sensory information from memory to the current movement, sends an error signal following the completion of the movement, and then modifies the schema based on the sensory feedback and knowledge of results. In **Box 2-2** recognition schema is applied to voice treatment.

With deliberate practice the individual uses recall and recognition schema to build stronger memory traces and to produce complex motor patterns more effectively. The selection process for the recall schema becomes more automatic as the movement pattern is assimilated and the individual's adjustment to changes in the environment and the real-time adjustments based on the recognition schema become faster and more efficient. In **Box 2-3** recognition schema is applied to treatment with a classroom teacher.

Schmidt and Lee's (2011) generalized motor program accounts for the ongoing changes in the environment in order for the patient

Box 2-1

Recall Schema During Voice Treatment

How is recall schema acquired? If, for example, your patient hyperadducts the vocal folds and uses abrupt onset of phonation consistently, you might introduce a technique to reduce medial compression of the vocal folds (voiceless consonants in initial position of single syllable words). With each repetition of an /h/ initiated word a memory trace remains, and as he accumulates these memory traces these residual perceptual traces become stronger and he builds recall schema. He can then use this recall schema to program the voice production system to produce voice with **less effort**. The traces might include the sensory information regarding the vocal tract configuration prior to the onset; the changes in speed, duration, and strength of the movements within the vocal subsystems; the sensory feedback during the /h/-initiated word; and, finally, the easy onset of voicing.

Box 2-2

Recognition Schema During Voice Treatment

As your patient attends to his voice he begins to compare the goal (easy manner of phonation) to his vocal behavior (recognition schema). He makes many subtle adjustments as he discovers the difference between effort and ease, and the balance and coordination necessary to achieve the effectiveness he seeks. As he refines his production through the recognition schema, his production becomes more efficient. The ultimate target—effective phonation—will remain elusive until he builds the requisite perceptual and motor traces (memories) that will eventually facilitate a more appropriate manner of phonation more consistently.

to adapt to the demands of a new context. Generalization of skills is explored within the generalized motor program model (**Box 2-4**).

Motor control of the voice production process is extremely complex, and requires not only the control to produce effective voice, but the skill and flexibility to make rapid, ongoing phonetic/phonemic transitions within a variety of linguistic contexts. The prosodic elements of voice production add complexity to the flow of this complex, precise motoric sequence of events. The cognitive, psychological, and **emotional states** that your patient brings to the process add yet another layer of complexity. Ultimately, the stresses in the environment (teaching, giving a presentation, or an opening night performance) are novel contexts that require an individual to include an infinite number of adaptations within himself. In general, we use little or no deliberate control of the voice when we speak and rely on the generalized motor program to adapt our motor patterns to meet the needs of the environment. Thus, during conversation, we do not overwhelm our cognitive resources by attending to each onset and offset of voicing, each change in pitch and loudness, and each variation in intonation and stress. We have found our patients to be not only

Box 2-3

Recall and Recognition Schema During Voice Treatment

A teacher in a noisy classroom, whose goal is to project his voice efficiently, may deliberately choose to use the abdominal control he practiced in therapy to cope with the persistent noise in his class (recall schema). In this case, he consciously estimates the sensory adjustments—the sustained, controlled exhalation, the openness of the throat, and the vibrations in the vocal tract—that will take place when he projects his voice efficiently to cope with this environmental challenge (recall schema). As he produces voice, he then implements recognition schema to compare his production with past experience and the sensory consequences of that outcome to evaluate his performance.

Box 2-4

Generalized Motor Program During Transfer

One of the challenges that actors face is moving a performance from the rehearsal studio to the stage. The actor relies on a strong generalized motor program based on prior sensorimotor experiences (e.g., rehearsing a monologue in a rehearsal studio) that facilitate the creation of a vocal character, and he then uses recognition schema to evaluate the accuracy of the performance (performing the monologue in a large theater, in the presence of an audience on opening night) under new conditions. Based on previous sensory experience making adjustments from a small rehearsal space to a large theater (recall and recognition schema), the performer makes several adjustments (e.g., use of **breath control**, sensory awareness of projection, and integration of relaxation techniques to optimize posture).

receptive to information regarding skill acquisition, but inquisitive and enthusiastic as they gain a better understanding of the motor patterns that affect movement.

Cognition

Schema theory is a powerful tool for describing motor learning and control and for explaining error detection and generalization to novel movements, but it does not take into account cognitive processes, hierarchies, or the practice of decision making (Sherwood & Lee, 2003). A discussion of motor learning would be incomplete without consideration of the relationship between motor learning and **cognition**: specifically attention, focus, memory, decision making, practice, and self-regulation.

Attention and Sensory Awareness

Attention, awareness, memory, and decision making are features of cognition and play a significant role in learning, whether it is cognitive or motor learning. The new voice patient typically has little cognitive or **sensory awareness** that he is using counterproductive compensation to improve the sound of his voice because he is ignoring the way his throat **feels**. He is devoted only to the sound of his voice, often feels no laryngeal discomfort, and rarely relies on kinesthetic feedback to regulate his manner of phonation. His limited understanding and narrow perspective provide little insight into the development of the voice problem or strategies that would be appropriate to address the problem. He may have tried to cope with vocal fatigue, limited pitch and loudness inflections, and perceived roughness by straining or speaking louder. These counterproductive strategies, coupled with a limited awareness of the effortful manner of phonation, or a belief that "pushing through" will achieve a better sound, often lead to phonotrauma.

Verdolini (2000) suggests that there is a distinction between attention and awareness. When your patient *attends* to your model of easy onset, when he attends, without evaluation, to the kinesthetic feedback he receives when he imitates your model, he is alert and ready to receive information without distraction from extraneous thoughts and self-criticism. He is present. He does not evaluate his output, does not question the **validity** of what he does or feels at that moment. He simply allows the larynx to do what it wants to do. He does not drive it or push it to produce an idealized sound. He remains alert to the sensations that come, but does not *demand* that they come. He is simply attending.

Your patient's attention to the sensations in his throat and head may prompt his realization that he has decreased vocal intensity, produced sound with less phonatory effort, or increased his sensory awareness of vibration in the head (**resonance**). This awareness may be experienced kinesthetically, acoustically, or cognitively. As the therapeutic process continues, your patient's awareness will shift between types of sensory feedback. He may rely on tactile feedback by placing his hands on his face to feel vibrations through the bridge of the nose, or place his hands on his abdomen to feel its expansion during an easy **inhalation**. Eventually, he may rely on the sensations in his lips, nose, and hard palate to monitor his performance. Over time, attention and awareness are strengthened and eventually leave a **procedural memory** trace that becomes easier to access and take advantage of as the hierarchy of your procedures becomes more complex (Lessac, 1997; Titze & Verdolini-Abbot, 2012; Verdolini, 2000).

Memory

Memory is a fundamental part of all learning, including motor learning. We recognize many types of memory including short-term memory, long-term memory, working memory, declarative or explicit memory (pertaining to direct recall of knowledge or past experience), and procedural or implicit memory. Verdolini (2000) proposes that attention and awareness are requisites to the development of procedural memory. *Procedural memory* is recognized as a primary component of motor learning and represents a memory that is formed without awareness of remembering, although it does require attention, repetition, and sensory awareness (Titze & Verdolini-Abbott, 2012). We build procedural memory with focus on and repetition of a movement, as well as alertness to the kinesthetic and proprioceptive features of the manner in which the movement was executed. In the realm of voice production, one might rely on procedural memory to imitate the cackle of the wicked witch from *The Wizard of Oz* or the forbidding, seductive voice and Transylvanian accent of Count Dracula.

Benefits of Deliberate Mental Practice

Closed- and open-loop and schema theories propose that motor learning takes place with repetition of a movement and the development of a memory trace. Recent evidence, however, suggests that motor learning may be enhanced *without* actual movement—the Olympic athlete, for example, who visualizes an ice-skating routine or the aerobatic pilot who visualizes a series of maneuvers in slow motion or real time capitalize on this learning strategy. The strength of the memory trace is enhanced when imagery and **mental practice** are combined with the sensory information from the motor practice of the intended behavior. Voice habilitation and rehabilitation take advantage of this synergistic effect by combining imagery and mental practice with specific vocal exercise. Most interesting is the suggestion that the use of **cognitive work** (imagery, mental practice, etc.), not only facilitates the development of a memory trace, but because cognitive effort increases during these processes both the underlying cognitive decision-making skills and motor learning are boosted. The male-to-female transgender voice client, for instance, uses imagery when she pictures herself wearing female clothing and speaking in a feminine voice as she walks into a room. She may spend a fair amount of time and cognitive energy using imagery before she feels comfortable enough to actually wear feminine clothing in public and use the voice and feminine gestures she has rehearsed.

The benefits of mental practice in the area of voice production may be derived from rehearsing an easy, effortless manner of phonation prior to the production of connected speech that increases in length and complexity. Mental practice appears to be more effective with tasks containing a high cognitive component (Gabriele, Hall, & Lee, 1989; Heuer, 1989). A newly acquired motor pattern is somewhat tenuous during the generalization phase of treatment because the patient must cope with the "How am I saying it" and "What am I saying" of an intended spoken message at the same time. It is virtually impossible, however, to split one's attention between this "how" and "what." As Schmidt and Lee (2011) suggest, if one were to attend to each and every phoneme, every phrase and prosodic change, as well as the content of the message, there would be no time for anything else, including the message. During the process of acquiring a new vocal behavior, a high degree of attention, concentration, and focus are necessary in order to learn the new motor pattern (i.e., easy, efficient manner of phonation), incorporate it within varying articulatory and prosodic contexts, and eventually transfer that vocal behavior to unfamiliar situations. During the final phase of generalization, these motor patterns will become increasingly consistent and automatic. Due to the high level of cognitive focus that your patient applies when he mentally rehearses these vocal techniques, learning and generalization are enhanced.

Blocked Versus Random Practice

Sherwood and Lee (2003) suggest that practice order, whether it is **blocked practice** (drill) or **random practice** (nonrepeating), affects learning. Blocked practice appears to be more effective earlier in treatment to enhance consistency of production (Shea, Lai, Wright, Immink, & Black, 2001), but random practice develops better error detection, self-recognition of accurate productions, retention of skill, and transfer of performance to novel situations (Green & Sherwood, 2000; Shea & Morgan, 1979; Wong, Whitehill, Ma, & Masters, 2013;

Wrisberg & Liu, 1991). In effect, random practice of a motor skill appears to develop a more durable schema with better retention and generalization of proficiency of the motor act (Sherwood & Lee, 2003). Random practice during the voice rehabilitation process might include varying phonemic context, cognitive and linguistic complexity, conversation partners, and communication environment while incorporating a specific vocal technique.

Fine-Tuning the Cognitive Load

When you begin the therapeutic process, you consider whether the patient is cognitively intact with respect to arousal, memory, attention, executive function, and can process abstract information. Typically, you take notice of whether cognition affects the patient's skill for following multi-step directions, whether he has difficulty attending to explanations and rationales for suggestions and techniques, and whether he remembers to practice. You know that adding pauses or delays, increasing linguistic complexity, and adding an audience will increase the cognitive load and possibly the difficulty learning specific, detailed information. It may not be common, however, to consider cognition as a facilitator of motor learning—that is, high levels of cognitive *work* can have a positive effect on motor learning.

It may not be intuitive that acquisition of new motor patterns may be facilitated or hindered by an increase or decrease in the cognitive work required for retention of a new behavior (Sherwood & Lee, 2011). Further, the timing (immediate or delayed) of motor practice and clinician feedback influence the type of learning, speed of actuation of a movement, and generalization of the new motor skill. The benefit a patient derives from imitating a voice model comes from his motor memory, cognitive-sensory rehearsal, translation of the memory into a motor plan, and, finally, execution of the model. In the early stages of therapy, you might model an *h*-initiated word (to decrease adduction and medial compression of the vocal folds), for instance, and ask your patient to copy the model immediately to facilitate consistency. As time goes by and his phonation becomes more stable, you may insert a delay between your model and his production. Inserting a pause between the model and the imitation increases the cognitive load, and this delay may facilitate better retention and generalization of the new movement pattern (Weeks, Hall, & Anderson, 1996).

As clinicians, we are all familiar with the notion that our feedback will reinforce a behavior. It may not be obvious that immediate clinician feedback pertaining to the effectiveness of a motor performance can actually *hinder* its long-term acquisition (Sherwood & Lee, 2003). If your patient were to produce a new vocal behavior following a delay in clinician feedback, for instance, he would be responsible for determining the appropriateness of the trial and making modifications on the next attempt. His cognitive load increases, and his immediate performance might suffer as he made trial-and-error attempts to reach the goal. Unexpectedly, however, his performance later in therapy would probably improve and be more consistent due to his semi-independent problem solving to find the most effective way to produce the new motor skill (Verdolini, 2000). Why does this happen? Sherwood and Lee (2011) suggest that when a clinician provides immediate feedback on all of the patient's attempts, the learner does not have any responsibility for error detection and the cognitive load is diminished. Although the immediate performance might improve following positive reinforcement from the clinician, the patient's independent performance may not develop as fully (Schmidt, 1991). When the clinician *delays* feedback, the learner has time to use sensory information to independently assess the efficiency of his production and his analysis can then be verified or critiqued by the clinician. This short delay adds cognitive load to the learning process and may facilitate generalization of the desired vocal behavior to future productions (Verdolini, 2000).

The Relationship Between Self-Regulation and the Cognitive Load

In voice therapy, most of our voice procedures require high levels of attention, focus, and concentration, which intensify the cognitive load. Although a high cognitive load may actually reinforce learning, however, it comes at a cost. The concentrated focus and attention required to modify a chronic, long-term habit may lead to mental fatigue, emotional stress, and frustration, which diminish the capacity for self-regulation and self-control (Vinney & Turkstra, 2013). As you work with your voice patient, you create an appropriate hierarchy of motor skills and cognitive challenges and continually adjust the complexity and difficulty of the procedures in order to mitigate the challenges to self-regulation by varying the motor and cognitive demands such that the new vocal motor patterns become consistent and integrated.

Self-regulation (self-control), as described in the cognitive psychology literature, pertains to one's capacity to monitor, modify, and control behavior, thinking, and emotion under stress and over time (Vinney & Turkstra, 2013; Vohs & Baumeister, 2004). Self-regulation is not static and varies depending on the person, his age, gender, personality, tendency to procrastinate, and the surrounding environment—all of these factors play a role in self-regulation. It is common for a patient under the stress of maintaining attention and concentration in order to understand and apply an abstract therapeutic procedure, for example, to exhibit signs of mental fatigue and frustration, which negatively affect performance. Although self-regulation is subject to depletion, manifesting in mental fatigue, distraction, frustration, decreased performance accuracy, and lack of adherence to practice, periods of rest and relaxation as well as activities that promote positive feelings often restore one's self-control and perseverance.

Vinney and Turkstra (2013) integrate the concept of self-regulation into voice therapy in an attempt to illuminate the problems associated with the acquisition, transfer, and maintenance of newly established motor patterns. When you include procedures at random levels of complexity to facilitate motor automaticity, the cognitive effort needed to attend to those behaviors will increase in the beginning and will eventually abate. If you and your patient decide, for instance, that he is ready to integrate resonant voice for two minutes, six times per day, in a conversation with a friendly listener, he is using an increased cognitive load to consciously integrate and solidify a motor technique that facilitates a more efficient vibratory pattern of the vocal folds. Over time, the cognitive effort and self-regulatory demands required to sustain this manner of phonation within the new context will decrease as the behavior becomes more automatic. Your observation skills will serve you well in these circumstances as you monitor the subtle changes in your patient's energy level, attentiveness, concentration, alertness, and possible overstimulation.

The impact of cognitive load and self-regulation on vocal health and coordination of the voice production subsystems are factors to consider as you guide your patient to integrate sensorimotor information and adhere to practice schedules and voice conservation protocols. Your awareness that your patient's fluctuations in self-control are common and expected during this process of change, and your attunement to these shifts, gives you the opportunity to accommodate to them by simplifying, maintaining the current level of complexity, or, when appropriate, increasing the complexity of the procedure in order to ensure the patient's readiness for change.

Physiological Model of Normal Speech Production

Motor learning theory, cognition, and hypothesis-driven approaches to the voice rehabilitation process incorporate the physiological underpinnings that contribute to a voice problem. Appreciation of both the underlying physiology responsible for clinically normal voice as well as the physiological changes that are associated with the voice problem will provide a more complete picture of voice rehabilitation. Constructs such as the transglottal pressure differential, phonation threshold pressure (Titze, 2001; Zemlin, 1998), back pressure (Chapman, 2012; Titze, 1994), the inertive vocal tract (Laukkanen, Titze, Hoffman, & Finnegan, 2008; Titze, 1994), **source-filter theory**, and the physiologic adjustments needed for changes in pitch and loudness can be used to rationalize the procedures you use to modify the configuration of the vocal tract in order to improve coordination among the vocal subsystems.

A good place to start the rehabilitation process is with a physiological definition of effective voice production, which is the long-term goal for your patient. As defined here, effective voice production refers to the optimal coordination among the respiratory, phonatory, resonation, and articulation subsystems of voice production for a given task. This definition is deceptively simple. "Effective voice production" encompasses the notions of ease, efficiency, **reliability**, and flexibility of phonation. The phrase *for a given task* suggests that the voice can be used dynamically to meet all of the challenges and expectations of the patient, whether it is during customary speech production, or production of unusual sounds, character voices, yodeling, or singing opera (based on the patient's inherent skill and knowledge level). The phrase *optimal coordination among the respiratory, phonatory, resonation, and articulation subsystems of voice production* refers to the physiological capability to negotiate adjustments in pitch, loudness, quality, intonation, and stress to meet the ever-changing needs of voice production.

Closely related to the definition of effective voice production is the notion of **freedom to act**. If you look at the spectrum between the body's most lax position and its stiffest, the position that allows for freedom to act resides between these extremes. Lessac (1997) uses the concept of freedom to act as an "energetic rest" or a "state of release" (p. 48) where the body is ready "to spring alertly into action" (p. 48) without strain or tension in the muscles. When the voice is produced effectively, it is free to negotiate broad ranges of pitch, loudness, and quality. There is a strong relationship between the freedom of the body to move and voice production (Dimon, 2011). This freedom involves a balance between expiratory drive and laryngeal resistance to cope with varying levels of vocal intensity, **fundamental frequency**, voice quality/**timbre**, and the ever-changing configuration of the vocal tract.

When you rely on a **physiological framework**, your treatment goals and procedures follow logically. If you note that your patient uses excessive loudness, for example, you incorporate a **physiological model** to modify this behavior. The physiological rationale suggests that the excessive loudness may be associated with increased expiratory drive and subglottal pressure, which lead to hyperadduction and increased stiffness of the vocal folds as well as sharp, effortful glottal closure during phonation. It is a logical step then to translate this approach into practice. Your goal, then, is to decrease the expiratory drive and medial compression of the vocal folds. There are several procedures that will achieve this goal, including the use of a confidential voice, which will decrease the excessive expiratory drive and subglottal pressure. The example in **Box 2-5** illustrates the application of the physiological model.

Box 2-5

Integration of Physiology and Hypothesis Development

Ms. B, a 27-year-old third grade public school teacher, was recently diagnosed with bilateral vocal fold nodules. She demonstrates moderate to severe dysphonia characterized by moderate roughness and breathiness, frequent abrupt initiations of phonation, severe stridency, and moderate inappropriate loudness with frequent voice and **pitch breaks**. She exhibits excessive expiratory drive and apparent, excessive extraneous muscle activity in the head, neck, and thorax. She reports that her voice is better in the morning, but complains that it deteriorates over the course of a teaching day that demands "speaking over noise" and the use of dynamic intonation patterns. Ms. B does not have access to a voice amplification system and is concerned that her teaching career is in jeopardy.

Given this information, you will develop several hypotheses to address the underlying physiological disturbances. You observe abrupt initiation of phonation and inappropriate vocal intensity. These phenomena suggest excessive expiratory drive, a significant buildup of subglottal pressure, and a high transglottal pressure differential. You recall that phonation onset relies on matching phonation threshold pressure (the minimum air pressure needed to initiate and sustain phonation) (Titze, 1988) and vocal fold biomechanics, including prephonatory glottal width, stiffness, medial surface thickness of the vocal folds, and mucosal wave velocity (Hirano, 1974; Titze, 1988). Given Ms. B's extreme loudness, you expect excessive vocal fold stiffness, medial compression, and a wide lateral excursion of the vocal folds during the vibratory cycle. You hypothesize that the increased expiratory drive, glottal width, vocal fold stiffening, increased thickness, and increased amplitude of vibration will generate greater friction between the vocal folds, which, in turn, will aggravate the existing laryngeal pathology.

The transglottal pressure differential describes the difference between the pressure below (subglottal) and the pressure above (supraglottal) the vocal folds. When the transglottal pressure differential is very high, the vocal folds may snap together with excessive force creating abrupt initiation of phonation and excessive loudness. Conversely, if we decrease the difference between the subglottal and supraglottal pressures (increase back pressure and inertance), the transglottal pressure differential will be reduced and medial compression of the vocal folds will diminish.

The Vocal Subsystems

At any time during assessment or treatment, your patient may turn to you and ask, "Why am I doing this exercise?" When your treatment plan is based on the physiology of voice production, you have a context from which to answer this question. The time you take to clarify the purpose of your procedures contributes to the partnership you hope to build during this process.

Physiology of Respiration

What do you feel when you breathe and how are these sensations linked to the underlying **physiology of respiration**? If you breathe quietly through your nose and attend to your breath, you may feel your chest and abdomen expand effortlessly as the air flows into your nose and then the easy collapse of your chest and abdomen as the air flows out through your nose during exhalation. This easy movement of air is related to **pleural linkage** (Hixon, Weismer, & Hoit, 2008).

Exhalation is the energy source for phonation. When we assess phonation, we evaluate the effectiveness and coordination of respiration and phonation. When we link our knowledge of the physiology of respiration with the sensations of inhalation and exhalation, the information becomes accessible in a more practical way so that you can assess the ease of respiration and explain the process to your patients.

Given the differences that exist among quiet breathing, breathing during exertion, speech breathing, and breathing for singing, it is essential that your hypotheses reflect the dynamic physiological adaptations that the vocal subsystems negotiate to maintain a balance among them. To that end, let us review the biomechanics of breathing and apply this information to hypothesis development and testing during assessment and treatment.

Pleural Linkage

"When I breathe should I feel my chest move?" Efficient inhalation and exhalation occur as an effortless exchange of air that takes place because of the linkage of the lungs to the chest wall. A thin, airtight membrane (visceral pleura) clings to the outside of the lungs, and a similar membrane (parietal pleura) attaches to the inside of the chest wall and upper side of the diaphragm and mediastinum. The space between the membranes is filled with intrapleural fluid, which acts very much like the tears in your eyes that wet your contact lenses and hold them in place with negative pressure, allowing the lenses to float without friction yet remain in place. Similarly, as illustrated in **Figure 2-2**, intrapleural fluid binds the chest wall to the lungs via negative pressure and transfers the movements of the chest wall directly to the lungs so that the lungs and chest wall act as a unit, allowing for frictionless movement of the lungs across the inside of the chest wall (pleural linkage). If you focus on the feeling in your chest during inhalation, you will become aware of this easy movement.

This dynamic pulmonary–chest wall unit moves as a result of the interaction of active (muscular) and passive (nonmuscular) forces. The *active* forces contributing to the inspiratory and expiratory cycles are variable depending on which muscles are in use and the interplay between them. The inhalatory muscular forces include the descent of the diaphragm to enlarge the thoracic space and the contraction of the external intercostal muscles to expand and elevate the chest wall. Exhalatory muscular forces are used primarily during forced exhalation and to control the airflow during sustained phonation with contraction of the internal intercostal muscles, transversus abdominis, external and internal obliques, and rectus abdominis with possible assistance from other thoracic muscles, muscles of the torso, and back.

The *passive* forces include elasticity, gravity, the surface tension of the fluid that lines the alveoli, and the natural recoil of cartilages and

Figure 2-2

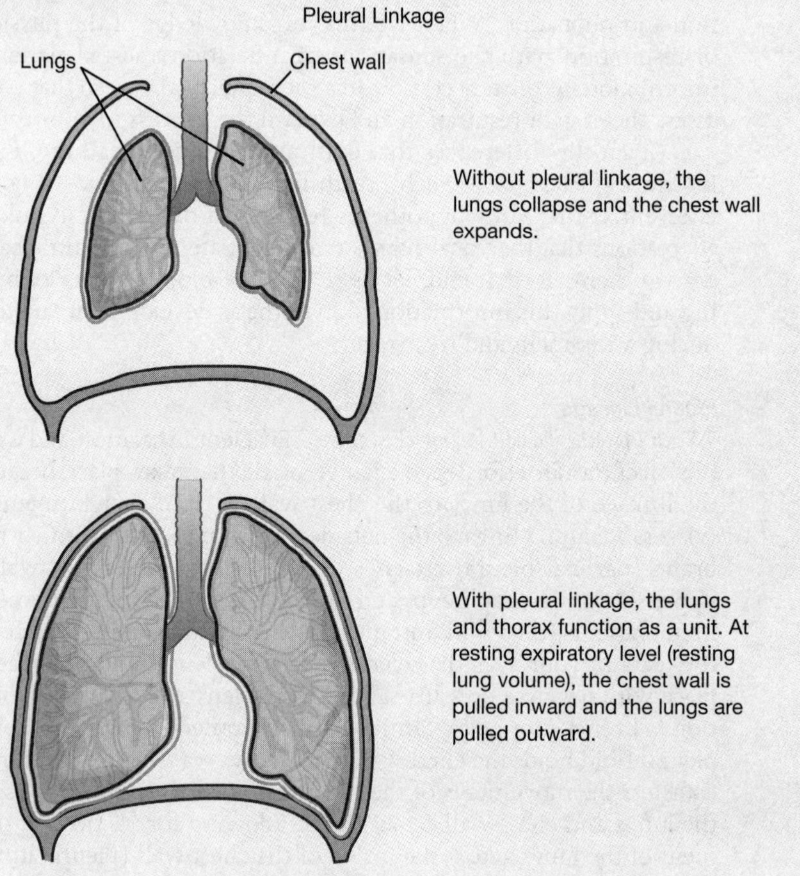
Pleural Linkage
Lungs
Chest wall
Without pleural linkage, the lungs collapse and the chest wall expands.
With pleural linkage, the lungs and thorax function as a unit. At resting expiratory level (resting lung volume), the chest wall is pulled inward and the lungs are pulled outward.

ligaments (Hixon & Hoit, 2005). An oppositional relationship exists between the lungs, which, because of elasticity, have a natural tendency to shrink (collapse), and the chest wall, which, by contrast, has a natural tendency to expand. The oppositional relationship between the lungs and chest wall creates a dynamic balance whereby the pull from the elastic recoil of the pulmonary–chest wall unit reduces the need for muscular activity during quiet breathing and breathing for speech (in the midrange of the system) (Figure 2-2).

Lung Volumes and Lung Capacities for Speech

"How do I know how much breath to take?" The quantity of air used for different activities such as quiet breathing, speaking, shouting, singing,

and blowing out candles varies considerably and a speaker needs the freedom to move effortlessly between the different lung volumes. It is useful to have a common nomenclature for the various air volumes in order to follow a patient's progress over time, compare one patient to another, and to discuss respiratory problems with other professionals. As we continue to provide a context for discussion of respiration, we will connect the **lung volumes** and **lung capacities** with the anatomy and physiology of respiration and draw your attention to the sensations you experience during inhalation and exhalation.

When we connect these sensations to the physiology related to the air moving in and out of the lungs, we may be more likely to identify varying breathing patterns in our patients. To begin the exploration, inhale deeply and hold your breath at the top of your inhalation. What physical sensations are you aware of as you reach the end of your inhalation? You will note that there is a limit to how much air you can inhale, and that your chest tightens as your inhalation nears its limit. Now try a maximum expiration by exhaling all of the air that you can move. Do you feel changes in your chest and vocal tract as you exhale, and do those feelings intensify as you reach the end of the expiratory cycle? During speech, we stay within the middle portion of this range because the passive respiratory forces are minimal in this range. You easily vary the size and speed of your inhalation depending on the loudness and length of the intended utterance by slightly increasing your inhalation when shouting or projecting your voice and by taking small quick breaths during a long monologue. During assessment, we carefully observe the patient's respiratory adjustments during various speech tasks and monitor respiratory patterns for possible shortness of breath, tightening in the thorax, or reversed inhalation patterns in order to obtain a clear understanding of the challenges that might inhibit an efficient coordination among the vocal subsystems.

Vital Capacity

"Am I taking enough air? I sometimes run out of breath. Should I take a bigger breath before I talk?" Typically, you avoid the extremes of inhalation and exhalation during customary speech because it takes so much muscular work to move air as you reach the limits of the respiratory system. It is most efficient to produce voice within the middle range where the oppositional relationship between the elasticity of the lungs and chest wall does most of the work (Titze & Verdolini-Abbott, 2012). During the evaluation we obtain the **vital capacity** (VC) because it provides insight into the strength of the respiratory muscles and the elasticity and compliance of the lung-chest wall unit. **Forced vital capacity** is a measure of all the air that can be forcibly exhaled following a maximum inhalation. Vital capacity decreases with age or disease, such as asthma or **chronic obstructive pulmonary disease (COPD)**,

but these changes are not significant to the production of speech. The vital capacity can decrease to so low a volume as to barely sustain life, and it will be sufficient to support speech (Aronson, 1990).

When assessing VC, you ask the patient to take in as much air as possible and then exhale all of the air into a spirometer. You then compare this to the normative data that accompanies the device. This measure varies, however, based on gender, as well as body size and position (standing or supine) during the maneuver. It is recommended that after you collect this data you consult a table of normative values to see if your patient's vital capacity is within normal limits.

Vital capacity is often divided into three components: tidal volume, inspiratory reserve volume, and expiratory reserve volume. The amount of air that is inhaled and exhaled easily during quiet breathing rests in the middle of the vital capacity range and is called **quiet tidal volume (QTV)**. This quantity of air (approximately 500 ml) is inhaled and exhaled primarily due to the oppositional relationship between the lungs and chest wall and requires little muscular effort. At the end of a tidal breath prior to inhalation, there is a fleeting moment when the elastic forces of inhalation and exhalation are at equilibrium and you can stop breathing without holding your breath. That state of equilibrium is referred to as **resting expiratory level (REL)** or **resting lung volume (RLV)**. When a healthy young adult wishes to take a fuller, deeper breath and exceed the inhalation for quiet tidal volume, he can inhale up to an additional 2500+ ml (**inspiratory reserve**). The maximum volume of air that he can exhale below resting expiratory level is referred to as **expiratory reserve volume** (an additional 900+ ml). Quiet tidal volume lies in the middle of our inhalation and exhalation range, thus providing flexibility when a deeper breath is needed to shout, sustain a singing note, or continue speaking after the tidal air has been depleted. During assessment, in addition to the VC data you collect, you will observe your patient while he sits quietly to determine if his breathing pattern appears effortless, rhythmical, and coordinated with the onset and sustained production of voice.

Relaxation-Pressure S-Curve

Relaxation pressure represents the pressures that are generated entirely by *passive* (elastic) forces generated by the lungs and chest wall, be they positive (atmospheric) or negative (subatmospheric). These pressures are developed in the pulmonary airway and lungs. We can analyze the relationship between the net passive and active respiratory forces (or pressures) using a relaxation-pressure curve. In **Figure 2-3**, the forward S-curve represents the passive (elastic) forces of the oppositional relationship between the lungs and chest wall unit. Remember that both inhalation and exhalation are reflected on the curve. In

Figure 2-3

Relaxation-Pressure S-Curve Diagram

This figure illustrates the passive forces of respiration with and without pleural linkage. The dotted lines represent passive forces that occur *without* pleural linkage. The solid line represents the passive forces that exist *with* pleural linkage.

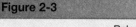

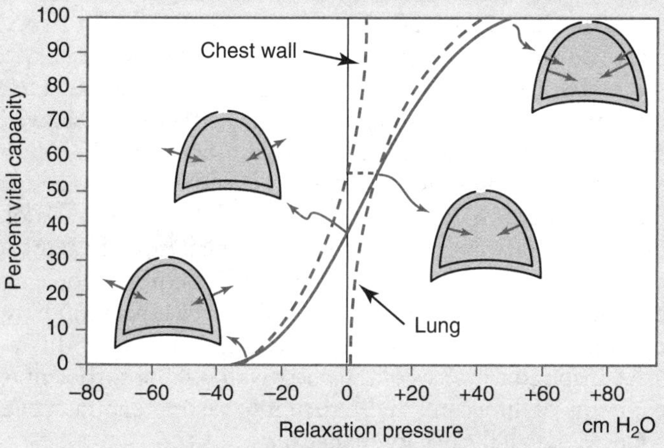

The relative strength and direction (inhalatory, exhalatory) of the passive forces of the chest wall–lung unit are shown by the length and direction of the arrows. Note that at ~60% VC the chest wall is at rest (Zemlin, 1998).

Modified from Zemlin, W.R. (1998). *Speech and Hearing Science: Anatomy and Physiology* (4th ed.). Needham Heights, MA: Allyn and Bacon. Reprinted by permission of Pearson Education, New York, NY.

Figure 2-3 inspiration is shown as you trace the curves upward and exhalation as you trace the curves downward.

Pressure Changes During a Vital Capacity Maneuver

"Sometimes when I talk it feels like I don't have enough air." When you study the relaxation-pressure S-curve, consider the passive elastic pressures that develop and are expended to control the flow of air in and out of the lungs, and you will notice that the respiratory pressures change

dramatically throughout the vital capacity range. During the process of inhalation for a vital capacity maneuver, the diaphragm and external intercostal muscles engage, expand the size of the chest wall unit and pull the lungs along to increase the internal lung volume, thus decreasing the pressure within the lungs in relation to atmospheric pressure. As the volume of air inside the lungs approaches 55% of vital capacity, passive expiratory forces increase and additional muscle activity is necessary to expand the chest wall as well as the lungs. The more that the chest wall–lung unit is stretched (as it approaches 100% vital capacity), the greater the muscular exertion required to continue inhalation.

As the lungs expand, the passive elastic forces of exhalation increase so that during exhalation above resting expiratory level, the passive, elastic recoil forces of the lungs alone are sufficient to return to the resting expiratory level (approximately 38% vital capacity). The high passive elastic forces of exhalation cause a rapid decrease in the size of the chest wall–lung unit, and if left unchecked result in a rapid release of air. Exhalation below resting expiratory level continues only if the muscles of exhalation are engaged. As the vital capacity approaches 0%, the exhalatory muscular forces exert their maximum force to contract the chest wall, and the passive elastic forces of inhalation have reached their limit. If all of the expiratory muscles release at this point, the passive inspiratory forces of the chest wall will be sufficient to expand the chest wall–lung unit and return it to resting expiratory level. This completes the vital capacity maneuver.

Quiet Tidal Breathing

When you study the relaxation-pressure S-curve, consider the active and passive pressures that are responsible for quiet tidal breathing (the amount of air that flows in and out when you are breathing at rest). From the S-curve in **Figure 2-4** you can see that the lower border of quiet tidal breathing rests at approximately 38% of vital capacity (located in the lower mid-third of the relaxation-pressure S-curve) (Zemlin, 1998) and the upper border is approximately 60% of vital capacity.

If you attend to your breathing cycles during quiet tidal volume, you may notice that you can pause momentarily at resting expiratory level without holding your breath. However, if you pause at the top of the cycle, you must hold your breath by either closing your glottis or stabilizing the chest wall. You can rest the respiratory mechanism for a moment at resting expiratory level without holding your breath because the passive elastic forces of inhalation and exhalation are in balance. The momentary pause at resting expiratory level is effortless and does not compromise phonation. You may observe this pause at resting expiratory level in patients, and then determine whether the patient is merely pausing before inhalation or is in fact holding his breath (closing the glottis). Closing the glottis before the onset of

Figure 2-4

Relaxation Pressure Curve Figure with Speech Tidal Volume Highlighted

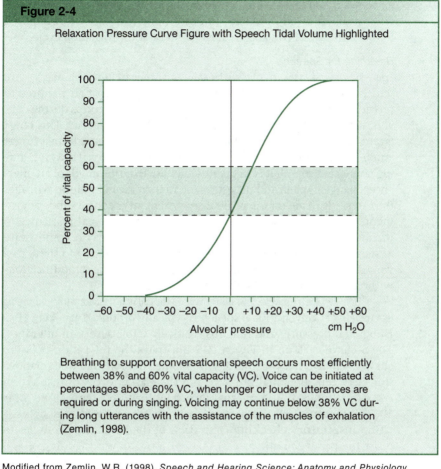

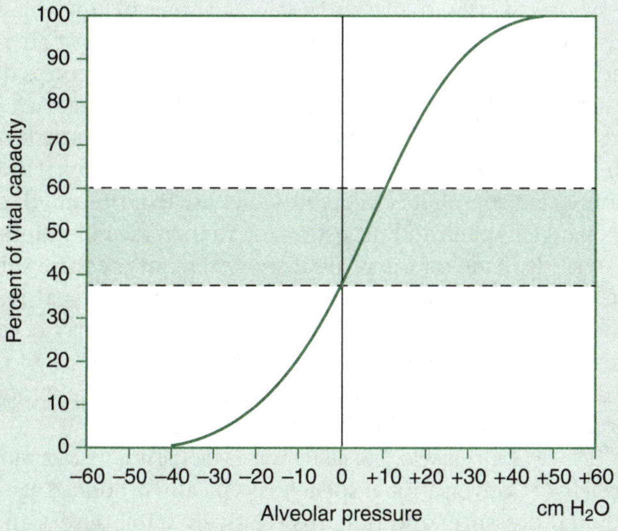

Breathing to support conversational speech occurs most efficiently between 38% and 60% vital capacity (VC). Voice can be initiated at percentages above 60% VC, when longer or louder utterances are required or during singing. Voicing may continue below 38% VC during long utterances with the assistance of the muscles of exhalation (Zemlin, 1998).

Modified from Zemlin, W.R. (1998). *Speech and Hearing Science: Anatomy and Physiology* (4th ed.). Needham Heights, MA: Allyn and Bacon. Reprinted by permission of Pearson Education, New York, NY.

phonation is an atypical pattern that occurs when patients make abrupt onsets of phonation and in those patients with adductor spasmodic dysphonia, who often hold their breath at various points in the respiratory cycle.

When you examine Figure 2-4 you will notice that quiet tidal volume is in the middle of the respiratory range, and the relaxation-pressure curve is steep in this range, suggesting that large quantities of air can be moved with little work. The curve flattens out toward the extremes, suggesting that as you approach the limits of the oppositional relationship between the lungs and chest wall unit the work required to move air increases. You can experience the contrast between the easy exchange of air during tidal volume and the effortful exchange at the extremes if you take several quiet breaths feeling the easy movement of chest wall, followed by a deep, full breath, noticing the effort required to move the air as you approach the limit of your inhalation cycle.

Breathing for Speech

"How do I know when to stop and take a breath?" The range of lung volumes within which speech is generally produced and the amount of air required to provide the necessary respiratory support for **breath groups** during conversation typically lies between 38% and 60% vital capacity. This range is similar to quiet tidal breathing and is the range in which the greatest amount of air can be moved for the least amount of work. However, during connected speech it is frequently the case that the length of an utterance, change in pitch and inflection, or an increase in loudness will alter the demands made on the respiratory system and require subtle adjustments in lung volume, alveolar pressure, and laryngeal resistance to maintain coordination among the subsystems. You may become aware of these adjustments and feel these changes by continuing to speak past your customary breath groups and attempt to make these modifications without tightening or stiffening the vocal tract.

"How do I keep my voice loud all the way to the end of a sentence without dropping into vocal fry?" Conversational speech is typically produced at ~7 cm H_2O (subglottal pressure) and remains relatively stable across an utterance. The S-curve cartoon in **Figure 2-5** illustrates the relaxation-pressure curve with alveolar pressure highlighted to demonstrate the relationship between subglottal pressure and the elastic forces of inspiration and expiration during connected speech. At the top of the S-curve (near 100% vital capacity), the passive elastic forces are excessive, necessitating **inspiratory checking** (activation of the inspiratory muscles to resist the passive elastic forces). As you move down the S-curve and vital capacity diminishes to approximately 55%, the passive expiratory forces are sufficient to maintain phonation. However, as you can see from the diagram, the passive expiratory forces become *insufficient* to sustain phonation as you approach and go below resting expiratory level (38% vital capacity). Consequently, the expiratory muscle forces (the internal intercostal, external obliques, and the rectus abdominis) must become active in order to maintain the steady exhalatory pressure that is necessary for continuation of long utterances (Hoit, 1995; Hoit, Palssman, Lansing, & Hixon, 1988). The engagement of the abdominal muscles becomes even more relevant when we increase vocal intensity to speak over noise or project the voice to a large audience.

Inspiratory Checking (Checking Action)

"Do I need a deeper breath to hold a note longer?" The complex relationship between the passive and active forces is well illustrated with a singer who requires a constant alveolar pressure during phonation. The singer faces many breathing challenges that require subtle adjustments, including the rapid

Figure 2-5

Relaxation-Pressure S-Curve During Maximum Phonation Time Maneuver

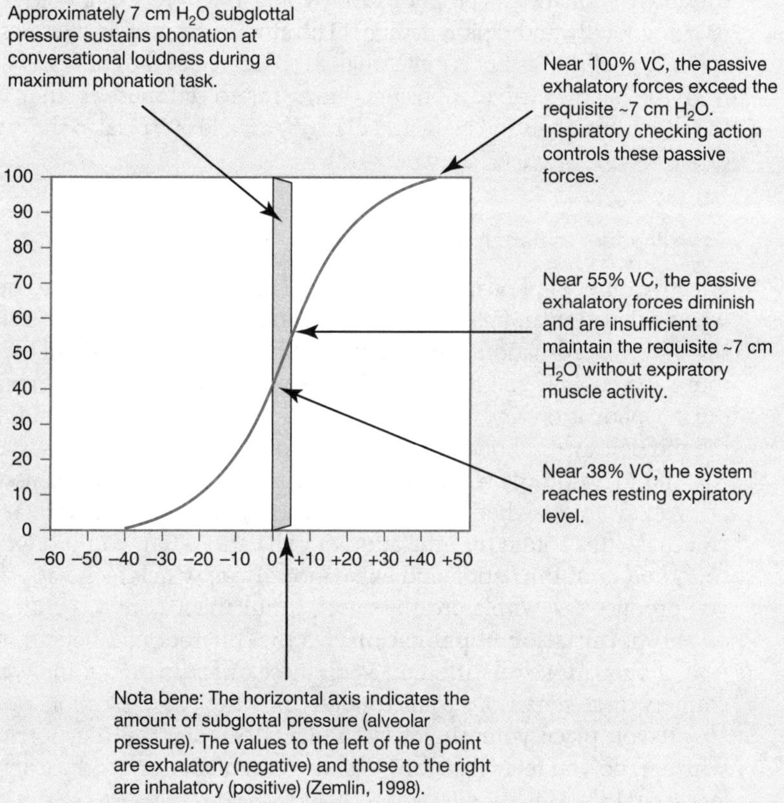
Approximately 7 cm H_2O subglottal pressure sustains phonation at conversational loudness during a maximum phonation task.
Near 100% VC, the passive exhalatory forces exceed the requisite ~7 cm H_2O. Inspiratory checking action controls these passive forces.
Near 55% VC, the passive exhalatory forces diminish and are insufficient to maintain the requisite ~7 cm H_2O without expiratory muscle activity.
Near 38% VC, the system reaches resting expiratory level.
100
90
80
70
60
50
40
30
20
10
0
−60 −50 −40 −30 −20 −10 0 +10 +20 +30 +40 +50
Nota bene: The horizontal axis indicates the amount of subglottal pressure (alveolar pressure). The values to the left of the 0 point are exhalatory (negative) and those to the right are inhalatory (positive) (Zemlin, 1998).

Modified from Zemlin, W.R. (1998). *Speech and Hearing Science: Anatomy and Physiology* (4th ed.). Needham Heights, MA: Allyn and Bacon. Reprinted by permission of Pearson Education, New York, NY.

intake of air before singing, sustained phonation, phrasing, stress, executing pitch and inflection variations, crescendo and decrescendo (**messa di voce**), maintaining a high **tessitura** (the average pitch of a song or part of a song), **vibrato**, and projecting to a large audience. The challenge becomes even greater when a singer must make these modifications without tightening or squeezing in the vocal tract (Titze, 1994). If he inhales very deeply (near 100% vital capacity), the elastic recoil forces will require that he use the muscles of inhalation to cope with and control the additional air pressure (**checking action**). The inspiratory musculature will remain contracted during the expiratory phase until he reaches the area where the passive elastic forces no longer exceed his requisite expiratory drive, at which point the internal intercostal muscles are engaged to extend exhalation and phonation. If the singer did not implement the checking action, the passive exhalatory forces at the top of the inhalation would remain unchecked and the rapid decrease in pressure would not support sustained phonation. The phonation would be more like a voiced sigh (starting loudly and rapidly fading). The amount of muscle energy spent at the level of the larynx is quite small as compared to the energy available from the bellows (rib cage, pleura, lungs, intercostal muscles, muscles of the abdominal wall and back, and diaphragm) and is crucial to the control of the sound source (Chapman, 2012).

Coordination: Initiation of Phonation

Effective onset of phonation during vowels and voiced consonants occurs when exhalation and phonation begin simultaneously. Your understanding of the coordination between respiration and phonation will become more accessible if you focus your attention on the sensations that occur during phonation and link these sensations to your understanding of the physiology of phonation. To begin this process, produce a sustained /a/ and focus on the sensations in your upper airway. What sensations are you aware of when you produce a series of short /a/, /a/, /a/? Do you make this sound on inhalation or exhalation? Can you produce the sound on both inhalation and exhalation? If so, which feels easier? Can you produce /a/ with a breathy onset, simultaneous onset (gentle), and an abrupt **initiation of phonation**? Do the different manners of initiation of phonation feel different? With these differences in mind we will connect these sensations to the underlying physiology of phonation.

If you place your finger at the level of your thyroid notch and whisper, do you feel vibration? When you **whisper** or produce a voiceless sound there is no phonation. A *delayed onset of phonation* occurs when the exhalation is initiated prior to the adduction of the vocal folds. This delayed onset occurs naturally in words that start with voiceless fricative sounds such as /h/ (turbulence at the level of the glottis) or /s/ (turbulence at the level of the teeth). A voiceless sound or whisper occurs when air flows through a constricted space, the air becomes turbulent, and energy is converted into noise. In voice therapy, we use a voiceless sigh or syllables and words that begin with voiceless sounds to decrease the adduction of the vocal folds and reduce laryngeal stiffness.

"You asked me to use a gentle onset. What does that feel like?" **Simultaneous initiation of phonation** is the effortless voicing that is a result of the synchronized initiation of exhalation and adduction of the vocal folds. It is one of the goals of most voice treatment programs and typically begins with words that begin with vowels. The vocal folds vibrate gently when phonation begins in this manner and they attain full closure after several cycles. The glide /j/ can be incorporated into the back pressure hierarchy to facilitate this easy vowel onset. The illustration in **Figure 2-6** depicts

Figure 2-6

Simultaneous Initiation of Vocal Fold Vibration and Exhalation During the First Cycle of Phonation

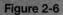

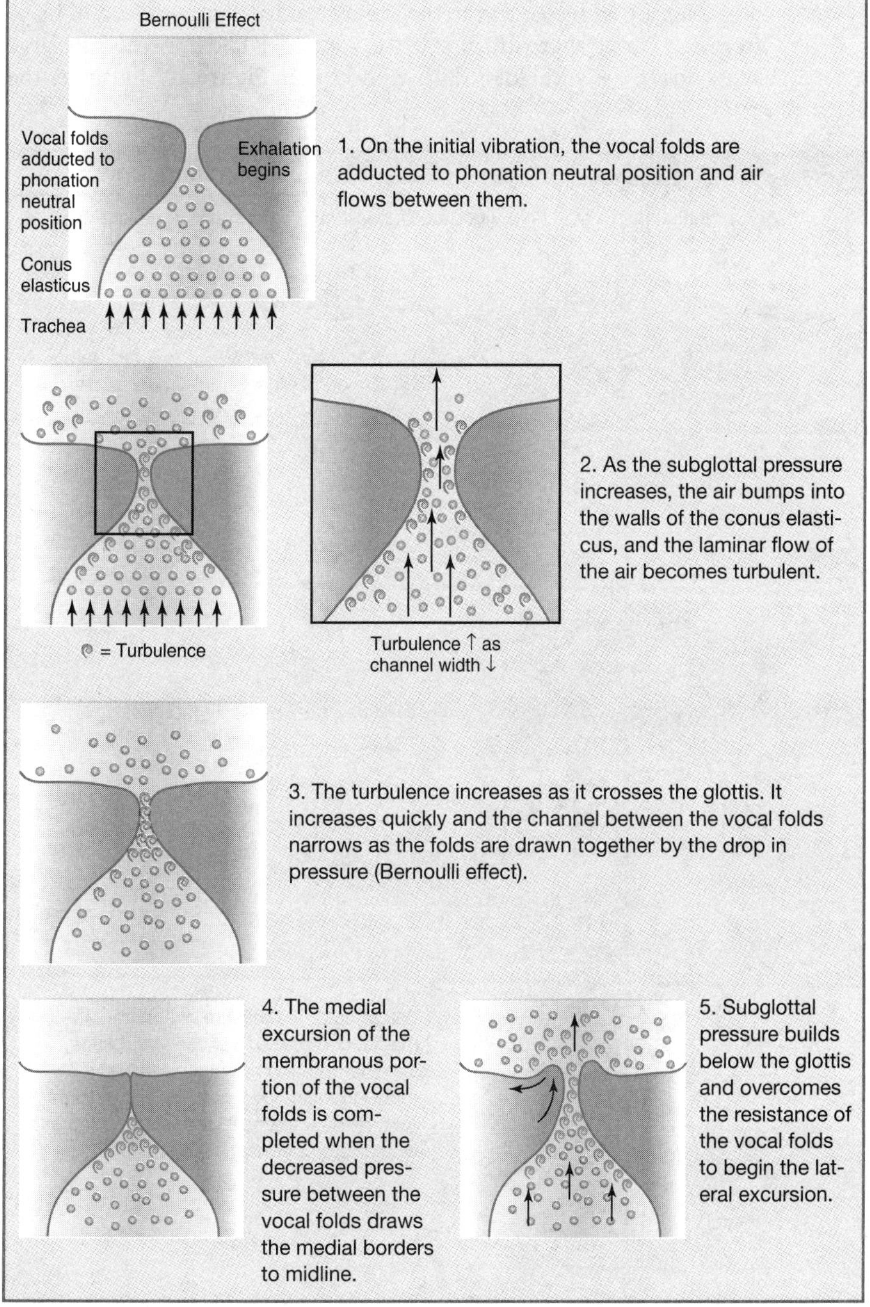
Bernoulli Effect
Vocal folds adducted to phonation neutral position
Exhalation begins
Conus elasticus
Trachea
1. On the initial vibration, the vocal folds are adducted to phonation neutral position and air flows between them.
= Turbulence
Turbulence ↑ as channel width ↓
2. As the subglottal pressure increases, the air bumps into the walls of the conus elasticus, and the laminar flow of the air becomes turbulent.
3. The turbulence increases as it crosses the glottis. It increases quickly and the channel between the vocal folds narrows as the folds are drawn together by the drop in pressure (Bernoulli effect).
4. The medial excursion of the membranous portion of the vocal folds is completed when the decreased pressure between the vocal folds draws the medial borders to midline.
5. Subglottal pressure builds below the glottis and overcomes the resistance of the vocal folds to begin the lateral excursion.

the simultaneous initiation of vibration on the first cycle of phonation. The voice flows without effort, and sound begins easily and smoothly. If you attend to the sensations in your throat during simultaneous initiation, you may feel a gentle buzzing. *Abrupt onset* of phonation occurs when the vocal folds are adducted *prior* to the onset of exhalation resulting in inappropriately strong approximation of the vocal folds and unnecessarily large excursions of the vocal folds during phonation. **Figure 2-7** illustrates the

Figure 2-7

Abrupt Initiation of Vocal Fold Vibration During the First Cycle of Phonation

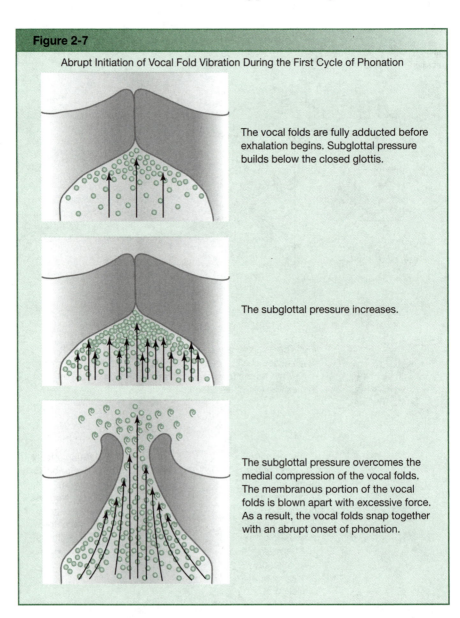

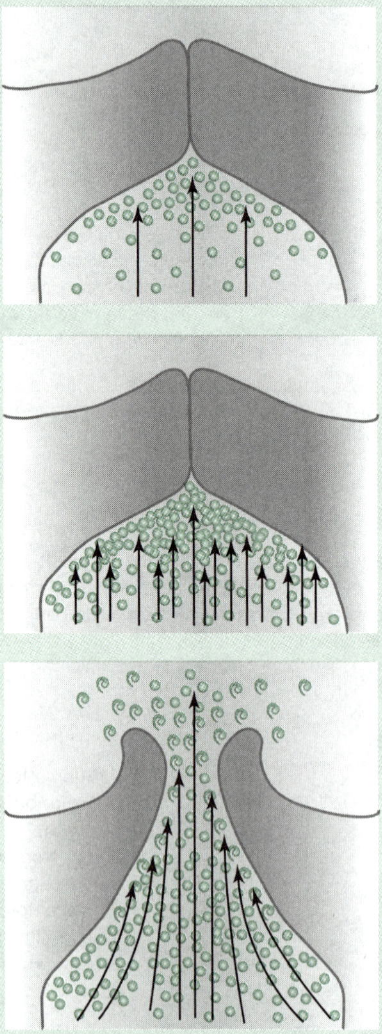

The vocal folds are fully adducted before exhalation begins. Subglottal pressure builds below the closed glottis.

The subglottal pressure increases.

The subglottal pressure overcomes the medial compression of the vocal folds. The membranous portion of the vocal folds is blown apart with excessive force. As a result, the vocal folds snap together with an abrupt onset of phonation.

abrupt initiation of vocal fold vibration during the first cycle of phonation. You can feel this strong burst at the initiation of phonation if you take a breath and hold it briefly before starting phonation. Over time, the effort and stress (excessive adduction, medial compression, and longitudinal stiffness of the vocal folds) may lead to phonotrauma. Many voice procedures focus on the reduction and elimination of this inefficient, effortful manner of phonation and replace it with a *simultaneous* initiation of phonation.

Myoelastic-Aerodynamic Theory of Voice Production

If we use the **myoelastic-aerodynamic theory of voice production** (Muller, 1843; van den Berg 1958) to describe a simultaneous onset of voicing, we describe a manner of phonation that may diminish phonotrauma and facilitate recovery of clinically normal voice production. In this state, the synchronized adduction of the vocal folds to phonation neutral position with a small space (~3 mm) between the vocal folds (Zemlin, 1998) and the coinciding initiation of exhalation result in simultaneous onset of voicing (Verdolini, Druker, Palmer, & Samawi, 1998). On the *initial* vibration, and as air passes through the narrow space between the vocal folds, the soft, compliant membranous portions of the vocal folds are sucked together by the **Bernoulli effect**. The cartilaginous portion of the vocal folds (the vocal processes of the arytenoid cartilages) remains in phonation neutral position (stabilized by the interarytenoid muscles). As the airflow continues, air pressure builds up below the closed glottis, and when the subglottal pressure exceeds 3 to 4 cm of H_2O (for quiet phonation) the membranous portions of the vocal folds begin their lateral excursion but the cartilaginous portions remain in phonation neutral position. This lateral excursion stretches the membranous tissue, and the theory suggests that the elasticity of the membranous tissue is sufficient to snap the vocal folds together and close the glottis to create the first glottal pulse. The frequency of vocal fold vibration is determined by vocal fold length in relation to its stiffness and mass.

Coordination: Pitch and Loudness Changes

"My husband says I sound like a robot when I practice. Is that the way it should be?" When we speak, we make dynamic changes in pitch and loudness to convey suprasegmental information about the mood and intent of the message. Changes in pitch occur primarily from adjustments in the length and stiffness of the vocal folds accompanied by the necessary fine-tuning of the subglottal pressure to match the stiffness in the folds. Due to the dynamic coordination and relationship between airflow/pressures and glottal resistance, the membranous portion of the folds vibrates at variable speeds and amplitudes of excursion making a broad range of pitch

and loudness possible. When individuals do not make active and appropriate changes in pitch and loudness, the voice becomes monotonous and disconnected, drawing negative attention to itself.

Your understanding of the physiology of pitch and loudness changes may be enhanced as you attend to the sensations in your vocal tract. As you move up and down a musical scale and focus on the vibrations behind your thyroid notch, you may feel a slight rising of the larynx, changes in the speed of vibration, and possibly the length or stiffness of the vocal folds. When an individual attends to these sensations, he uses sensory feedback to identify effort and makes appropriate modifications that permit changes in pitch and loudness more effectively. When you observe inappropriate pitch for a patient's age or gender, you consider whether this difference is a function of an inappropriate manner of phonation or changes in structure (edema, atrophy, scarring) that precipitated an inappropriate manner of phonation. Regardless of the cause, effective treatment focuses on decreasing this effortful production.

"Are you telling me that I should talk quietly all the time?" Habituated and excessive loudness during connected speech is a common symptom associated with voice problems. Inappropriate loudness is a result of excessive expiratory drive (subglottal pressure), medial compression, and stiffness of the vocal folds. You may ask your patient to attend to these sensations in order to decrease effortful phonation and loudness. When voice is produced quietly, the subglottal air pressure and medial compression of the vocal folds decrease. Many voice treatment procedures capitalize on this phenomenon in the early phases of therapy to enhance and reinforce a reduction in phonatory effort and decrease the transglottal pressure differential simply by using quieter phonation (confidential voice). Of course, quiet phonation is not the ultimate goal of therapy, and over time the patient learns to increase vocal intensity by exploiting the effect of back pressure/inertance.

Given that loudness is, in part, determined by subglottal air pressure, we will follow the air pressures from below the glottis (subglottal pressure), through the glottis (transglottal pressure), to above the glottis (supraglottal pressure). If we begin below the glottis, *subglottal pressure* is controlled by changing the pattern of respiratory muscle activation and vocal fold resistance, and is increased and decreased to change the loudness of phonation. If you say "taxi" quietly and then shout "taxi," you will notice that you use a fuller breath when you shout (increase your subglottal pressure). You automatically change your *subglottal pressure* when you modify the loudness of your voice. The minimum subglottal pressure required to initiate quiet phonation is 3 to 4 cm H_2O pressure, while 7 to 8 cm H_2O of subglottal pressure generates and maintains conversational loudness, and 10+ cm H_2O is used to generate a shout. This automatic coordination of subglottal pressure with phonation depends on the volume of air in the lungs, the elastic recoil of the chest wall, the control and grounding from the external intercostal and the abdominal muscles, in coordination with the medial compression (resistance) of the vocal folds.

If you consider that air pressure increases when the airflow is blocked, it is obvious that *subglottal pressure* is generated when the flow of air from the lungs is restricted at the level of the glottis. You can feel this pressure when you close your glottis to hold your breath. You will hear (and possibly feel) the result of this pressure when you produce voice with an abrupt initiation of phonation. In therapy we work to actively coordinate the air pressures (expiratory drive, subglottal pressure, transglottal pressure differential, and supraglottal pressure) and phonatory pressures (adduction, medial compression, and stiffening of the folds) to facilitate easy, efficient phonation.

Self-Sustained Oscillation of the Vocal Folds

Fant (1970) developed the linear source-filter theory of voice production to describe a two-step process that transforms the buzz created at the level of the vocal folds into speech sounds based on the resonant properties of the vocal tract **(Table 2-2)**. This resonance (energy) within the vocal tract can be defined in both clinical (sensations of vibration in the head and neck) and scientific terms (sympathetic vibration of the air in the vocal tract).

Titze (1994) postulated that the myoelastic-aerodynamic theory and the negative pressure created between the vocal folds by the Bernoulli effect are not sufficient to explain the continuing oscillation of the vocal folds. Expanding upon Fant's linear source-filter theory, he developed a nonlinear interactive source-filter hypothesis that incorporates the inertive reactance (sluggish response) of the air column in the vocal tract with the airflow and pressures at the level of the glottis to facilitate **self-sustained oscillation** (**Table 2-3**).

Table 2-2 Inertance

Linear Source-Filter Theory
Filter (vocal tract)
↑
Source (vocal folds)

Table 2-3 Inertance

Nonlinear Source-Filter Theory
Filter (vocal tract) + Inertive Reactance
↑↓
Source (vocal folds)

Titze (1994) suggests that some of the **acoustic energy** moving through the vocal tract is reflected back to the vocal folds to sustain continuous vibration and amplify the loudness of the laryngeal sound. He proposes that self-oscillation of the membranous folds is assisted by the inertia (sluggishness) of the air column in the vocal tract. If we track the air from the lungs toward the mouth, we can better understand this response. As the glottis opens and the airflow through the glottis increases, a positive pressure is created below the stationary air column in the vocal tract. This positive pressure above the vocal folds facilitates the opening of the glottis. As air continues through the glottis, the air in the vocal tract overcomes the inertia and begins to move toward the mouth. When the elastic recoil of the vocal folds closes the glottis (air stops moving through the glottis), the momentum of the air toward the mouth continues due to inertia. This continued, upward movement of air in the vocal tract creates an asymmetry and a small drop in the pressure immediately above and between the vocal folds. This resulting pressure drop facilitates closure of the glottis (Titze, 1994). The sluggishness of the air column above the glottis (**inertance**) is illustrated in **Figure 2-8**.

As we said earlier, the self-sustained vibration of the vocal folds requires an additional component: the **inertia** (delay) of the air column in the vocal tract (Titze & Verdolini-Abbott, 2012). The delay between the oscillation of the vocal folds and the movement of the supraglottal air results in a push-pull relationship that facilitates medial and lateral movement of the vocal folds. When the push-pull forces

Figure 2-8

Inertance

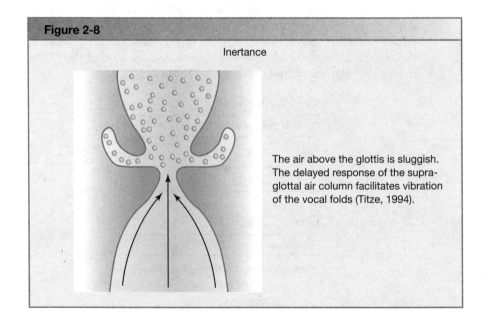

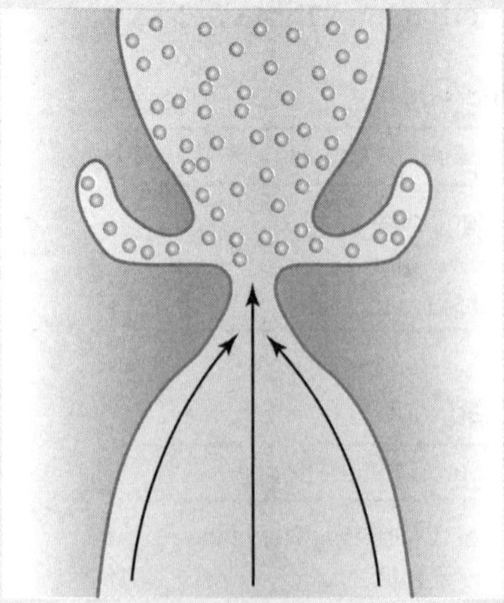

The air above the glottis is sluggish. The delayed response of the supraglottal air column facilitates vibration of the vocal folds (Titze, 1994).

are out of phase by one-quarter of a cycle, the supraglottal push-pull force works most efficiently. Titze proposes that inertive reactance (the degree of interaction and feedback of energy from the vocal tract to vocal folds) is regulated by the size, length, and shape of the vocal tract, and that it enhances resonance (the interaction between the vocal tract and the vocal folds), thus maximizing the perception of vibratory feedback.

Resonance

"I feel the vibrations in my nose, but what does that mean?" The vibration of the vocal folds produces sound waves that travel through and excite the air column in the vocal tract to create resonance. These vibrations can be felt as sensations in the nose, lips, hard palate, pharynx, and larynx. The reduction of extraneous muscle activity in the head and neck (e.g., releasing the lips, tongue, and jaw) enhances the strength of these vibrations, thus enhancing the vibratory feedback. Resonance is most apparent on nasal sounds (/m/, /n/, and /η/) but can also be felt to a lesser degree on vowels and some continuant phonemes (/r/, /v/, /∂/, /3/, /z/, /j/). When your patient consciously attends to these sensations he is capitalizing on the air column in the vocal tract to enhance self-oscillation of the vocal folds and the back pressure phenomenon.

Articulation

The source-filter theory recognizes the process by which the sound generated at the glottis is then shaped and modified by the vocal tract. When we produce consonants and vowels the pressure builds below the place of articulation, and the manner of articulation determines the degree of occlusion in the vocal tract. In American English the primary manners of phonation are plosives (highest back pressure) (/p/, /b/, /t/, /d/, /k/, /g/), affricatives (/tʃ/, /d3/), fricatives (/f/, /v/, /s/, /z/, /h/, /ʃ/, /3/, /θ/, /∂/), nasals (/m/, /n/, /η/), glides and semivowels (/w/, /r/, /l/, /j/), and approximately 20 vowels and diphthongs (minimal back pressure) (Borden, Harris, & Raphael, 2007).

Back Pressure: Coordination of Respiration, Phonation, and Resonation/Articulation

"Why do you have me say phrases that have certain sounds?" During connected speech the high back pressure associated with plosives, affricates, fricatives, and nasals creates a semi-occluded vocal tract and inertive reactance. As we briefly described in the *Introduction and Clinical Orientation* chapter, back pressure/resistance represents the increase in pressure above the vocal folds (supraglottal pressure) that is generated by

resistance to the flow of air above the glottis, resulting in a decrease in the collision forces between the vocal folds. When you produce a vowel, the vocal tract is open and there is little or no resistance to the flow of air above the glottis. In this state, the supraglottal pressure is equal to atmospheric pressure—hence, very little back pressure/resistance. In contrast, when you produce a bilabial voiced plosive—/bʌ/, /bʌ/, /bʌ/—you will feel pressure increase behind your lips (supraglottal or back pressure/resistance). The implosion of the /b/ generates so much back pressure/resistance that the vibrations of the larynx actually stop momentarily.

Essential to the concept of back pressure/resistance is the **transglottal pressure drop (differential)**, which describes the pressure difference between the supraglottal and subglottal pressures, which occurs as the air flows through the glottis, contributing to the force with which the vocal folds adduct during the vibratory oscillations. This elevated supraglottal pressure/resistance generates higher supraglottal pressure and diminishes the airflow across the glottis (transglottal pressure differential) by creating an opposing force throughout the vocal tract (**Pascal's law**). The back pressure/resistance exerts a force on the top of the vocal folds and pushes the membranous portions slightly apart. The air pressure between the folds decreases, thus diminishing the lateral and medial excursion of the vocal folds. This process is illustrated in **Figure 2-9**.

"Why do you want me to feel buzzing on my lips and fingers when I say /u/ through the straw?" When the transglottal pressure drop is excessively elevated the vocal folds snap together with great force. In therapy we create procedures to decrease the transglottal pressure drop in order to avoid these counterproductive, extreme collision forces. To that end, we develop a hierarchy of techniques that capitalize on the semi-occluded vocal tract by lengthening and narrowing the tract with phonation through straws of varying diameters, an airway reflex maneuver, Puffy Cheeks Exercise, or production of voiced consonants that generate a high intraoral pressure (e.g., /b/, /m/, /n/). These procedures serve the purposes of voice rehabilitation well because they both prevent laryngeal injury and maintain vocal fold health.

Physiology of Counterproductive Compensation

"Sometimes my voice sounds clearer if I talk louder." Patients frequently attempt to cope with their vocal symptoms by pushing the subsystems of voice production to work harder in an effort to overcome their dysphonia and produce a better, clearer, louder sound that they feel is closer to their "normal" voice. Some patients will be more aware of their compensatory behaviors and will acknowledge the effort they are using to produce voice. When you probe your patient's kinesthetic awareness of

Figure 2-9

Back Pressure

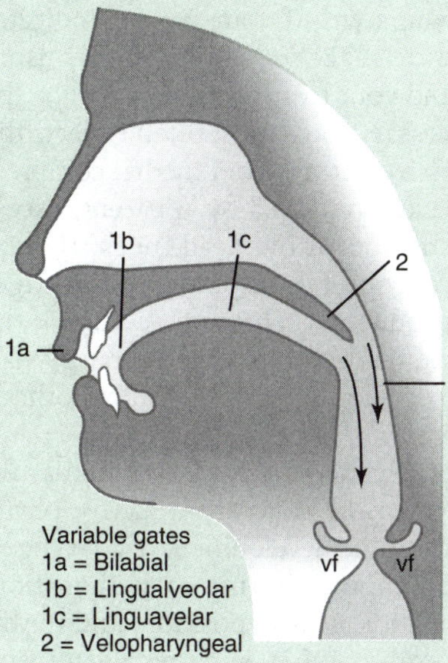

When the articulators move to narrow or close the vocal tract (articulation of consonants) the flow of air is slowed and pressure is reflected from this constriction toward the glottis.

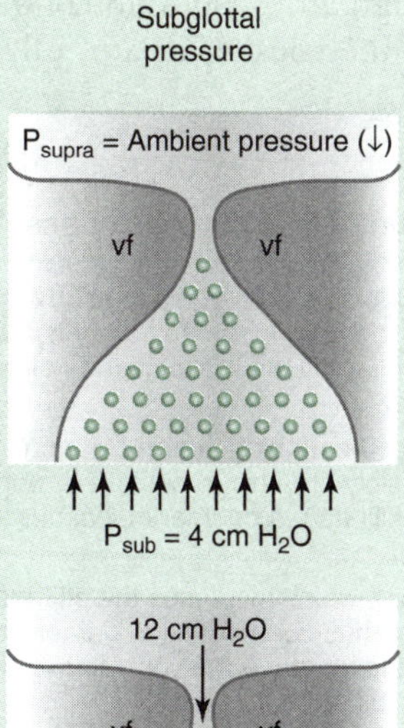

The back pressure is variable due to the amount of constriction above the glottis. During the production of vowels, the back pressure is minimal (equal to the ambient pressure in the room) due to the open vocal tract. During the production of vowels, the transglottal pressure drop (pressure drop across the glottis) equals the subglottal pressure.

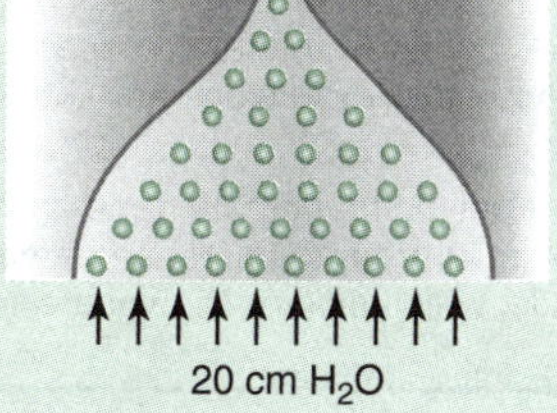

During production of stop consonants, the vocal tract is blocked and pressure builds up behind the articulators, resulting in an increase in supraglottal pressure (back pressure) and a simultaneous decrease in the transglottal pressure drop. Since the pressure above the glottis is higher than ambient pressure, the transglottal pressure will decrease. During the production of a consonant, for example, with a subglottal pressure of 20 cm H_2O and supraglottal pressure of 12, the transglottal pressure drop would equal 8 cm H_2O.

the degree of effort he feels when producing voice, you hope to learn more about his perspective regarding listening versus feeling as well as the acuity of his perceptions. You use **physiological empathy** when you compare his effort levels to your own. If your patient indicates that he is using a great deal of effort to make sound, he is likely using counterproductive compensation, and your treatment focus will be the reduction of that effort. This unnecessary force most often reflects the use of excess expiratory drive, excessive stiffness and medial compression of the vocal folds, and may be accompanied by apparent, excessive, and generalized muscle contraction in the head, neck, thorax, shoulders, and back. Further, if you observe respiratory challenges (and you identify them as counterproductive behaviors because of the differences between those behaviors and customary respiratory patterns), you can use that evidence to develop a physiological hypothesis that addresses the behavioral changes you hope to facilitate.

Before describing the common characteristics of dysphonia, we will offer several hypotheses related to the counterproductive physiological patterns that may contribute to the development of a laryngeal pathology and the symptoms of dysphonia. During easy phonation, the vocal folds are adducted to phonation neutral position, and in this position a small space (~3 mm) (Zemlin, 1998) exists between them. *Simultaneous* onset of exhalation results in small excursions of the vocal folds and reduced impact stress (Verdolini, 2000). In contrast, during an effortful manner of phonation the vocal folds are fully adducted,

Table 2-4 Hypotheses for Development of Counterproductive Compensation

- The patient has excessive mucus on the vocal folds due to allergies or **reflux**. The extra mucus damps vibration and contributes to perceived roughness. To compensate for the vocal change he coughs and clears his throat and increases the amplitude of the excursions and the force with which the glottis closes.
- The patient has vocal fold swelling due to prolonged coughing, throat clearing, or loud talking. Consequently, his voice is rough and possibly breathy. To achieve a more uniform vibration along the length of the vocal fold and facilitate a smoother mucosal wave, he stiffens the vocal folds to produce a clearer sound.
- The patient has a small, unilateral nodule or **polyp**, which increases the stiffness on and around the lesion and reduces the mucosal wave, thus contributing to perceived roughness. To achieve a more uniform vibration along the length of the vocal fold and facilitate a smoother mucosal wave, he stiffens both vocal folds.
- The patient has a nodule or polyp on the vocal fold that increases the mass and stiffness on the vocal fold. He increases his expiratory drive to cope with the increased stiffness and weight of the vocal fold, which increases the vibratory excursions and the force with which the glottis closes.
- The patient has bilateral (striking zone) nodules or polyps that create gaps anterior and posterior to the lesion, often resulting in breathiness. In order to decrease air wastage, he increases medial compression of the vocal folds, which stiffens the vocal folds and decreases the breathy quality.

and the arytenoid cartilages are squeezed together *prior* to the onset of exhalation. This pattern leads to increased excursions and medial compression of the vocal folds during vibration. **Table 2-4** provides several hypotheses that explore the development of counterproductive compensation.

A patient may often demonstrate immediate improvement in his voice quality when he implements a maladaptive behavior. When these patterns become habituated, the collision forces and mechanical stress on the vocal folds will likely exacerbate the voice problem. As this cycle continues, the patient further increases vocal fold stiffness, expiratory drive, and the amplitude of the vocal fold excursions. This relentless cycle of increasingly effortful voice production leads to further deformation of and friction between the vocal folds, thus aggravating the existing voice problem.

Underlying Physiology and Characteristics of Dysphonia

Regardless of the etiology of a voice problem, some of the most common characteristics of dysphonia are roughness, breathiness, abrupt initiation of phonation, pressed phonation, limited pitch and loudness ranges, excessive loudness, stridency, and aphonia (intermittent or continuous). A patient with a vocal fold paresis or paralysis (hypofunctional disorder), for example, may demonstrate a pattern of phonation similar to a patient diagnosed with **muscle tension dysphonia** associated with nodules or polyps (hyperfunctional dysphonia). *Consequently, the perceptual voice symptoms are not sufficient to distinguish the underlying physiology.* In the following section, we link some common vocal symptoms to possible underlying physiological changes. The symptoms reflect the counterproductive strategies typically implemented to manage symptoms and produce voice at any cost.

Roughness

Rough, hoarse, and raspy are often used synonymously to describe a voice that reflects aperiodicity in the vibration of the vocal folds, noise in the spectrum, and a low harmonics-to-noise ratio. Roughness suggests changes in the weight and/or stiffness within or between the vocal folds, which may lead to asynchronous and/or asymmetrical vocal fold patterns of vibration. Edema, vocal fold nodules, polyps, polypoid degeneration, Reinke's edema, papilloma, ankylosis of the cricoarytenoid joint, sulcus vocalis, vocal fold scarring, and carcinoma are common examples of pathologies associated with roughness. Individuals whose voice problem is associated with hyperfunction often attempt to decrease roughness and improve the clarity of the voice by hyperadducting the vocal folds and increasing expiratory drive.

Breathiness

A breathy voice is produced with excessive airflow through the glottis, and is often associated with reduced loudness. When airflow exceeds 400 milliliters per second, voice may be perceived as breathy (Grillo & Verdolini, 2008). Breathiness often occurs when air leaks through the small gaps anterior and posterior to a lesion on the medial border of the vocal fold (nodule or polyp). In the case of glottal insufficiency or vocal fold bowing, breathiness is the most salient characteristic. A unilateral vocal fold paralysis may lead to air wastage when one vocal fold fails to adduct to midline and the glottis is not completely sealed. In the case of a vocal fold paralysis, a patient may produce fewer words per breath group than expected or may become dizzy and hyperventilate as a result of air wastage and a disrupted inhalatory/exhalatory pattern. Ankylosis of the cricoarytenoid joint (associated with arthritis), often observed in older patients or those with Lupus, is also associated with breathiness, in this case due to lack of movement of the arytenoid cartilage and incomplete glottal closure. On the other hand, the mild breathiness that is sometimes a consequence of a posterior chink (often observed in women) is not considered a voice problem (Aronson & Bless, 2009).

Abrupt Initiation of Phonation

When the vocal folds are adducted or hyperadducted and stiffened *before* the exhalation phase begins, several counterproductive patterns are set in motion. Excessive stiffness may also be present in the vocal tract. As you will recall, phonation may begin with a breathy (air escapes prior to phonation), simultaneous (exhalation and phonation are synchronized), or abrupt onset. In the case of abrupt initiation, the vocal folds are stiffer than necessary and subglottal pressure is high before phonation begins, often triggering an increase in respiratory driving forces. Abrupt onset, frequently accompanied by stridency, can be associated with vocal pathologies that are the consequence of chronic, counterproductive patterns of phonation. Abrupt initiations are rather common in American English, although they have no linguistic significance in our language and usually occur less frequently and to a less extreme degree when voice is produced effectively.

Pressed Phonation

A pressed manner of phonation is characterized by excessive stiffness and medial compression of the vocal folds, high subglottal pressures (up to 21 cm of H_2O), limited airflow, and possible subglottal and supralaryngeal constriction (Grillo & Verdolini, 2008; Titze & Verdolini-Abbott, 2012). Over time, the long closed phase that is also associated with pressed phonation may be detrimental to the vocal fold tissue, and this prolonged mechanical stress may lead to phonotrauma.

It would not be unusual for a patient who has been diagnosed with vocal fold nodules, polyps, or edema to demonstrate a pressed manner of phonation in an attempt to compensate for the phonatory limitations that the lesion has imposed on the laryngeal system. A pressed voice is often a counterproductive strategy unconsciously used to enhance acoustic and harmonic energy and increase loudness. Constriction of the subglottal or supraglottal airway may be more acoustically efficient, but it is physiologically detrimental to **vocal longevity** given the high degree of effort it requires. Patient awareness of increased effort is quite variable, especially when this manner of phonation has been habituated over months and even years. Pressed phonation may have a link to abrupt initiation of voicing and hypernasality if velopharyngeal insufficiency is present and the patient attempts to compensate for the leakage of air through the velopharyngeal port (Kosowski, Weathers, Wolfswinkel, & Ridgway, 2012; McWilliams, 1991; McWilliams, Morris, & Shelton, 1984).

Stridency

A strident voice is associated with increased expiratory drive, hyperadduction, and increased stiffness of the vocal folds, as well as excessive supraglottal constriction throughout the vocal tract. Repeated use of this manner of phonation often leads to a laryngeal pathology (nodules, polyps, contact ulcer, edema, and hyperemia). A strident voice may actually be a maladaptive strategy to reduce breathiness and roughness and cope with limitations in loudness. It may be accompanied by abrupt initiation of phonation. On the other hand, an actor may choose stridency to portray a character (e.g., the wicked witch in *The Wizard of Oz*) in a play, and in that case will capitalize on the vocal tract to achieve this effect without stiffening or causing injury. to the larynx.

Limited Pitch and Loudness Ranges

The possible physiological patterns associated with limited pitch and loudness ranges include excessive, passive stiffness or incomplete adduction of the vocal folds, velopharyngeal port insufficiency, or lack of coordination between the vocal tract and vocal fold vibration. These changes diminish the dynamic ranges for loudness and pitch at both extremes. With excessive, passive stiffness in the vocal folds, the flexibility needed to increase and decrease pitch is limited. These limitations may develop following prolonged effortful voice production or may be of neurological (vocal fold paralysis) or psychological origin (prepubescent dysphonia). Singers may complain of a restricted pitch range (e.g., a difficulty producing an efficient **glissando**), difficulty sustaining a high tessitura (average pitch of a song or aria), and difficulty producing an efficient *messa di voce* (i.e., gradual crescendo and diminuendo).

Intermittent Aphonia

Sudden, unplanned, and momentary voice breaks (i.e., **intermittent aphonia**) may occur in response to many pathologies that passively stiffen the vocal folds, including edema, vocal fold nodules, polyps, polypoid degeneration, sulcus vocalis, and carcinoma, or when a neurological problem weakens a vocal fold and renders it flaccid (unilateral vocal fold paresis/paralysis). Short, sudden unintended cessation of phonation may occur when respiratory drive is insufficient to generate the necessary subglottal pressure (~3 to 4 cm H_2O) to initiate and sustain phonation, or when there is a mismatch between subglottal pressure and the adduction, stiffness, and mass characteristics of the vocal folds. The rapid changes that take place during articulation, voiced to unvoiced, pitch and **loudness inflection**, and changes in the quality/timbre, for example, involve a dynamic balance among the respiratory, phonatory, and resonation subsystems. This balance may be disrupted when these linguistic/prosodic demands overload the minimal, requisite coordination among these subsystems.

Continuous Aphonia

When aphonia is continuous, perceived as a whisper or mimed speech, it may be of short or long duration. The aphonia may reflect a viral or bacterial infection; the effects of chronic, accelerating effort; a single traumatic laryngeal injury; a psychogenic problem; or the absence of a larynx. When the aphonia is of psychological origin, the larynx may appear completely normal without edema or changes in mass. If the absence of voicing relates to infection, it is common to observe edematous, stiffened, and inflamed vocal folds. The physiological patterns associated with continuous aphonia, observed in bilateral vocal fold paralysis, with high respiratory drive, insufficient adduction of the vocal folds, flaccidity, and mismatch of vocal fold stiffness with the expiratory drive, make phonation unlikely. Patients who have **abductor spasmodic dysphonia** may demonstrate periods of aphonia owing to unplanned and involuntary abduction of the vocal folds.

Summary

A clinician usually incorporates several models simultaneously, even within a particular session, in order to cope with the challenges that arise and the disparate problems a patient introduces. Theoretical constructs offer a perspective from which you will develop a treatment program. We have discussed several theories in this chapter, and anticipate that they will provide a beginning framework for reflection on the treatment process and the development of an appropriate hierarchy of goals and procedures. These theories are meant to act as a reference point as you embark on the development of your long- and short-term goals.

References

Adams, J.A. (1971). A closed-loop theory of motor learning. *Journal of Motor Behavior, 3*, 111–149.

Angsuwarangsee, T., and Morrison, M. (2002). Extrinsic laryngeal muscular tension in patients with voice disorders. *Journal of Voice, 16*, 333–343.

Aronson, A. (1990). *Clinical voice disorders: An interdisciplinary approach*. New York, NY: Brian C. Decker.

Aronson, A.E., and Bless, D. (2009). *Clinical voice disorders: An interdisciplinary approach*. New York, NY: Thieme.

Bernstein, N.A. (1967). *The coordination and regulation of movements*. Oxford, England: Pergamon Press.

Borden, G.J., Harris, K.S., and Raphael, L.J. (2007). *Speech science primer: Physiology, acoustics and perception of speech* (5th ed.). Baltimore, MD: Lippincott Williams and Wilkins.

Bowen, J.L. (2006). Educational strategies to promote clinical diagnostic reasoning. *New England Journal of Medicine, 355*, 2217–2225.

Chan, A.K., McCabe, P., and Madill, C.J. (2013). The implementation of evidence-based practice in the management of adults with functional voice disorders: A national survey of speech-language pathologists. *International Journal of Speech-Language Pathology, 15*(3), 334–344.

Chapman, J. (2012). *Singing and teaching singing: A holistic approach to classical voice* (2nd ed.). San Diego, CA: Plural.

Dimon, T. (2011). *Your body, your voice: The key to natural singing and speaking*. Berkeley, CA: North Atlantic Books.

Fairbanks, G. (1954). Systematic research in experimental phonetics: A theory of the speech mechanism as a servosystem. *Journal of Speech and Hearing Disorders, 19*(2), 133–139.

Fant, G. (1970). *Acoustic theory of speech production*. The Hague, Netherlands: Monton.

Franco, D., Martins, F., Andrea, M., Fragoso, I., Carrao, L., and Teles, J. (2014). Is the sagittal postural alignment different in normal and dysphonic adult speakers? *Journal of Voice, 28*(4), 523.e1–523.e8.

Gabriele, T.E., Hall, C.R., and Lee, T.D. (1989). Cognition in motor learning: Imagery effects on contextual interference. *Human Movement Science, 8*, 227–245.

Green, S., and Sherwood, D.E. (2000). The benefits of random variable practice for accuracy and temporal error detection in a rapid aiming task. *Research Quarterly Exercise Sport, 71*(4), 398–402.

Greene, P.H. (1972). Problems of organization of motor systems. In R. Rosen and F.M. Snell (Eds.), *Progress in theoretical biology* (Vol. 2) (pp. 304-338). New York, NY: Academic Press.

Grillo, E.U., and Verdolini, K. (2008). Evidence for distinguishing pressed, normal, resonant, and breathy voice qualities by laryngeal resistance and vocal efficiency in vocally trained subjects. *Journal of Voice, 22*(5), 546–552.

Heuer, H. (1989). A multiple-representations approach to mental practice of motor skills. In B.D. Kirkcaldy (Ed.), *Normalities and abnormalities in human movement* (pp. 36–57). Basel, Switzerland: Karger.

Hirano, M. (1974). Morphological structure of the vocal fold as a vibrator and its variations. *Folia Phoniatrica, 26*, 89–94.

Hixon, J.T., and Hoit, J.D. (2005). *Evaluation and management of speech breathing disorders: Principles and methods.* Tucson, AZ: Redington Brown.

Hixon, J.T., Weismer, G., and Hoit, J.D. (2008). *Preclinical speech science: Anatomy, physiology, acoustics, perception.* San Diego, CA: Plural.

Hoit, J.D. (1995). Influence of body position on breathing and its implications for the evaluation of treatment of speech and voice disorders. *Journal of Voice, 9*, 341–347.

Hoit, J.D., Palssman, B.L., Lansing, R.W., and Hixon, T.J. (1988). Abdominal muscle activity during speech production. *Journal of Applied Physiology, 65*, 2656–2664.

Kent, R. (2006). Evidençe-based practice in communication disorders: Progress not perfection. *Language, Science and Hearing Services in Schools, 37*, 268–270.

Kosowski, T.R., Weathers, W.M., Wolfswinkel, E.M., and Ridgway, E.B. (2012). Cleft palate. *Seminars in Plastic Surgery, 26*(4), 164–169.

Kuhn, T.S. (Ed.). (1970). *The structure of the scientific revolution* (2nd ed., Vol. 2). Chicago, Ill: University of Chicago Press.

Laukkanen, A.M., Titze, I.R., Hoffman, H., and Finnegan, E. (2008). Effects of a semi-occluded vocal tract on laryngeal muscle activity and glottal adduction in a single female subject. *Folia Phoniatrica et Logopedica, 60*, 298–311.

Lessac, A. (1997). *The use and training of the human voice: A practical approach to speech and voice dynamics* (3rd ed.). Santa Monica, CA: McGraw-Hill.

Mandin, H., Jones, A., Woloschuk, W., and Harasym, P. (1997). Helping students learn to think like experts when solving clinical problems. *Academic Medicine, 72*(3), 173–179.

Maxwell, D.L., and Satake, E. (2006). *Research and statistical methods in communication sciences and disorders.* Boston, MA: Thomson/Delmar.

McWilliams, B.J. (1991). Submucous clefts of the palate: How likely are they to be symptomatic? *Cleft Palate Craniofacial Journal, 28*, 247–251.

McWilliams, B.J., Morris, H., and Shelton, R. (1984). *Cleft palate speech.* Burlington, Ontario: BC Decker.

Muller, J. (1843). Cit. by Grutzner, P. (1879). *Physiologie der stimme und sprache. Handbuch der physiology*, 1, Berlin.

Ratner, N.B. (2006). Evidence-based practice: An examination of its ramification for the practice of speech-language pathology. *Language, Speech, and Hearing in Schools*, *37*, 257–267.

Schmidt, R.A. (1975). *Motor skills*. New York, NY: Harper and Row.

Schmidt, R.A. (1976). Movement education and the schema theory. In E. Crawford (Ed.), *Report of the 1976 conference June 3–8*. Cedar Falls, IA: National Association for Physical Education of College Women.

Schmidt, R.A. (1991). Frequent augmented feedback can degrade learning: Evidence and interpretations. In J. Requin and G.E. Stelmach (Eds.), *Tutorials in motor neuroscience* (pp. 59–75). Dordrecht, Netherlands: Kluwer.

Schmidt, R.A., and Lee, T.D. (2011). *Motor control and learning: A behavioral emphasis* (5th ed.). Champaign, IL: Human Kinetics.

Shea, C.H., Lai, Q., Wright, D.L., Immink, M., and Black, C. (2001). Consistent and variable practice conditions: Effects on relative timing and absolute timing. *Journal of Motor Behavior*, 33, 139–152.

Shea, C.H., and Morgan, R.I. (1979). Contextual interference effects on the acquisition, retention, and transfer of a motor skill. *Journal of Experimental Psychology: Human Learning and Memory*, 5, 179–187.

Sherwood, D.E., and Lee, T.D. (2003). Schema theory: Critical review and implications for the role of cognition in a new theory of motor learning. *Research Quarterly for Exercise and Sport*, *74*, 376–382.

Silman, S., Silverman, C.A., Emmer, M.B., and Gelfand, S.A. (1993). Effects of prolonged lack of amplification on speech-recognition performance: Preliminary findings. *Journal of Rehabilitation and Research Development*, 30(3), 326–332.

Titze, I.R. (1988). The physics of small amplitude oscillation of the vocal folds. *Journal of the Acoustical Society of America*, 83(4), 1536–1552.

Titze, I.R. (1994). *Principles of voice production*. Denver, CO: National Center for Voice and Speech.

Titze, I.R. (2001). Acoustic interpretation of resonant voice. *Journal of Voice*, 15(4), 519–528.

Titze, I.R., and Verdolini-Abbott, K.V. (2012). *Vocology: The science and practice of voice rehabilitation*. Salt Lake City, UT: The National Center for Voice and Speech.

van den Berg, J.W. (1958). Myoelastic aerodynamic theory of voice production. *Journal of Speech and Hearing Science*, *I*, 227–244.

Verdolini, K. (2000). *The vocal vision: Views on voice by 24 leading teachers, coaches and directors*. New York, NY: Applause Books.

Verdolini, K., Druker, D.G., Palmer, P.M., and Samawi, H. (1998). Laryngeal adduction in resonant voice. *Journal of Voice*, 12(3), 315–327.

Vinney, L.A., and Turkstra, L.S. (2013). The role of self-regulation in voice therapy. *Journal of Voice*, 27(3), 390.e1–390.e11.

Vohs, K.D., and Baumeister, R.F. (2004). Ego depletion, self-control, and choice. In T. Pyszczynski (Ed.), *Handbook of experimental existential psychology* (pp. 398–410). New York, NY: Guildford Press.

Weeks, D.L., Hall, A.K., and Anderson, L.P. (1996). A comparison of imitation strategies in observational learning of action patterns. *Journal of Motor Behavior, 28*, 348–358.

Whiting, H.T. (1984). *Human motor actions: Bernstein reassessed*. Amsterdam, Netherlands: Elsevier.

Wong, A.W., Whitehill, T.L., Ma, E.P., and Masters, R. (2013). Effects of practice schedules on speech motor learning. *International Journal of Speech Language Pathology, 15*(5), 511–523.

Wrisberg, C.A., and Liu, Z. (1991). The effect of contextual variety on the practice, retention, and transfer of an applied motor skill. *Research Quarterly for Exercise and Sport, 62*, 406–412.

Zemlin, W.R. (1998). *Speech and hearing science: Anatomy and physiology* (4th ed.). Needham Heights, MA: Allyn and Bacon.

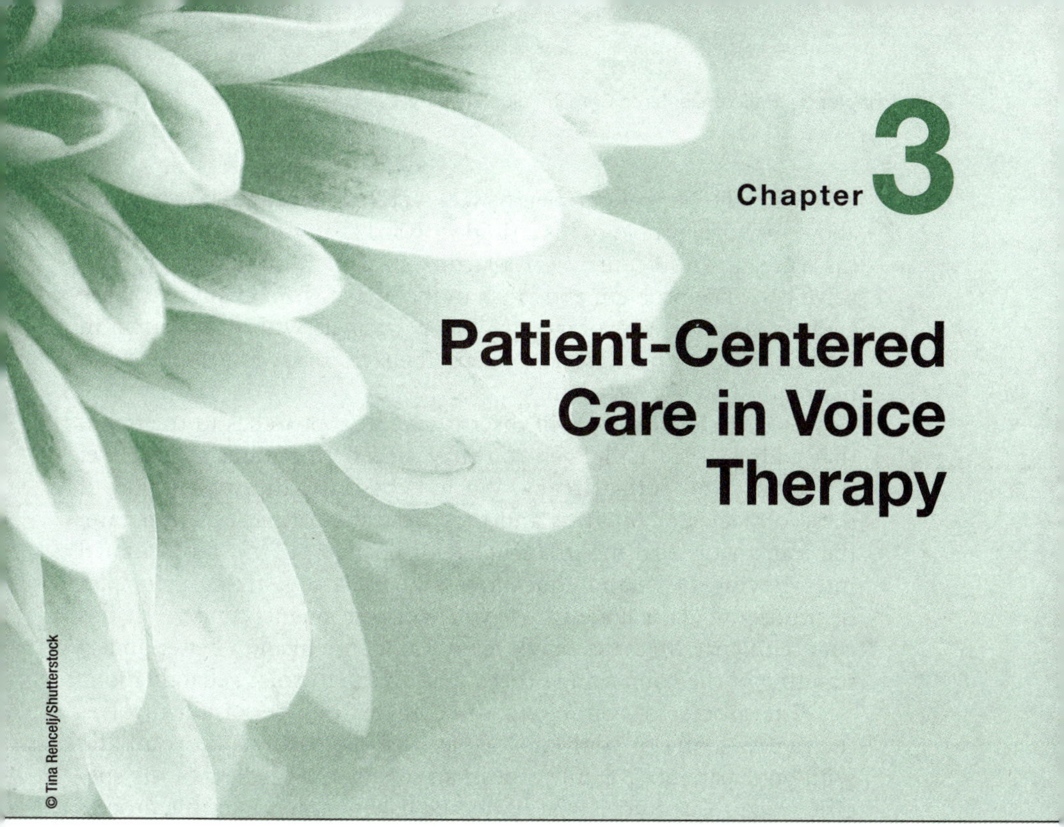

Chapter 3

Patient-Centered Care in Voice Therapy

"I began with an open question, 'Tell me about your voice problem.'"

How do I help my patient to change? He doesn't focus on the things I suggest. When I ask him how a procedure *felt*, he says it *sounded* bad. He tells me he is motivated, but he doesn't use deliberate practice. He always has an excuse and says that he is going to practice. What is going wrong? What is wrong with him? What is wrong with me?

The purpose of therapy is to do something different—to change (Yalom, 2009). It's easy to say, but… hard to do. If a patient could change his manner of phonation on his own, using his intuition and inner resources, he would not need your help as a speech-language pathologist. Your skills in counseling, your therapeutic repertoire, and your perceptual skills will facilitate his openness to the changes he needs to consider as he begins to make sound in an easier and more efficient way. The process begins with **active listening**—how he feels about his voice problem, his attitude toward changing the way he uses his voice, and co-occurring risk factors. Bear in mind that you cannot solve his voice problem and you cannot "make" him change. You are a *partner* in the process of change. You participate with your patient in finding solutions to counterproductive behaviors that contribute to and maintain the voice problem.

In this chapter, we will discuss several approaches to treatment that address the challenges you may face with patient **adherence**, resistance, and **self-efficacy**. We will begin with a discussion of these obstacles to progress and then describe patient-centered care, the transtheoretical model of behavior change (TTM), motivational interviewing (MI), and education as possible organizing principles of counseling. Our hope is that you will continue to explore various counseling paradigms as you develop confidence in and a better understanding of the counseling process pertaining to voice rehabilitation.

The process of counseling is a complex one because it involves the interweaving of your knowledge with the partnership you build with your patient. It is inherent in all sessions, regardless of the specific voice-related goals you have established. You begin this process when you meet your patient for the first time. As you begin therapy, the relationship you develop will hopefully encourage your patient to take risks, try new ways of producing his voice (despite feelings of awkwardness), and then feel confident enough to generalize the techniques he developed with you to his social and work situations.

How Do You Prepare to Meet Your Patient's Needs?

The ancient Greek aphorism "know thyself" is probably familiar to you, but how does it apply to clinical competence in the area of voice? Martin (1983) suggests that counseling skills emerge with practice, and an intrinsic part of that development is the exploration of your own responses to feelings of apprehension, anxiety, and self-doubt as a voice clinician. It will be useful, then, to maintain an open and ongoing discussion with your supervisor or a colleague to support you as you explore these feelings and work through moments of indecision during the preparation of your sessions. There will be times when your patient is aware of your trepidation and uncertainty, but it may be helpful to realize that your feelings are a reflection of your conscientious attitude as you strive to meet this challenge with competence. You are capable of conveying respect, listening without judgment, and appreciating another individual's response to a problem.

Cultural Humility

As citizens of the twenty-first century, we envision a society that values and respects cultural differences and is enriched by the music, food, customs, and the language and idioms of the world community. Unfortunately and all too often, fear, ignorance, and prejudice undermine society's response to those who represent "the other." If we minimize the import and impact of cultural differences on an individual's citizenship in society, we fall prey to our own biases and cultural ethnocentricity.

Our profession and the **American-Speech-Language-Hearing Association's (ASHA) principles of ethics** charge us to welcome all individuals, irrespective of age, race, religion, ethnicity, national origin, politics, gender identity, or sexual orientation. **Cultural humility** (Alsharif, 2012; Brennan, Barnsteiner, Siantz, Cotter, & Everett, 2012; Gruppen, 2014; Kutob et al., 2013) calls for our recognition and appreciation of the values held by other cultures, an acknowledgment that, while our perspectives may differ, they are of equal significance, and that we do not practice cultural imperialism. The notion of a cultural positive regard in a therapeutic relationship warrants emphasis and reiteration. Only when this humility exists can the clinician develop a person-centered collaboration with individuals who do not share the same culture. As with all areas of specialty in the communicative sciences, however, the voice clinician must acknowledge any reservations or biases that might negatively affect the client-clinician partnership and adjust appropriately in order to provide therapy in a way that respects and honors the patient's cultural background.

What Is Patient-Centered Therapy?

The practice of medicine and other disciplines has begun to incorporate the patient as a partner in the treatment process. This change in perspective to include the patient's insights, knowledge, expectations, fears, etc. in the treatment process grew out of a patient-centered model developed over 60 years ago. Carl Rogers (1946, 1951) introduced the concept of patient-centered care within the psychotherapeutic process to capitalize on the idea that the patient is the expert and has the capacity to actively participate in solving his problems. This underlying framework acknowledges the patient's autonomy and provides an environment of respect and **empathy** that fosters change. Over time, the original model was modified to include other disciplines such as nursing, medicine, and very recently, speech-language pathology (DiLollo & Favreau, 2010; Geller & Foley, 2009; Leahy & Walsh, 2008; Luterman, 2008; Manning, 2010). Stewart et al. (1995) modified and expanded the concept of **patient-centered therapy** to be more specific and included "(1) exploring both the disease and the illness experience, (2) understanding the whole person, (3) finding common ground, (4) incorporating prevention and health promotion, (5) enhancing the patient-doctor relationship, [and] (6) being realistic" (pp. 24–25) regarding what changes are feasible given the presenting problem. These concepts work best when integrated into both the diagnostic evaluation and ongoing treatment.

Patient-centered care emphasizes not only the importance of including the patient in the decision-making process regarding therapeutic intervention, but the need to determine the compatibility of treatment options with the patient's personal perspective. Attention to patient self-efficacy (one's belief in one's capacity to change) (Bandura, 1986), concerns, preferences, and attitudes is central to the successful creation of a partnership with your patient. When you develop practice schedules and home exercises, for instance, if the patient is not comfortable with the exercises or practice schedule, adherence to the therapeutic program will be threatened, thus slowing the recovery process (Messer, 2004). A patient's lack of confidence or comfort with a procedure can lead to halfhearted attempts to perform exercises, lack of adherence to practice, and eventually discontinuation of treatment.

Several studies have suggested that patients are more receptive to following a treatment regimen when they have a voice in the treatment process (Stemple, 2000; van Leer & Connor, 2010; van Leer, Hapner, & Connor, 2008). Moreover, the burden of sole ownership for the treatment process and treatment decisions is shared in a patient-centered partnership. This paradigmatic shift moves the responsibility for change to the patient, thus reducing the pressure you feel to be the expert, and increasing the patient's participation in the process.

What Is Active Listening?

How do you include the patient in the **decision-making process**? The first step is to actively listen and attend to the patient's narrative, showing interest by affirming with a nod, asking follow-up questions, and asking if the patient has more information to offer. If you observe excessive effort and loudness during the interview, you and the patient will problem solve to generate ideas that address reduction of effort in situations that require increased levels of vocal intensity. If the patient reveals that he "always speaks loudly," further exploration of what "always" means, as well as your explanation of the effect of prolonged loudness on the larynx, may lead to a cooperative brain-storming effort to change this habit, which sets the stage for the partnership you hope to create. Similarly, if you ask the patient to describe what he feels in his throat before and after a straw phonation procedure, you have included him as a partner in the search for procedures that he feels work for him, or to which he does not respond. If he says, "My throat feels more relaxed after that exercise," you have information about his kinesthetic awareness and a possible option for decreasing laryngeal stiffness. This aspect of patient-centered care facilitates not only the inclusion of the patient as expert, but the development of an individualized treatment program that will promote patient self-efficacy.

What Is Empathy?

You may not realize how much insight you already have into the impact of a voice problem on one's communication skills. When you were in school, you may have worried whether your voice would project during class presentations, debates, chorus, and plays. You may have developed laryngitis after yelling at a game, rehearsing for a school show, or performing as a cheerleader, or had difficulty talking when you had a sore throat. Hopefully, your voice disturbance was transitory, but it may have provided a glimpse into the frustration and emotional turmoil that a voice disorder can cause in one's life. Moreover, you may have had a family member who had spasmodic dysphonia, vocal fold paralysis, nodules, or a polyp and shared their feelings of shame, embarrassment, and frustration. It may be that as a child or teenager you participated in therapy and understand from a very personal perspective how frustrating and challenging it can be to live with a problem and work to resolve it. More recently, you may have observed treatment sessions, possibly shadowed the treating student clinician, or even participated in voice therapy yourself. These experiences can be called upon as part of the foundation that prepares you for your role as a voice clinician.

What Is Accurate Empathy?

These previous experiences provide a starting place to develop the accurate, or evocative, empathy (Martin, 1983; Rogers, 1975) you will need when you work with a patient who has a voice problem. Remember, as a voice clinician your goal is not to feel what the patient is feeling, but to develop an accurate understanding and appreciation of the patient's response to the problem. "It is extraordinarily difficult to know really what the other feels; far too often we project our own feelings onto the other" (Yalom, 2009, p. 21). If you see a patient in the same way that you see your family member or yourself, you will be less effective as a clinician. It is not your job to feel sad. In the context of voice rehabilitation you will use "evocative empathy," which allows you not only "to appreciate the patient's experience" of the voice problem (Yalom, 2009, p. 18), but to demonstrate a "positive, unconditional regard"

(Rogers, 1961, p. 47) for him. Accurate empathy will provide the freedom you need to manage your anxiety and self-conscious attention by focusing on "the person rather than the task" (Grosch, Medvene, & Wolcott, 2008, p. 24). You begin with your respect for the patient's perception of his voice problem and his desire to improve his voice.

It's Not Personal

Imagine that you are about to begin an evaluation with a voice patient. You introduce yourself, and she bursts into tears. This scenario may seem extremely unlikely to you, but rest assured we have experienced this difficult situation numerous times. There are many such examples of patients' despair and loss of emotional control as they anticipate the opportunity to relate their story to an empathetic listener. When this happens, your first response may be helplessness and a feeling of being overwhelmed. An alternative first meeting might involve a very angry patient, who rages against the otolaryngologist who, he believes, severed the recurrent laryngeal nerve leaving him severely breathy, winded, and incapable of working as a salesperson.

A new patient who expresses extreme frustration and distrusts the process of voice therapy altogether because previous voice rehabilitation "did not help at all," can make you feel defensive and required to prove that you are, indeed, an expert. How do you respond to these strong feelings without invoking persuasion to convince your patient to participate in this new voice therapy relationship? It would not be surprising if you felt that the patient's anger and frustration are aimed directly at you. His emotions, however, reflect his anxiety, fear, and desperation from the abyss of "why me?" and have nothing to do with you. The answer to your dilemma is simple, yet hard to do. Listen with "accurate sensitivity" (Martin, 1983, p. 9) and acknowledge his feelings.

Situations with strong emotions may make you uncomfortable, and that discomfort may propel you into action. You may want to do something—to give the patient advice, to help him feel better, or to fix his problem—but you may feel incompetent and wonder how you will solve his voice problem. Fortunately, this is not your job. The role of the voice clinician is to create a partnership that allows the patient to tap his capacity (Rogers, 1959) to modify his manner of phonation in order to meet the challenge of integrating a more effective coordination among the vocal subsystems. As experience leads to a clearer definition of your role as a voice clinician, your need to fix, to save, or to solve the patient's problem will fade and be replaced by a recognition of your role as active listener and partner in the voice rehabilitation process.

The dialogues throughout this text include the clinician's thought process (*italicized*) as the clinician formulates a response that is appropriate to the patient's readiness for change. These subtle shifts provide data related to the patient's capacity to modify counterproductive vocal behaviors. **Dialogue 3-1** incorporates both a **client-centered approach** (open-ended questions, acknowledgment of the patient's perspective) and, when appropriate, an evidence-based practice model (provision of information and education).

Dialogue 3-1
Excerpt from Initial Assessment

I began, "Tell me about your voice problem." (Open-ended question)

Ms. A almost barked, "I don't have a voice problem. My boss thinks I need to fix my voice. He said that if I don't sound better when I answer the phone, he'll fire me."

Startled by the obvious agitation in her response, and hoping to dissipate her strong reaction, I listened closely and noted her rigid body posture and severely rough, strident voice. "That's frustrating. It sounds like you don't feel you have a choice."

Glaring at me and stiffening her jaw, "It is none of his business, and I don't need to be here. There's nothing wrong with my voice."

I recognized that she was angry, and I knew that it would interfere with her receptivity to suggestions related to change. "Can you tell me what is going on?"

With a hint of softening in her voice and upper body, "He is a jerk. I have worked at the hospital for six years. I do a good job. Why is he being so mean?"

I noted the subtle change in her voice, and continued using accurate empathy hoping to dissipate more of her anger. "You are in a tough spot." *My response appeared to soothe her.*

Softening even more, Ms. A said, "People understand me well enough. You understand me."

With the knowledge that my genuine interest in her voice might engage her in the evaluation, I said, "Yes, I do. Do you ever notice any changes in your voice, even during the day when you are working?"

With surprise, "What do you mean?"

I perceived her rising pitch and slight lean forward, and I realized that her curiosity had opened a channel of communication. I explained, "Well, if you are answering the phone all day it is easy for your throat to get tired and feel a little sore or tight. Has that ever happened?"

She leaned forward and spoke in a quieter voice, "Is that important?"

I was relieved when she expressed her interest. "If you are talking a lot and using a lot of effort, it can cause problems over time, and it can become more difficult to talk with your friends at restaurants, on the phone, and over noise."

Ms. A said, "Now that you mention it, I have noticed that after work I don't want to talk any more. It feels like too much work. I've started avoiding going to restaurants with my friends and cutting phone conversations short."

In Dialogue 3-1, the clinician shifted the focus from the patient's anger with her employer to her manner of phonation and its impact on her vocal performance. The clinician attempted to validate the patient's feelings and introduce the subject of her manner of phonation. This patient-centered response acknowledges the patient's feelings and establishes a supportive environment that encourages the patient to engage in the initial consultation. If the clinician had ignored the patient's feelings, it is possible that her focus would remain on her anger with her boss and she would decide against therapy despite the threat of lost employment.

Scope of Practice

It is not unusual for even an experienced clinician to sometimes feel that it is his job to save the patient, especially when patients express anxiety, depression, or feelings of helplessness. However, these symptoms may require a referral to an outside specialist. Although accurate empathy is appropriate and reflects your appreciation of the impact of these issues on the voice patient, **psychotherapy** is outside the realm of expertise for a speech-language pathologist. We acknowledge these symptoms and explore how the patient is coping with these issues. Is he in psychotherapy? Is he on medication? Is a referral to a psychotherapist relevant? We always consider the relative impact of co-occurring problems on the patient's manner of phonation. If, for instance, a bulimic patient is regurgitating six or seven times per day, he will likely show laryngeal consequences associated with exposure to gastric acid and strenuous laryngeal valving. It would be appropriate to discuss the relationship between the patient's voice, the frequent regurgitation, and its impact on the outcome of therapy, and to recommend that he consult the appropriate professional to assess the underlying problem. It is often surprising how receptive patients can be to a referral to a counselor or psychotherapist because their suffering is so oppressive they welcome a suggestion that provides a course of action.

Eight Mantras for a New Clinician

Given that it is normal, typical, and expected that you will be anxious, self-conscious and possibly overwhelmed by the self-perceived expectations you have for your first therapy sessions, we will offer a few basic premises you might include in your thinking as you prepare for these first encounters. They provide a starting point, a basic set of counseling principles that we have integrated in our approach to voice rehabilitation, regardless of the models and therapeutic techniques we have chosen to use over the years.

1. It is impossible to remember and implement *everything* you have learned in your coursework.
2. Your skills will improve as you gain more experience.
3. Listen to the patient's account of his voice problem. Be *in the present*, explore, and ask for more information regarding his perspective.
4. Every patient is unique.
5. Remember that you do not empathize with the patient in the way you do with family and friends in your personal life.
6. You cannot persuade or convince anyone of anything.
7. No technique or model works for every patient.
8. It is okay to say, "I don't know."

Who Is My Patient?

You will work with many patients who come to you from various social and cultural backgrounds, professions, and outlooks on life. The elite voice user; professional voice user; the homemaker with three children; the 80-year-old retiree; the individual with concomitant problems such as acid reflux; the patient who is self-referred or comes to you under doctor's orders; the transsexual client; the person who works in a noisy environment; the patient with logorrhea; the individual with spasmodic dysphonia (SD), and the list goes on. Although their presenting problems may be different, they share a common goal—to modify and improve the use of their voice. They may react to the voice problem in different ways and come with varying degrees of self-awareness, proprioceptive and kinesthetic sensitivity, knowledge related to the voice, past experience with success or failure with change (self-efficacy), and readiness to make change. How do you provide effective voice rehabilitation in the face of so much variability? The answer lies in a patient-centered approach, which allows you to respect and adjust to the needs, expectations, and perspective of the patient.

What Is Adherence?

Although voice rehabilitation is the gold standard for the resolution of many voice problems, resistance to change and adherence to voice programs remain the most common challenges we all face as we guide our patients through the rehabilitation process. Adherence to physician referral to voice therapy (38% do not follow through), follow-up with the therapist after the assessment (47% do not follow through), and completion of treatment (65% do not complete treatment) remain dishearteningly poor (Hapner, Portone-Maira, & Johns III, 2009; Smith, Kempster, & Sims, 2010). These statistics may surprise you, but they are in line with adherence to treatment regimens for otolaryngology, gastroenterology, and psychology (Portone, Johns III, & Hapner, 2008). Several studies recognize that there are many complex variables that contribute to patients' adherence or nonadherence to treatment. Attending four or more therapy sessions and shorter delays between referral and onset of treatment have been correlated with perseverance for completing voice treatment (Hapner et al., 2009). Interestingly, in a study of 13 female patients with vocal fold nodules, Verdolini-Marston, Burke, Lessac, Glaze, and Caldwell (1995) found that adherence was a stronger factor in determining outcome than specific treatment approaches. How do we, as speech-language pathologists, enhance adherence?

The determining factors that contribute to your patient's perseverance in voice therapy are individualistic, complex, and variable. Given that each patient is unique and comes to the therapy experience with specific expectations, differing levels of education pertaining to voice production, and prior success or failure with previous attempts to make behavioral changes, adherence to the process of voice rehabilitation is an ongoing, omnipresent dilemma that all clinicians and patients face. The clinician and patient view adherence from different perspectives. From the patient's viewpoint there are several internal and external barriers to making a commitment to change. Van Leer and Connor (2010) identified three major themes that emerged from interviews with patients regarding adherence: "voice therapy is hard" (p. 461), "make it happen" (p. 464), and "the clinician-patient match matters" (p 465). These themes may coexist and present themselves over the course of treatment as patients grapple with ambivalence related to change.

The first theme of patient adherence that van Leer and Connor (2010) identified is "voice therapy is hard" (p. 461). You may remember when you were first introduced to the voice exercises that would become part of your repertoire, and you struggled to feel and then integrate them into your kinesthetic memory, that you felt awkward, possibly embarrassed, and even burdened by the demands of deliberate practice in order to make them appropriate clinical models for your patient. You may have felt that deliberate practice was unnecessary—even felt reluctant and awkward as you practiced, until you rationalized the techniques from a physiological perspective. Imagine your new patient, suddenly confronted by the need for regular, scheduled practice of vocal techniques that have little or no obvious meaning. He feels uncertainty regarding the need for and appropriateness of outside practice (which may lead to feelings of failure and poor perseverance), and impatient with the constant and seemingly relentless need to attend to his voice. His family and friends react to the modified voice as affected or phony, and his expectations for a quick and straightforward remedy to the voice problem have been dashed (van Leer & Connor, 2010). When you consider these factors you will understand only a few of the obstacles that your voice patient must face in order to reach his goals. It is especially challenging to establish a new motor pattern and sensory awareness that allows for "interpreting sensory (acoustic-kinesthetic) feedback" (van Leer & Connor, 2010, p. 467), which is necessary for the development of resonance and flow phonation. As van Leer and Connor (2010) further suggest, the acquisition of new motor patterns for phonation is different from other motor skills because the immediate outcome is difficult to measure, and these patterns are foreign and uncharacteristic to the average speaker who most often does not attend to the voice. Furthermore, the seemingly subtle adjustment you ask your patient to make from an auditory to a kinesthetic focus represents a dramatic and challenging paradigmatic shift.

Van Leer and Connor's (2010) second theme of adherence is "make it happen" (p. 464). Self-motivation is an intrinsic aspect of this theme as your patient finds his own connections between his goals and the possible environmental obstacles met daily in order to speak over noise, maintain a regular practice regimen, and incorporate the vocal techniques developed in therapy. Patients who are active in finding solutions to problematic voice situations often elicit support from their peers to facilitate adherence to treatment, practice, and generalization. The authors found that a group interaction offers just such an opportunity, not only for peer modeling, feedback, and learning from others, but for emotional support, empathy, and mutual concern. The authors' recent experience leading a voice group brought these benefits into high relief as participants found that peer interaction strengthened their resolve. The struggles described by the newer members to modify effortful manner of phonation and sustain the motivation necessary to persevere in the treatment process were addressed by a more seasoned participant, who understood and empathized with their difficulties. When she became a role model, her own resolve to monitor her practice schedule and to generalize techniques to social and work situations became stronger.

The third and final theme is "the clinician-patient match matters" (van Leer & Connor, 2010, p. 465). According to van Leer and Connor (2010), the match between patient and therapist consists of two intersecting components: agreement regarding the goals and procedures of treatment, and the relationship between the patient and the clinician. Your patient's confidence in you, the effort you make to include him in setting goals, as well as the specific adaptations of your procedures represent critical factors in strengthening his self-efficacy as he wrestles with the need for change and his readiness for change (see **Dialogue 3-2**). One of our underlying hypotheses in this text is that your clinical model of efficient voice production has a profound effect on the therapeutic endeavor. Our emphasis here, however, is the effect of the clinician-patient relationship on your patient's adherence to voice rehabilitation. The feedback you provide (e.g., kinesthetics, physiology, motor patterns, education, counseling, strategies) and your attempts to make procedures specific to the individual patient provide an implicit support of their efforts and are crucial to the ongoing adherence necessary for a successful outcome.

Dialogue 3-2
Excerpt from the Fourth Therapy Session

At the start of the session I asked, "How did your practice go this week?" (Open-ended question)

With downcast eyes, Mr. B sheepishly said, "Well, we were on vacation this week, and I guess that it should have given me more time to practice, but it didn't."

Noting his quiet voice and recognizing his embarrassment and sense of failure, I replied, "Sounds like you thought about it, but something got in the way." (Reflective listening)

Looking down, "Yes, it feels like a burden, and I don't like to do things on a schedule."

As I listened carefully, I became aware that he was speaking with a quieter voice. Again, recognizing his frustration with the need for practice and his embarrassment over his failure to follow through, "Yes, it is very difficult to add something to an already full schedule, especially when you just want to relax." (Affirming)

Making eye contact and nodding, Mr. B said, "Yes, I just wanted to have a good time this week. We were staying with some friends whom we hadn't seen for a long time, so it was just talk, talk, talk, and my throat started to feel sore. I did try to talk less and listen more because of that."

I noticed that he was speaking with less effort, and I decided to focus on his success rather than belabor his sense of failure. "That's great! So you used a couple of strategies to help yourself and you are using some right now!" (Affirming)

Maintaining eye contact and smiling, Mr. B said, "Oh yeah, I didn't realize that. Before I came here I'd have just kept talking even though my throat hurt."

I knew that his responses would guide me, and so I continued to observe closely. As he spoke, the effort in his voice continued to diminish and he began to use confidential voice (one of our goals). Smiling and emphasizing his success, I suggested, "Using strategies to conserve your voice is practice, isn't it?" (Affirming) Do you realize that you have begun to use confidential voice?" (Physiological awareness)

Resistance

It is easy to think of resistance as a "problem," but if you accept resistance as a normal component of change, you will not take it personally. You will thus be freer to cope objectively with this inevitable part of therapy. The challenge of patient resistance is directly related to adherence, and it occurs in all therapeutic interactions, including voice rehabilitation. The form that resistance takes varies, not only between individuals but over time and at different stages of the therapeutic process. The patient who dismisses therapy because he has no experience with the process or lacks information regarding its value, the individual who expects immediate results ("How long is this going to take?"), the "traveling" (Cooper, 1974, p. 146) patient who has worked with several clinicians without success, the patient who expects change without deliberate practice, and those whose progress is unusually swift but ephemeral represent examples of individuals whose resistance negatively affects progress.

What Is Self-Efficacy?

Bandura (1986) describes self-efficacy as one's confidence in one's capacity to successfully complete a task and persevere in the face of adversity. Self-efficacy is central to an individual's perseverance in and adherence to therapeutic intervention, whether it is weight loss, cessation of smoking, management of illnesses such as diabetes and multiple sclerosis, or an entrenched motor pattern (van Leer et al., 2008; Hu et al., 2012). An implicit component of self-efficacy is the investment of the patient's efforts and his expectations regarding the outcome from those efforts. Bandura suggests that self-efficacy is not static and fluctuates as the person experiences success or failure. Those with higher self-efficacy may need less help or support as they move through the treatment process, but those with low self-efficacy will require more external support. Early in the treatment process, when the patient has little experience attending to and modifying his voice, he may need more support. Certainly, as patients make progress and recognize their success, their tenacity will increase despite the obstacles that are inevitable during any process of change. Van Leer et al. (2008) describe four sources of self-efficacy. These are "**mastery experience**, **vicarious experience**, **verbal persuasion**, and **emotional-physiological state**" (p. 690).

Mastery Experience

During your early therapy sessions, it will be useful to introduce techniques that can be easily mastered by your patient so that he feels successful and realizes that he can change his behavior. Confidential voice, voice conservation, and increase in hydration may be implemented easily and offer the opportunity for immediate success and a sense of vocal control. Techniques that are within your patient's reach, both psychologically and physiologically, will maximize the successful implementation of your recommended modifications and enhance self-efficacy. If your patient feels overwhelmed by the procedures or changes you propose, if he has difficulty executing the procedures appropriately, or his previous experiences have been negative ones, his feelings of self-efficacy may be threatened.

Vicarious Experience

Bandura (1986) suggests that even simple techniques such as imitating vocal procedures can prompt a variety of emotional responses based on the success of the procedure. As clinicians, we often demonstrate procedures in treatment and ask the patient to use physiological empathy to imitate our model. When the patient matches your model of confidential voice, he is using vicarious experience to modify his manner of phonation. This straightforward technique easily lends itself to the feeling of "if they can do it, I can do it" (van Leer et al., 2008, p. 690). However, a more physiologically complex and somewhat abstract procedure like a singing scale might elicit feelings of inadequacy (you are the expert), and the skill required to match your easy manner of phonation is difficult to achieve. The patient's personal self-efficacy may be compromised in such a situation. Your sensitivity to your patient's confidence level as he attempts to incorporate unfamiliar techniques and the flexibility you need to adjust the hierarchy of treatment accordingly are critical at these times.

Verbal Persuasion

Evidence suggests that verbal persuasion is less effective than either mastery or vicarious experience (Bandura, 1986). When you use verbal persuasion to support your patient's efforts, his previous success or failure in other areas of change may facilitate or impede your efforts and the result may not be related to persuasion at all (van Leer et al., 2008). Rollnick and Miller (1995) emphasize the tendency for patients to become more resistant to change with direct verbal persuasion. Finally, counseling by persuasion makes the voice clinician responsible for change; the patient becomes a passive receiver who agrees with your suggestion but does not really internalize it, and he is less likely to initiate independent problem solving or decision making (Luterman, 2008). When acid reflux contributes to the patient's voice problem, for instance, clinicians often encourage diet modification.

Verbal persuasion may include statements like, "Even though it is difficult right now, it will get easier as you go on." This straightforward attempt to motivate patients is often an appealing one, but evidence suggests that it is not effective and may even hinder progress in therapy.

The use of persuasion may temporarily bring about adherence, but in our experience patients who seemingly agree to the clinician's recommendation/argument most often do not follow through because persuasion is, at best, temporary and artificial. As Zuckoff (2012) so aptly states, "These patients display what I've called the 'bobble-head effect': the more the clinician speaks, the more the patient nods, typically without expressing anything other than blanket agreement" (p. 518). If you unconsciously react adversely to your patient's resistance, or if friends or family respond negatively to the patient's attempts to change the manner of phonation, self-efficacy will be threatened. Your honest acknowledgment of how difficult it is to change will open the door for change more effectively than well-rehearsed agreements.

Physiological-Psychological State

The patient's physiological and psychological well-being also provide information pertaining to self-efficacy (van Leer et al., 2008). Patients who are singers, dancers, or athletes may be accustomed to relying on sensory feedback to monitor the body in motion, but the average speaker is not. Because individuals most often monitor the voice by listening, and success in voice therapy is more integrated when the patient uses kinesthetic feedback, the patient may complain of awkwardness, embarrassment, and uneasiness ("psychological clumsiness") (van Leer et al., 2008, p. 692) associated with changing his manner of assessing and monitoring his voice production. The concept and sensation of *less effort* may feel foreign. It is common for male-to-female transsexual individuals, for instance, to report that they feel ambivalent and uncomfortable using a more feminine voice because it does not yet feel authentic. Discovery of an effective voice that matches one's persona and meets all of one's needs is an uneven process and may manifest as self-criticism, reticence to incorporate new techniques, and distrust of the authenticity of the emerging voice.

How Do I Assess Self-Efficacy?

It is useful, as part of your initial assessment to ask your patient to complete a self-efficacy scale. The patient indicates the response that best describes the extent to which the statement describes his self-efficacy. The General Self-Efficacy Scale (GSES) (Schwarzer & Jerusalem, 1995) is used specifically with individuals who have voice disorders to identify general characteristics that facilitate or hinder personal effort and commitment to the voice rehabilitation process. Hu et al. (2012) developed the Disease-Specific Self-Efficacy in Spasmodic Dysphonia (SE-SD) to identify the specific factors that threaten self-efficacy for these individuals. These self-efficacy assessments provide valuable information regarding your patient's self-esteem, optimism, and perseverance in the face of frustration. Certainly, patients' feelings of self-efficacy will fluctuate over the course of therapy, requiring that you adjust and modify your responses and choice of procedures.

Personal Self-Efficacy

Thus far, we have discussed self-efficacy as it pertains to your patient, but how is this concept relevant to you as a voice clinician? Your feelings of confidence in your accurate conveyance of information and the provision of an appropriate clinical model contribute to your personal self-efficacy. It takes time to build your confidence, competence, flexibility, and creativity. With this in mind, your expectations will be more realistic, thus making it possible for you to work with what you have now.

A Vocabulary for Change

We will now introduce several possible approaches to the counseling aspects of voice rehabilitation. Of course, it is understood that no theory or model works for all patients or for any one patient all the time. But the clinician's belief that the resolution of a voice problem and maintenance of change are possible only with the recognition of the importance of the patient's preferences, needs, expectations, and self-knowledge (Rogers, 1959) is implicit in our framework for voice therapy.

Transtheoretical Model

Over the course of voice therapy you receive a great deal of information from your patient. It may be useful, therefore, to use a model that provides a vocabulary to organize the phenomena you observe, to provide a reference for understanding the patient's perspective, and to monitor his readiness for change. The **transtheoretical model (TTM)** (van Leer et al., 2008) provides such a vocabulary for the clinician and has been widely used to enhance lifestyle changes, such as stress-management, increased physical activity, cessation of smoking, alcoholism, and obesity. It is not meant to be a specific therapeutic technique, but rather represents theoretical groupings of readiness for change. The original TTM included four stages: "(1) contemplation, (2) decision, (3) action, and (4) maintenance" (Prochaska & DiClemente, 1984, p. 21). In 2008 van Leer, Hapner, and Connor applied TTM to voice therapy, modified the stages to include *precontemplation*, and then linked those stages to voice rehabilitation. Progression through stages is not necessarily linear (Velicer, Norman, Fava, & Prochaska, 1999; van Leer et al., 2008), and patients can move forward or backward through the different stages. The transtheoretical model provides a useful framework that will draw your attention to specific areas of ambivalence and fluctuation in your patient's readiness for change. When there is a disparity between an individual's readiness for change and the clinician's procedures, resistance may increase. When you are aware of the potential for this mismatch you will introduce procedures that are commensurate with your patient's readiness and skill level (Dijkstra, Conijn, & De Vries, 2006).

Stage 1: Precontemplation

Patients in the **precontemplation stage** may not know or recognize that change is possible, or may realize that change is possible, but do not have a desire to change. Those who are unaware of the voice problem do not recognize the negative impact a disturbed voice has on others, the consequences of effortful production on the vocal folds, and see no reason to change their manner of phonation. Others who are aware of the voice problem may include those who like the way the voice sounds (despite the effort required to produce it), the attention and livelihood it brings (e.g., the character actor or singer who is associated with a signature that is detrimental to his vocal health) (Cooper, 1974), and those who work in noisy environments, smoke cigarettes, drink alcohol, habitually speak loudly and with effort, but are not ready or willing to contemplate change. Dialogue 3-1 provides an illustration of a possible interaction between the clinician and a patient who is in the precontemplation stage. The patient claims that she has no voice problem and it is only the threat of losing her job that brought her to the voice evaluation.

Stage 2: Contemplation

Although patients who are in the **contemplation stage** are considering change, they remain ambivalent between rationales for change and reasons to postpone change. A patient who habitually uses an effortful, inappropriately loud voice might say, "I just couldn't speak quietly. I went to a party and dinner was served with loud jazz music in the background. I know that I feel better when I don't talk so loudly." Or, "I couldn't practice when I was on vacation. We were so busy. I know my throat feels better after I practice." It is clear from these statements that the patient remains ambivalent about changing his behavior.

He continues to wrestle with his recognition of the need for change and whether it is possible for him to make that change. It may be counterproductive to begin direct therapy while the patient continues to struggle with these conflicting mindsets, but this struggle does not necessarily foreshadow failure. Explore the modifications the patient feels he might realistically attempt; ask him to keep a journal of situations during which he has success; identify one concrete, realistic goal that feels attainable. It may be difficult for the patient to acknowledge, given his ambivalence, that this is not the most appropriate time for him to begin the challenge of voice therapy. You will want to assure your patient that this reservation is perfectly reasonable and that it may be in his best interest to postpone this undertaking to a time when he feels more confident that he can participate in this partnership more actively.

Stage 3: Preparation

The **preparation stage** is usually a time when patients demonstrate an awareness of the problem, indicate their need to modify the vocal behavior, verbalize their commitment to change, and prepare to make a change (Levinson, Cohen, Brady, & Duffy, 2001). This stage provides an opportunity for you to begin to problem solve with your patient and implement strategies to maintain a practice schedule, consider necessary lifestyle changes, and introduce techniques to decrease phonatory effort (van Leer et al., 2008). Your patient might say, "I've figured out some good times for me to practice." "I will be on vacation for two weeks and I can talk quietly while I'm away." "I've noticed that my throat burns and I cough after I talk in a funny voice to the kids. I've started having the kids make the animal voices." "I'm going to look for a new job that is quieter than the bar where I work now." This is a time when you want to acknowledge your patient's successful efforts to change his vocal behavior. You might reinforce his feelings of success by acknowledging his active participation in the process and his demonstrated capacity to take responsibility for change. The two of you can build on his success and jointly brainstorm additional changes in the hierarchy of techniques that reduce effort.

Stage 4: Action

During the **action stage**, patients actively participate in the process of making changes in their manner of voice production. During this time your patient will develop the skills he needs to produce voice efficiently and ultimately generalize those skills to his daily life. Your insight and support during this time of change are invaluable in order to facilitate consistency in appropriate manner of phonation. It is not unusual for patients to struggle to identify and hold on to the ephemeral, kinesthetic awareness needed for independent modification of effort and carryover of ease. Now is the time to work together to build a hierarchy of more difficult situations within which he will incorporate the techniques he has learned in treatment. Your patient might say, "I noticed that I was pressing when I was talking at a loud party, so I started to use my resonant voice," or "I've started doing deliberate sneak practices of /mhm/ to relax my throat when I'm talking to my friends," or "Sometimes it's hard to focus on how my throat feels while I'm so involved in what I'm saying." This last statement requires reassurance from you that it is extremely difficult to think about what you are saying and how you are saying it at the same time, especially before the techniques developed in therapy are more firmly established.

Stage 5: Maintenance

Your patient's final goal in the therapeutic process is to maintain an efficient and easy manner of phonation during spontaneous speech, and to recognize and modify phonation when he encounters vocal difficulty. When your patient has reached a point in treatment when he says, "I was at a loud bar last night and used my resonant voice for hours and my throat feels great," he is describing maintenance. An actor who must modify the timbre of his voice for a role might say, "I had complete control of that 'wicked witch' voice during the performance. I've never been able to sustain that before and my throat felt great." A parent who says, "I was reading the story of 'The Three Bears' to my daughter, and I made all of the different voices easily," has achieved maintenance. At this point you will want to acknowledge your patient's progress and the control he has in a variety of challenging speaking situations. However, maintenance is rarely a smooth process. Relapse is expected during the **maintenance stage** of voice rehabilitation. It is not unusual for actors who assume roles that require changes in vocal timbre, professional voice users who speak over prolonged periods, or parents who deal with stressful situations with children to relapse (Levinson et al., 2001; Prochaska & DiClemente, 1984; van Leer et al., 2008). These events can disturb the patient's sense of self-efficacy. You will want to assure your patient not only that your door is always open but that it is normal, given life's stresses and constantly changing demands that represent risks to vocal health (e.g., colds, allergies, talking over noise, life events), to experience relapse. These experiences can be fruitful as patients realize that they have the tools to cope with these stressors.

TTM and Resistance

Given that TTM provides broad categories that identify the patient's level of readiness for change, you can use this model to identify and cope with your patient's resistance. Resistance may occur when there has been a mismatch between the patient's stage of change and a therapeutic procedure (Dijkstra et al., 2006). Resistance that follows the introduction of a procedure too early in the treatment process, however, is a consequence of the clinician's failure to consider and correlate the patient's current level of kinesthetic awareness and readiness for change with the procedures. This is not a fatal error, however. The TTM model provides a framework that will help you recognize when a mismatch between the procedure and the patient's readiness has occurred in order for you to make the necessary corrective adjustments to the treatment hierarchy.

The inclination to label the patient as resistant when he does not cooperate with the clinician's recommendations or choice of procedure is a natural one because of the frustration the patient's resistance may elicit in you, but you will have more success if you focus on his level of readiness and match your therapy to his level of comfort. It is our professional responsibility to coordinate the treatment strategies we use with the patient's readiness to participate in them (Chanut, Brown, & Dongier, 2005). That is not to say that resistance does not exist, but that you can strive to create the best environment for change by creating a client-centered, supportive, and respectful approach. If you recognize that resistance is a natural part of the process, and that it is not static, it may be easier for you to adjust your goals and procedures as resistance varies over the course of treatment.

There is a strong connection between the principles of Rogers' client-centered model (1942) of therapy, TTM, and motivational interviewing, all of which place the patient at the center of the decision-making process. We have found that **motivational interviewing** also recognizes the obstacles that confront the patient and create ambivalence during his effort to change long-standing vocal behaviors. As you gain confidence, you will probably combine elements from these and other approaches in order to build the collaboration that is critical to patient-centered therapy.

What Is Motivational Interviewing?

Adherence, resistance: the two faces of motivation. As Zuckoff (2012) plaintively asks, "Why won't my patients do what's good for them?"(p. 514). He answers the question by recognizing the importance of ambivalence during the process of change: fluctuations in readiness, priorities, values, concerns, and self-efficacy. Your patient may demonstrate resistance in voice therapy complaining about time constraints for practice, the difficulty of deliberate practice, dissatisfaction with particular exercises, or questions pertaining to the efficacy of therapy itself (Behrman, 2006). When we view resistance through the lens of motivational interviewing (MI), it becomes an assessment of the effectiveness of the therapeutic relationship rather than a dismissive appraisal of a character flaw in the patient (Chanut et al., 2005).

Motivational interviewing has been widely used to facilitate change and increase adherence. It has been effective for addressing problems related to addiction (alcoholism, smoking, and substance abuse) (Graeber, Moyers, Griffith, Guajardo, & Tonigan, 2003), obesity (Zuckoff, 2012), eating disorders (Zuckoff, 2012), obsessive-compulsive disorder (Simpson, Zuckoff, Page, Franklin, & Foa, 2008), and adherence to medication regimens (Broers et al., 2005). More recently, MI has been adapted to enhance adherence in voice therapy, placing a strong emphasis on the inclusion of the patient in a collaborative relationship with the clinician. Moyers and Rollnick (2002) describe four principles that provide the foundation for MI as an approach to clinician–patient interaction: "express empathy," "develop discrepancy," "support self-efficacy," and "roll with resistance" (p. 186). However, the spirit of MI contains a "quietly directive" (Rollnick & Miller, 1995, p. 332) component, which supports your patient as he struggles with ambivalence and encourages his openness to change and as he strives to achieve his goals.

How can you use MI to address your patient's ambivalence? An awareness of your communication style and vocabulary, even during your first meeting with your patient, can have a profound effect on his readiness or resistance to change. Open-ended questions (encourage patient's verbal exploration), affirmation (recognition of patient effort, support), reflective listening (moving the dialogue forward by interpretation of the patient's communicative intent), accurate empathy (appreciation of patient's perspective), conveyance of optimism, genuineness (authenticity), warmth, change talk (eliciting patient participation in self-management), and partnership reflect the spirit of MI (Behrman, 2006; Zuckoff, 2012). At times it may feel as though you cannot think of an appropriate response to your patient's frustration. **Table 3-1** provides a sample of several possible situation-related responses that a clinician might use while integrating MI. In the following table, the clinician applies the principles of MI to respond to the same patient utterance.

The essence of motivational interviewing involves listening to the patient to understand and respect his perspective in order to enhance his self-efficacy (Rollnick & Miller, 1995). When your patient expresses his ambivalence, he is telling you that he is conflicted. He feels there is a need to change, he has a desire to change, but he wonders if he can, if it is too difficult, if it will take too long, and whether the changes recommended will, in fact, lead to his desired goal. The subtle, shaping style encouraged by MI allows your patient to take responsibility for his progress through the steps of change toward a voice that is produced with less effort.

Table 3-1 Motivational Interviewing

Set-up: Clinician and patient are working toward establishment of awareness of resonance in the **mask** (i.e., the nose, facial plates, and hard palate) during quiet production of /mhm/ (with a slight downward inflection) followed by a short phrase using a nasal phoneme to enhance resonance ("my oh my").

The clinician models the exercise "/mhm/, /mhm/ (breath) my oh my" (chosen because of the nasal resonance). Following the clinician's model, the patient produces "/mhm/, /mhm/" with a resonant sound and exhibits a mild reduction in effort and roughness during the phrase. The clinician is pleased by the improvement, but the patient responds negatively to the remaining roughness during the phrase. He says, *"I give that one a 'C.' It sounded ugly."* Below are a variety of possible clinician responses to the patient's statement based on the principles of motivational interviewing.

MI Principles	Strategies	Sample Clinician Responses
Express empathy	***Reflective listening***	**Patient**: "/mhm/, /mhm/ (easy breath) my oh my. I give that one a 'C.' It sounded ugly." **Clinician**: "It's disappointing that it wasn't perfect."
	Summarizing	**Patient**: "/mhm/, /mhm/ (easy breath) my oh my. I give that one a 'C.' It sounded ugly." **Clinician**: "We've been focusing on feeling vibrations in your nose, lips, and the roof of your mouth for two weeks, and it's frustrating that your voice is not where you want it to be."
	Affirmation	**Patient**: "/mhm/, /mhm/ (easy breath) my oh my. I give that one a 'C.' It sounded ugly." **Clinician**: "It's frustrating when you're trying so hard to access a feeling and it continues to elude you."
Develop discrepancy	***Reflective listening***	**Patient**: "/mhm/, /mhm/ (easy breath) my oh my. I give that one a 'C.' It sounded ugly." **Clinician**: "You are right that your voice was rough, but did you feel vibrations in your nose, lips, or the roof of your mouth?"
	Summarizing	**Patient**: "/mhm/, /mhm/ (easy breath) my oh my. I give that one a 'C.' It sounded ugly." **Clinician**: "You have been working on enhancing resonance with /mhm/ and have told me that you feel more buzz. Now that we have moved on to connected speech, what can you do to increase your focus on what you feel rather than what you hear?"
	Increase cognitive dissonance	**Patient**: "/mhm/, /mhm/ (easy breath) my oh my. I give that one a 'C.' It sounded ugly." **Clinician**: "Are you focusing on the vibrations or on the sound?"
	Open questions	**Patient**: "/mhm/, /mhm/ (easy breath) my oh my. I give that one a 'C.' It sounded ugly." **Clinician**: "What were you focusing on?"

Table 3-1 Motivational Interviewing

MI Principles	Strategies	Sample Clinician Responses
Support self-efficacy	***Directive component***	**Patient**: "/mhm/, /mhm/ (easy breath) my oh my. I give that one a 'C.' It sounded ugly." **Clinician**: "Earlier, you produced some of the phrases with ease and flow, and you noticed that you felt vibrations in your lips and nose. Were you aware of these sensations on this attempt?"
	Affirmation of self-efficacy	**Patient**: "/mhm/, /mhm/ (easy breath) my oh my. I give that one a 'C.' It sounded ugly." **Clinician**: "I know that it is difficult to focus on these small vibrations. You have already made many changes. Let's try it again."
	Unwavering optimism	**Patient**: "/mhm/, /mhm/ (easy breath) my oh my. I give that one a 'C.' It sounded ugly." **Clinician**: "It is difficult to change your manner of phonation. It takes time and lots of focus. I have seen you focus on resonance when we do the /mhm/ by itself, so I know you can do phrases too."
Roll with resistance	***Reflective listening***	**Patient**: "/mhm/, /mhm/ (easy breath) my oh my. I give that one a 'C.' It sounded ugly." **Clinician**: "Yeah, there is still some roughness. Let's see if focusing even more on what you feel helps."
	Affirmation	**Patient**: "/mhm/, /mhm/ (easy breath) my oh my. I give that one a 'C.' It sounded ugly." **Clinician**: "It's normal to feel frustrated by this. Therapy is hard and it's difficult to change the way you make sound."
	Consider patient's degree of problem recognition	**Patient**: "/mhm/, /mhm/ (easy breath) my oh my. I give that one a 'C.' It sounded ugly." **Clinician**: "The problem developed because you pushed for a better sound. What do you think would be a better way to approach the problem?"
	Encourages patient to advocate for change	**Patient**: "/mhm/, /mhm/ (easy breath) my oh my. I give that one a 'C.' It sounded ugly." **Clinician**: "You're right. What can you do to make sound more easily?"

Patient Education

As speech-language pathologists we are usually most comfortable providing education (the **biomedical model**) (Luterman, 2008), and there are certainly times when it is appropriate to do so, especially during the process of voice modification when the patient has questions about the underlying physiology of easy voice production. In fact, some patients respond more positively to an educational approach than a client-centered one. Nevertheless, when the patient is receptive, a patient-centered attitude is usually more effective when combined with the educational model.

The partnership you build with your patient, and the confidence and support you provide during this collaborative relationship, place you in an excellent position to be the provider of information relevant to the presenting voice disorder, its underlying physiology, manifestations, and the prognosis for return to clinically normal voice production. Your patient may come with misconceptions about the causes and consequences of the voice problem, and it will be your responsibility to provide information that not only educates, but contributes to his ultimate incorporation of the strategies and techniques the two of you develop together. The educational aspect of treatment becomes especially pertinent when patients are asymptomatic and are unable to rationalize or explain to themselves how it is possible that they have a problem, but do not feel it (Gold & McClung, 2006).

The atmosphere within which information is provided plays a significant role in your patient's willingness to accept and implement your recommendations, whether related to the cessation of smoking, the importance of hydration, voice conservation, the existing voice disorder and its consequences, or the relevance of a regular practice schedule. Your accepting, nonjudgmental attitude, encouraging the patient to ask questions and voice concerns, may be a decisive factor in his adherence to the voice rehabilitation program and the likelihood that he will integrate and act on the information you provide. The support of a collaborative and trusting relationship is vital to the ultimate goal of treatment, self-management, and generalization of effective voice production.

Silent Moments

Clinicians can be uncomfortable with silent moments. They struggle to fill each one and worry that they do not have enough procedures to fill the hour of therapy. However, these silent moments may be some of the most telling ones in the therapy sessions because they give the patient time to process... time to think... time to integrate... time to change. The patient may break the silence with an insight into his manner of phonation and ways to modify effort, or transfer effective voice production to the workplace and social milieu. Try not to rush to fill the silent moments... it can be surprising and rewarding to see how the patient fills them. This is client-centered therapy.

Summary

The success of any rehabilitation program rests, to a great extent, on the partnership that has been developed between the patient and the clinician. Listening with cultural humility in a nonjudgmental fashion, to understand, to recognize another's perspective and autonomy, and to create an environment of unconditional regard begin with your willingness to learn to listen openly and actively, and to be willing to share the responsibility for rehabilitation with the patient (Rogers, 1961; Spillers, 2007). If you accept that no one technique or perspective works for all patients, that you alone cannot solve or fix the patient's voice problem, that some issues are outside of your scope of practice, and that there will be patients who doubt the efficacy of therapy, you will be free to focus outside yourself and on the best way to help the unique, specific individual sitting in front of you.

The models we have described in this chapter can be useful as you begin to work with your voice patient because they provide a context for recognizing and facilitating your patient's readiness for change. As with all models, the counseling strategies we have described have limitations. Finally, despite your best efforts, there will be patients who do not follow through with therapy, whose lack of adherence to practice does not diminish, who do not respond to any of the procedures developed during treatment, and with whom you will feel you have failed. We have all experienced the disappointment and frustration that come from an unsuccessful outcome and question how we might have done things differently. But those questions are the questions of a good clinician... one who keeps searching for a more effective way to facilitate change and is never complacent.

References

Alsharif, N.Z. (2012). Cultural humility and interprofessional education and practice: A winning combination. *American Journal of Pharmacological Education, 76*(7), 120.

Bandura, A. (1986). *Social foundations of thought and actions: A social cognitive theory.* Englewood Cliffs, NJ: Prentice Hall.

Behrman, A. (2006). Facilitating behavioral change in voice therapy: The relevance of motivational interviewing. *American Journal of Speech-Language Pathology, 15*, 215–225.

Brennan, A.M., Barnsteiner, J., Siantz, M.L., Cotter, V.T., and Everett, J. (2012). Lesbian, gay, bisexual, transgendered, or intersexed content for nursing curricula. *Journal of Professional Nursing, 28*(2), 96–104.

Broers, S., Smets, E., Bindels, P., Evertsz, F.B., Calff, M., and de Haes, H. (2005). Training general practitioners in behavior change counseling to improve asthma medication adherence. *Patient Education Counseling, 58*(3), 279–287.

Chanut, F., Brown, T.G., and Dongier, M. (2005). Motivational interviewing and clinical psychiatry. *Canadian Journal of Psychiatry, 11*, 715–721.

Cooper, M. (1974). *Modern techniques of vocal rehabilitation.* Springfield, IL: Charles C. Thomas.

Dijkstra, A., Conijn, B., and De Vries, H. (2006). A match-mismatch test of a stage model of behavior change in tobacco smoking. *Addiction, 101*(7), 1035–1043.

DiLollo, A., and Favreau, C. (2010). Person-centered care and speech and language therapy. *Seminar Speech Language, 31*, 90–97.

Geller, E., and Foley, G.M. (2009). Broadening the "ports of entry" for speech-language pathologists: A relational and reflective model for clinical supervision. *American Journal of Speech Language Pathology, 18*, 22–41.

Gold, D.T., and McClung, B. (2006). Approaches to patient education: Emphasizing the long-term value of compliance and persistence. *American Journal of Medicine, 119*(4A), 325–375.

Graeber, D.A., Moyers, T.B., Griffith, G., Guajardo, E., and Tonigan, S. (2003). A pilot study comparing motivational interviewing and an educational intervention in patients with schizophrenia and alcohol use disorders. *Journal of Community Mental Health, 39*(3), 189–202.

Grosch, K., Medvene, L., and Wolcott, H. (2008). Person-centered caregiving instruction for geriatric nursing assistant students: Development and evaluation. *Journal of Gerontological Nursing, 34*(8), 23–31.

Gruppen, L.D. (2014). Humility and respect: Core values in medical education. *Medical Education, 48*(1), 53–58.

Hapner, E., Portone-Maira, C., and Johns, M.M., III. (2009). A study of voice therapy dropout. *Journal of Voice, 23*(3), 337–340.

Hu, A., Isetti, D., Hillel, A.D., Waugh, P., Comstock, B., and Meyer, T.K. (2012). Disease-specific self-efficacy in spasmodic dysphonia patients. *Otolaryngology—Head and Neck Surgery, 148*(3), 450–455.

Kutob, R.M., Bormanis, J., Crago, M., Harris, J.M., Jr., Senf, J., and Shisslak, C.M. (2013). Cultural competence education for practicing physicians: Lessons in cultural humility, nonjudgmental behaviors, and health beliefs elicitation. *Journal of Continuing Education and Health Professions, 33*(3), 164–173.

Leahy, M.M., and Walsh, I.P. (2008). Talk in interaction in the speech-language pathology clinic. *Topics in Language Disorders, 28*(3), 229–241.

Levinson, W., Cohen, M.S., Brady, D., and Duffy, F.D. (2001). To change or not to change: "Sounds like you have a dilemma." *Annals of Internal Medicine, 135*(5), 386–391.

Luterman, D.M. (2008). *Counseling persons with communication disorders and their families* (5th ed.). Austin, TX: Pro-ed.

Manning, W.H. (2010). *Clinical decision making in fluency disorders* (3rd ed.). Clifton Park, NY: Delmar.

Martin, D.G. (1983). *Counseling and therapy skills.* Prospect Heights, IL: Waveland Press.

Messer, S.B. (2004). Evidence-based practice: Beyond empirically supported treatments. *Professional Psychology, 35*, 580–588.

Moyers, T.B., and Rollnick, S. (2002). A motivational interviewing perspective on resistance in psychotherapy. *Journal of Clinical Psychology, 58*(2), 185–193.

Portone, C., Johns, M.M., III, and Hapner, E.R. (2008). A review of patient adherence to the recommendation for voice therapy. *Journal of Voice, 22*(2), 192–196.

Prochaska, J.O., and DiClemente, C.C. (1984). *The transtheoretical approach: Crossing traditional boundaries of therapy.* Homewood, IL: Dow Jones-Irwin.

Rogers, C.R. (1942). *Counseling and psychotherapy.* Boston, MA: Houghton Mifflin.

Rogers, C.R. (1946). Significant aspects of client-centered therapy. *American Psychologist, 1*, 415–422.

Rogers, C.R. (1951). *Client-centered therapy: Its current practice, implications, and theory.* Boston, MA: Houghton Mifflin.

Rogers, C.R. (1959). A theory of therapy, personality, and interpersonal relationships as developed in the client-centered framework. In S. Koch (Ed.), *Psychology: The study of science (Vol. 3): Formulation of the person and the social content* (pp. 184–256). New York, NY: McGraw-Hill.

Rogers, C.R. (1961). *On becoming a person: A therapist's view of psychotherapy.* Boston, MA: Houghton Mifflin.

Rogers, C.R. (1975). Empathic: An unappreciated way of being. *Counseling Psychologist, 5*, 2–10.

Rollnick, A., and Miller, W.R. (1995). What is motivational interviewing? *Behavioural and Cognitive Psychotherapy, 23*, 325–334.

Schwarzer, R., & Jerusalem, M. (1995). Generalized self-efficacy scale. In J. Weinman, S. Wright, & M. Johnston, *Measures in health psychology: A user's portfolio. Causal and control beliefs* (pp. 35–37). Windsor, UK: NFER-NELSON.

Simpson, H.B., Zuckoff, A., Page, J.R., Franklin, M.E., and Foa, E.B. (2008). Adding motivational interviewing to exposure and ritual prevention for obsessive-compulsive disorder: An open pilot trial. *Cognitive Behavioural Therapy, 17*, 38–49.

Smith, B.E., Kempster, G.B., and Sims, H.S. (2010). Patient factors related to voice therapy attendance and outcomes. *Journal of Voice, 24*(6), 694–701.

Spillers, C.S. (2007). An existential framework for understanding the counseling needs of clients. *American Journal of Speech-Language Pathology, 16*(3), 191–197.

Stemple, J.C. (2000). *Voice therapy: Clinical studies* (2nd ed.). San Diego, CA: Singular Thomson.

Stewart, M., Brown, J.B., Weston, W.W., McWhinney, I.R., McWilliam, C.L., and Freeman, T.R. (1995). *Patient-centered medicine: Transforming the clinical method.* Thousand Oaks, CA: Sage.

van Leer, E., and Connor, N.P. (2010). Patient perceptions of voice therapy adherence. *Journal of Voice, 24*(4), 458–469.

van Leer, E., Hapner, E.R., and Connor, N.P. (2008). Transtheoretical model of health behavior change applied to voice therapy. *Journal of Voice, 22*(6), 688–698.

Velicer, W.F., Norman, G.J., Fava, J.L., and Prochaska, J.O. (1999). Testing 40 predictions from the transtheoretical model. *Addictive Behavior, 24*(4), 455–469.

Verdolini-Marston, K., Burke, M.K., Lessac, A., Glaze, L., and Caldwell, E. (1995). Preliminary study of two methods of treatment for laryngeal nodules. *Journal of Voice, 9*(1), 74–85.

Yalom, I. (2009). *The gift of therapy: An open letter to a new generation of therapists and their patients.* New York, NY: Harper Collins.

Zuckoff, A. (2012). "Why won't my patients do what's good for them?" Motivational interviewing and treatment adherence. *Surgery for Obesity and Related Diseases, 8,* 514–521.

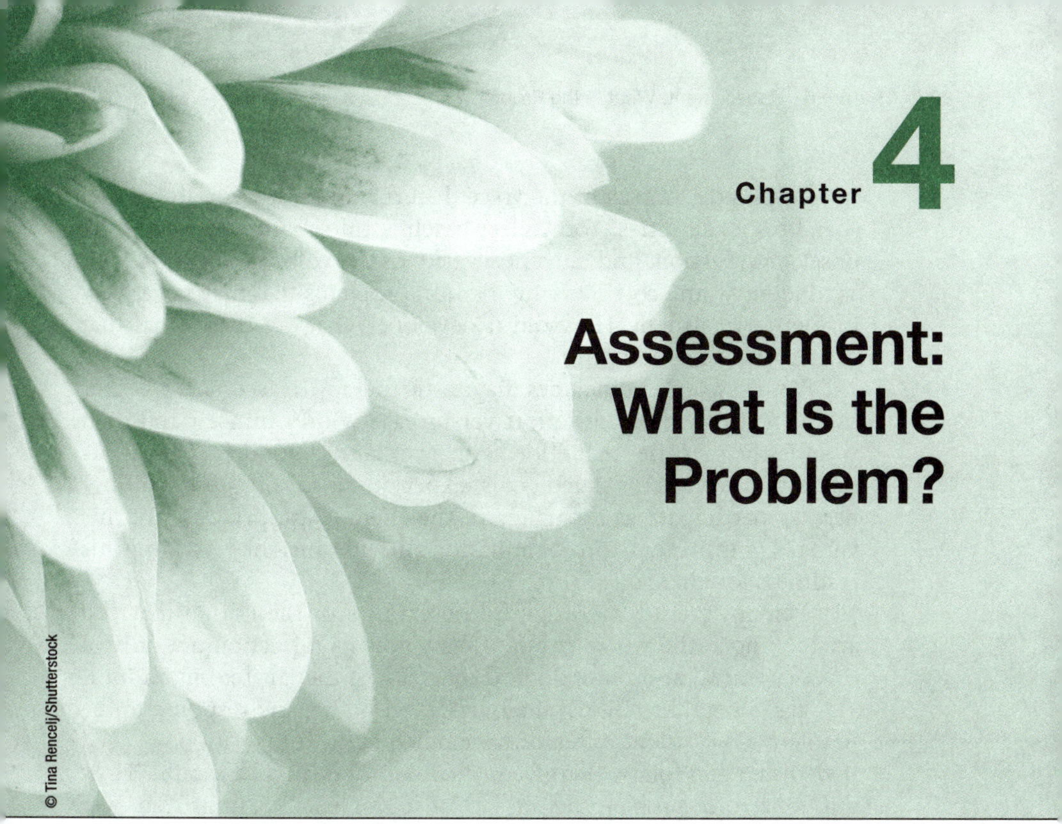

Chapter 4

Assessment: What Is the Problem?

"Rather than being an interpreter, the scientist who embraces a new paradigm is like the man wearing inverting lenses. Confronting the same constellation of objects as before and knowing that he does so, he nevertheless finds them transformed through and through in many of their details."
(Kuhn, 1970, p. 122)

Why Is a Voice Assessment Necessary?

As speech-language pathologists, we assume that voice therapy begins with a voice evaluation. However, if the patient comes with a diagnosis from an otolaryngologist, why do you need to do a voice assessment? Why is the physician's assessment and diagnosis insufficient to begin treatment? The purpose of your initial consultation is, first and foremost, to begin a collaboration with your patient that provides insight into the impact of the voice disturbance on his vocational and social responsibilities. You collect baseline information to clarify the onset, progression, and current severity of the voice problem, as well as to identify any co-occurring medical problems that may negatively influence treatment. How did it develop? What are the factors that exacerbate the condition?

Your assessment includes diagnostic therapy to ascertain whether the patient discriminates effort versus ease within himself and then whether he modifies that effort with your clinical models. This information, as well as his stated goals, expectations for progress, willingness to participate as a partner in the therapeutic process, and his verbal commitment to rehabilitation provide insight regarding his readiness for change.

Perhaps the key to insightful observation is the notion that you are looking at the whole person. The voice is a reflection not only of the anatomical and physiological integrity of the larynx but an individual's general health, psychological well-being, and response to the problem. Our patients often provide much of the information we need if we listen and follow their lead. Small prompts might include, "How did your voice problem begin?" "Has it worsened or improved over time?" "What makes your symptoms improve or worsen?" "How does the voice problem affect your life?" "Is there anything else I should know?"

Assessment is an ongoing process that continues as your patient makes changes and as goals and procedures are modified to match his current level of skill acquisition. You will integrate your perceptual analysis (what you see, hear, and feel) with the case history information, and the data from objective results in order to develop hypotheses regarding the physiological underpinnings of the voice problem and then determine the most appropriate place to begin the voice rehabilitation process.

How Do I Become an Active Listener?

Listening is an art (Barbara, 1968; Martin, 1983). Allowing a patient to tell his story without interruption or direction and following up with gentle probes to make certain that you understand his account sets the tone for a patient-centered evaluation. It is a given that at a certain level the patient knows more about his problem than you do because he lives with it. Although he does not have your training, knowledge, or professional language, and he may not specifically articulate the symptoms of his voice problem, he does know how his throat feels, he knows how the voice problem affects his life and career, and he has been living with the frustrations that accompany the voice problem for, possibly, a considerable time. He may have used a variety of techniques to cope with the changes in his voice (e.g., drinking throat tea, lowering or raising his pitch, limiting talking, or increasing or reducing loudness), and the effectiveness or ineffectiveness of these strategies have motivated him to seek voice therapy. He is the expert. With gentle probes you create the possibility "of entering the client's internal frame of reference" (Rogers, 1951, p. 36). When you enter this partnership with cultural humility, respect the patient's insights, and recognize that he has the capacity to change, you set the tone for an interactive therapeutic process. Initially, you may feel awkward maintaining this unscripted dialogue, but an interactive format not only facilitates an equal partnership, it creates an opportunity for the clinician to gather relevant information that might be lost with a more scripted and directive approach.

An open-ended question at the beginning of an assessment is often enough to elicit a descriptive narrative that provides much of the necessary information regarding the history and development of the patient's voice problem. "Tell me about your voice problem" may elicit a narrative during which the patient unknowingly reveals his understanding of the laryngeal pathology, his insight into the voice problem, his level of sophistication regarding medical concerns, his emotional response to the voice problem, its impact on his everyday life, and his goals. He says, "I can't project my voice." "My voice gets tired." "People ask me to repeat." "My voice cuts out on me." "I have a break in the **passaggio**." "My pitch range is limited." These statements suggest that, although the patient has not specifically designated his goals, he does know what they are. In a patient-centered approach, you integrate the narrative with your knowledge base to find a theme that facilitates the development of goals that will address the underlying physiological, medical, and emotional components of the problem. Of course, there are times when a patient does not respond to an open-ended approach to assessment and needs prompts and additional questions to provide a more complete picture of how the voice problem manifests itself.

Active listening immediately takes one's attention away from the self and provides a more patient-focused objective for the clinician (Rogers, 1951). You may feel uncomfortable asking questions that go beyond those listed on the case history form and self-assessment instruments. The adjustment away from *self*, however, may replace your self-consciousness with curiosity, concern for, and interest in the patient. For instance, basic questions on the assessment form regarding allergies may not be explored if you learn that the patient is or is not taking an allergy medication. However, relevant follow-up questions will provide more insight. "What are your allergy symptoms?"

"Are the allergies seasonal or do they occur all the time?" "Do you have any other allergies?" "How long have you had them?" "When do you take the medication?" "How does the medication make you feel?" "Does it dry you out?" All of these questions express a genuine interest in the patient and provide a beginning body of relevant medical information.

The patient's description of his response to the voice problem may reveal his attitude regarding the need for voice rehabilitation and, indirectly, indicate his willingness or lack thereof to participate in this process and change the behaviors that have negatively affected his voice production. Is the patient self-referred? Did his employer coerce him to address his voice problem? Did an otolaryngologist refer him? In an ideal world, all patients would be eager to make changes and improve their voices. But not all are ready for change, and it is critical for you to realize that, despite the patient's initial resistance to change, attitudes are not necessarily fixed, and your response can have a profound effect on his willingness to participate in this new venture.

As the patient provides his narrative, your attention remains focused on extracting and then integrating pertinent information into a cohesive framework. It may be difficult to decide what is relevant. The **Voice Evaluation Form** found in Appendix 1 provides an inventory of specific categories of information that may prove useful in organizing such a framework, but it is only a starting point for obtaining the history. There are often topics that require additional exploration. If, for instance, the patient reports that he stopped smoking recently, it is helpful to know when he started smoking, the number of cigarettes he smoked each day, whether this is the first time he has tried to stop smoking, and what made him stop now. These questions may provide insight into self-efficacy and candidacy for rehabilitation. The patient may have tried, unsuccessfully, to stop smoking several times in the past, and may lack confidence that he can change long-standing behaviors and habits. It may not be necessary, on the other hand, to ask a patient to elaborate on information regarding the successful cessation of smoking 30 years ago. You may feel that these questions are intrusive and hesitate to ask follow-up questions, but this line of inquiry tells you about the patient's response to previous attempts to change and his current self-efficacy with respect to change. If you recognize that your questions represent your interest in the patient and his problem, you may feel more comfortable exploring these issues further. As you will see in **Dialogue 4-1**, patients are often more forthcoming than you might expect, especially when it is clear that your questions are relevant to their concerns.

Dialogue 4-1
Excerpt from Initial Assessment

Broaching a sensitive topic with a nonjudgmental attitude and wanting to know more about his self-efficacy, I asked, "Do you smoke?"

Mr. C stated in a confident tone with a friendly nod, "I stopped smoking last week."

With full recognition of the commitment needed to quit and genuinely pleased with his success, "Congratulations! It can be difficult to stop. How did you do it?"

Smiling, "Well, I've tried many times but always started again. This time I've been coughing, and I am afraid something may be wrong with my throat. So I used some suggestions from the American Cancer Society."

I noticed his rough, breathy voice quality and his sense of satisfaction that he had stopped smoking. I nodded and thought that his attempt to stop smoking suggested that he was in the active stage of change (transtheoretical model) (Prochaska & DiClenente, 1984), *and that he was motivated to make change now. This was a positive indicator for candidacy.* "Which recommendations helped you?"

Smiling and nodding, Mr. C replied, "They have all sorts of strategies for making it harder to smoke. One of them is wrapping your cigarettes in paper and putting a rubber band around the paper so that it is more difficult to get a cigarette out of the pack. It made me more aware of how many cigarettes I was smoking."

I noted his organized approach to making change as well as a subtle decrease in the effort in his voice, and I was convinced that we could use his apparent willingness to change (cessation of smoking) to reinforce his commitment to improving his voice, "Do you notice that your throat feels better now? Is it less dry?"

After a short pause, Mr. C responded, "Actually, it feels a bit worse. I seem to have a lot of mucus, and I need to clear my throat more."

I was pleased that he was aware of these changes, and I recognized that the attention to this sensation in his throat might facilitate his awareness of resonance and easy phonation, so I took the opportunity to provide some information, "That is a good thing and typical of what people feel when they first stop smoking. The cilia that clean the lungs and trachea are starting to work so it feels like you are making more mucus. Your mucus should decrease over time."

He continued, "Really? I had no idea." *I noticed that his voice was quieter.*

"When did you start smoking?"

Mr. C shook his head and said, "When I was 15."

I observed that his vocal quality was less pressed and continued to gather relevant information with an open, supportive tone, "How much did you smoke?"

He sighed, "At least two packs a day, and I loved it."

As I studied him closely, I realized how difficult it had been for him to stop smoking and realized that it had taken a great deal of self-efficacy to make this change. "It must have been very hard to give it up! How long did your previous attempts to stop smoking last?"

Mr. C smiled at my question and leaned back, "Well, I stopped once for six months, and the last time I stopped for a year."

Knowing that it often takes several attempts to stop, I recognized his statement of commitment to the process of change. I continued to detect a drop in vocal effort and recognized that the therapeutic partnership had begun. I said, "Well, you seem to have found a useful strategy. Are you aware that you are using an easier way of talking right now? Does your throat feel different?"

Setting the Tone for Therapy

The words you use in therapy may have a disproportionate impact on the patient, and at times the impact is unexpected and unwanted. These words shape the therapeutic relationship into a collaborative one or a clinician-led, dependent one. Your words can inspire the patient to greater self-efficacy and adherence. A patient may return to you weeks or even years later and quote a phrase that you used. You may be surprised by the reference and startled that the patient remembered your exact words. He may have used these words to guide him when he was insecure about the effectiveness of his voice, ambivalent about using deliberate practice, or concerned about protecting his voice.

Some words have multiple meanings and may lead to misunderstanding. When you choose a word with a specific idea in mind, the patient may misinterpret your meaning. The more precise the vocabulary, the clearer and more precise your instructions will be for the use of deliberate practice and carryover of newly learned skills. The words in **Box 4-1** represent alternate descriptors for language that is often used in therapy when providing education and feedback to patients.

Voice Evaluation Form

The Voice Evaluation Form in Appendix 1 provides a framework for asking appropriate questions regarding the laryngeal diagnosis, laryngeal surgery, the onset of the problem, other pertinent medical history, and daily voice use. It suggests various self-assessment questionnaires that may be helpful for identifying specific information about the impact of the voice problem on the patient's daily life. The patient's responses

Box 4-1

Alternative Clinical Vocabulary

Words with Negative Connotations	Precise Words with Neutral Connotations
Abuse (vocal abuse): Doing something to harm oneself (e.g., drug abuse, bulimia)	Effort, push, strain, tight, scratchy, sore
Misuse (vocal misuse): Doing harm (e.g., frequent throat clearing, prolonged shouting)	See above
Relax: I should take a vacation and my voice will come back; relax your muscles	Release, let go, no effort, no pushing, no strain, no tightness
Voice feels (how your voice feels)	The voice does not have sensation. One can feel the *throat, jaw, tongue*, vibrations in the *nose* and *mouth*, and the flow of *air* across the *tongue*
Able to (able to produce an easy sound): Either a patient makes a sound or does not...you do not know what he is able to do	Patient *did not* produce an easy sound; patient demonstrated an easy sound
Listen/sound (listen to the sound): Having a patient listen to his voice may not be the best way to modify the voice	Feel, attend to the sensations in the larynx and vocal tract, feel the vibrations in the facial mask
Incorrect (negative self evaluation)	Effortful, pressed, tight

to these questions will provide information regarding the factors that influenced the development or continuation of the voice problem. Further exploration will be necessary in order to clarify the relationship between these potential risk factors and this patient's voice disturbance.

Medical Diagnosis

Ideally, before you meet your patient you have obtained information about the laryngeal diagnosis and the patient's complaint. Although it seldom happens, patients do occasionally come to the consultation without referral information. You may have no diagnosis, no case history information, and begin only with the information you derive from your first meeting. If the patient comes to the initial consultation without a diagnosis or case history, you may complete the voice evaluation, but you must refer the patient for a laryngeal examination before you begin therapy. Moreover, your voice evaluation may give the patient the support he needs to follow up with a laryngeal examination. If the patient has seen his primary care physician, who is not an otolaryngologist, the patient's diagnosis may be vague, and a referral to a specialist is indicated. It is also possible that you evaluate the patient following a laryngeal examination (by an otolaryngologist) that revealed no medical pathology. This circumstance may arise if there is an unobservable laryngeal lesion (too small for visualization), muscle tension dysphonia, a suspected neurological disorder (spasmodic dysphonia), or no laryngeal pathology. The absence of a medical diagnosis, however, does not obviate the necessity for a voice evaluation.

Patients are often quite anxious about a laryngeal diagnosis, given their limited knowledge and experience in the area of vocal pathology, and it becomes your responsibility to describe and clarify the otolaryngologist's examination results. They may need reassurance that the nodule, polyp, or cyst is benign. They may be curious about how it developed, how long it will take to resolve, whether it will recur, and even if it is contagious. A strong knowledge base allows you to answer these questions accurately and describe the rehabilitation process in a way that is both realistic and encouraging. Your patient's **prognosis** for recovery of normal vocal function is influenced by many factors, including but not limited to the laryngeal pathology and its effect on the vocal folds. For instance, the prognosis for recovery of clinically normal voice for an individual with vocal nodules might be excellent, but the prognosis for return to clinically normal voice following surgery to excise a cancerous lesion might be only fair to poor. If you are uncertain about a specific diagnosis, it is within your scope of practice to research the voice pathology and contact the referring physician to ensure that you have accurate and appropriate information. Your passive knowledge in the area of wound healing, should surgery be indicated, is relevant here as you continue therapy with your patient following his surgery.

View the *Consultation: Description of Voice Problem* video. During the voice evaluation of this speech pathology student/singer, she describes the origin and progression of her voice problem and its impact on her career. The clinician creates an environment that facilitates the patient's willingness to reveal the relevant information.

Risk Factors

During the assessment you will identify possible **risk factors** that may be associated with the onset of the voice problem or have exacerbated its symptoms. The onset of the voice problem may have coincided with a specific event or series of stressful events that precipitated a gradual or sudden deterioration in voice production. A history of surgery that required general sedation and intubation prior to the onset of the voice problem, for instance, suggests that if the intubation was difficult or prolonged, it might have irritated and inflamed the vocal folds or dislocated the cricoarytenoid joint. Chronic health problems, such as asthma, allergies, chronic cough, and reflux, as well as neurological disorders must be considered during your evaluation as possible exacerbating factors. Further, long-term use of medications, smoking, and/or recreational drug use may thicken secretions and dry the mucosal lining of the larynx. A family history of similar voice problems provides useful information regarding the habitual speaking environment and its impact on your patient's manner of phonation.

Collaboration

Your work with other professionals may include referral to or collaboration with one or more of the following: otolaryngologists, neurologists, primary care physicians, osteopaths, psychiatrists, psychologists, social workers, physical therapists, occupational therapists, music therapists, nutritionists, vocal coaches, voice teachers, etc. It is necessary to acknowledge when a problem is not within your scope of practice and requires a referral. The patient who has ongoing, intractable, and chronic reflux, for instance, may need referral to a gastroenterologist, and one whose responses to therapy are inconsistent and appear arbitrary may need referral to a psychotherapist. The patient who demonstrates dysphonia, as well as a mask-like facial countenance with limited movement (face and/or body) may need a referral to a neurologist.

Therapy provided within a unified, cohesive team will be more effective than if you work without professional collaboration. It is, therefore, a good idea to request permission from the patient and then communicate with the other professionals in your patient's life in order to provide the best possible care. At the very least, you will want to talk with the referring otolaryngologist to explore the medical treatment plan. Most professionals participate enthusiastically in the collaborative relationship. If the patient is reluctant to include other professionals in your relationship, you must honor his wishes. It is not unusual, for example, for singers to fear reprisals if their voice teacher or conservatory professors know that a voice problem exists. Although it is in the student's best interest that these professionals are aware of the singer's problem, it is not within our scope to inform without the patient's consent.

Sensitive Questions

There are times when you will feel uncomfortable asking questions that are sensitive because they are both personal and may have legal ramifications. How to ask questions regarding substance abuse, for instance, may be difficult and intimidate you as a new voice therapist. Be direct, matter-of-fact, and nonjudgmental when you pose these questions. **Dialogue 4-2** illustrates one possible way to handle a delicate situation. If you are concerned about this area of inquiry, practice and rehearsal with a peer may alleviate your anxiety and allow for a more natural interaction.

Dialogue 4-2
Excerpt from Initial Assessment

In a straightforward, matter-of-fact tone, "Do you use recreational drugs, and if so, which ones?"

Mr. D replied, "I smoke pot on weekends."

Through close observation, I assessed the severity of his moderately low-pitched, rough voice and asked follow-up questions to expand my understanding of the interaction of possible contributing factors to his voice disorder, "How much do you smoke?"

Mr. D paused and then continued, "It depends on what I am doing. I don't smoke every day, but if I'm having a party, I may share 2 to 3 joints."

I noted the consistency of his rough voice and wanted to know if he was aware of any sensory changes that can result from smoking marijuana. "Do you notice that your throat feels dry or burns after smoking?"

Mr. D immediately rejoined, "Now that you mention it, my throat does feel dry and burny. I get hungry, and I eat and drink a lot."

How Does the Patient Use His Voice?

It is not possible to know your patient's expectations of the therapy process unless you ask him. The items listed in the Voice Evaluation Form may guide your questions. Is he a professional voice user? Does he use the telephone extensively? Does he lecture? Your questions may raise his awareness of his voice use. He may not be aware that speaking in a noisy environment for prolonged periods, for example, may place a strain on his voice.

We use specific, self-administered questionnaires to elicit information about voice use and to raise the patient's awareness. At times, individuals will remember additional information or share details they did not consider related when they completed a self-administered questionnaire. The Voice Handicap Index (VHI) (Rosen, Lee, Osborne, Zullo, & Murry, 2004), the Voice-Related Quality of Life (V-RQOL) (Hogikyan & Sethuraman, 1999), General Self-Efficacy Scale (GSES) (Schwarzer & Jerusalem, 1995), and the **Reflux Symptom Index (RSI)** (Belafsky, Postma, & Koufman, 2002) are useful tools that estimate the relative impact of the voice problem on the patient's personal life and occupation.

What Is Direct Observation?

Thus far, you have obtained information that reflects the history and medical nature of the problem from the patient's perspective. During the second part of your assessment you will shift your focus to the perceptual, aerodynamic, and acoustic measurements of the voice symptoms. At the end of the evaluation, after you have collected all of your data, you will combine the patient's descriptions, your direct observations, your knowledge of his specific pathology, and your understanding of laryngeal anatomy and physiology to form an integrated **diagnostic hypothesis**.

How Does Posture Affect Manner of Phonation?

What do you notice about the patient? Is the patient's posture stiff or effortlessly supported by the appropriate alignment of the head and torso (Franco et al., 2014)? Are his breathing patterns rapid, labored, or shallow? As you continue your observation, you want to note signs of extraneous muscle activity in the head, neck, and thorax (Angsuwarangsee & Morrison, 2002). You might observe clenching of the jaw, furrowing between the eyebrows, and/or stiffening in the neck and thorax. These observations are essential to a multidimensional assessment because restrictions in the head, neck, and torso may negatively affect the manner of phonation. Stiffness in the structures adjacent to the larynx can radiate to the larynx itself, exacerbating (possible) preexisting intrinsic muscle tightness (Dimon, 2011). Similarly, stiffening of the chest wall may negatively affect respiratory efficiency. The patient who uses excessive movement or stiffness in the upper thorax, shallow breathing, or suboptimal posture may limit the quantity of air available for phonation and compromise the efficient coordination between respiration and phonation (Franco et al., 2014).

The Importance of the Patient's Self-Perception

The perceptual assessment is the gold standard of voice assessment. This statement suggests that it is the clinician who perceives the characteristics of the patient's voice quality, pitch, and loudness. However, it is the *patient's* perception of his voice that brought him to your examination room. His **self-perception** of roughness, breathiness, and effort offer valuable insight into his kinesthetic and auditory awareness. Not only are you using *your* perceptual skills to evaluate your patient's voice quality, but your *patient* comes to you with perceptions about his voice that are often accurate and emotionally charged. Patients regularly make judgments that are based on what they feel (effort), as well as what they hear (roughness, breathiness). When you listen actively, the patient's perceptions provide critical information that promotes a patient-centered approach, which will focus on the patient's experience with and perspective on the voice problem.

The Clinician's Perceptual Assessment

Your perceptual analysis of the patient's voice allows you to determine the characteristics and severity of the voice disorder in relation to the patient's response, the degree to which it interferes with communication, and the patient's skill in modifying his manner of phonation. Your perceptual assessment of pitch, loudness, and quality is more central to the patient's concerns than the instrumental assessment because the measurements obtained with instrumentation do not speak to the patient's frame of reference (Aronson & Bless, 2009; Carding, Carlson, Epstein, Mathieson, & Shewell, 2000). However, while perceptual measures allow us to monitor therapeutic changes, certain challenges limit the effectiveness of the perceptual evaluation. We remain aware of these limitations in order to reduce bias and unreliability, given that perceptual analysis is subjective and based on your **internal assessment** of appropriateness of voice quality. Moreover, all voice clinicians do not follow the same protocol or use a standard vocabulary to describe voice characteristics, and the choice of rating scale varies among clinicians. Variability in perceptual assessment exists, not only within and between clinicians, but between the clinician and the patient due to several factors, including the exposure that the clinician has had to voice problems, the tendency of patients to focus more on what they hear than what they feel, and their limited exposure to dysphonia (Bassich & Ludlow 1986; Gerratt, Kreiman, Antonanzas-Barroso, & Berke, 1993). Finally, the distinction between what is considered normal or abnormal voice quality exists, in part, on a continuum, and is confounded by the absence of hard and fast guidelines for what is *normal* and what is *problematic*. These labels change based on the context within which the voice is produced, the skill and expectation of the patient, and the structure of the larynx.

How Do I Rate Dysphonia?

Perceptual assessment is a three-part process that begins when you respond to the impact of the overall severity of the dysphonia on the patient. His reaction leads to a number of questions you can ask yourself: "How severe is the dysphonia?" "Does the voice problem negatively affect speech production?" "How much negative attention does the voice draw to itself?" "Is the patient's voice audible?" When you have rated the overall severity of the voice problem, you will then determine which specific characteristics represent the patient's dysphonia. As you refer to the symptoms listed on the Voice Evaluation Form in Appendix 1, you will rate the characteristics and severity of your patient's dysphonia by asking the following questions for each symptom: "Do I hear roughness?" "Do I hear breathiness?" You now ask, "Is the roughness and breathiness mild, mild to moderate, moderate, moderate to severe, or severe?" In this way, you describe not only the overall severity of the dysphonia, but you identify the severity of each individual characteristic as it contributes to the overall severity rating of dysphonia. If you use a framework such as the Voice Evaluation Form in Appendix 1 to guide your assessment of the perceptual characteristics of the patient's voice quality and severity of dysphonia, your perceptual assessment will be less challenging.

The Application of Perceptual, Aerodynamic, and Acoustic Information

Perceptual, aerodynamic, and acoustic analyses can be used to develop hypotheses about the underlying anatomy and physiology of the vocal folds (source), the response of the mucosa to laryngeal pathology, expiratory control, and the influence of vocal tract configuration (the filter) on the voice. As you collect your data, several factors may influence the reliability and validity of the information you obtain from these measures. You may remember that reliability refers to the consistency or precision of a measurement, and validity is defined as the degree to which the instrument "measures what it purports to measure" (Ventry, Schiavetti, & Denson, 1986, p. 87). It is possible, for example, that during testing your patient may not produce voice in his customary manner due to anxiety, self-consciousness, or his desire to give you his best performance. He may (or may not) fatigue as the session progresses. In any case, you will repeat many of your test procedures at least three times to ensure that you have a representative sample of his typical performance. In addition, you consider your patient's cognitive and hearing status as you decide which data you wish to collect and how you will provide directions while you conduct your assessment. Your specific directions, your ongoing encouragement during each task, and your appropriate demonstration of the tasks will facilitate the patient's optimum performance. Of course, you want to make certain that your equipment has been suitably calibrated, and that you have done a biological calibration to verify that the equipment is working, thereby reducing any interruption due to breakdown of the equipment.

Aerodynamic Assessment

Respiratory function testing is an integral part of the evaluation process that provides information pertaining to the coordination between the respiratory and phonatory subsystems. The voice disorder, the available equipment, and the sophistication of your skills and training determine the complexity of your **aerodynamic assessment**. Clinically relevant measures of volume, flow, and pressure can be captured in several ways. However, these values must be interpreted carefully. When obtaining forced vital capacity information, for instance, it is not unusual for patients to shorten the exhalation phase before they have exhaled all of the air possible. It is crucial, therefore, that all endurance tasks (e.g., vital capacity, **s/z ratio, maximum phonation time**) be demonstrated prior to patient performance, and that your patient be encouraged (verbally and/or with gestures) to persevere during the trials.

The maximum phonation time and the s/z ratio, both of which indirectly measure the integrity and efficiency of the respiratory system and the larynx, are popular and easy to obtain without sophisticated equipment (Speyer et al., 2010). Nonetheless, these measures may be highly variable and subject to a practice effect (Stone, 1983), given that multiple trials are typically expected for these procedures. Variability can be caused by both positive and negative compensations. If your patient is a singer, he may efficiently use inspiratory checking to decrease airflow and increase the duration of the /s/, /z/, and /a/ sounds (Behrman, 2007). Furthermore, increases or decreases in vocal intensity may influence your values. Increased intensity, for instance, requires an increase in subglottal pressure and may shorten the maximum phonation time (Gelfer & Pazera, 2006).

There are many counterproductive ways to achieve a clinically normal maximum phonation time and s/z ratio. If your patient increases medial compression and stiffness of the vocal folds, and/or if there is excessive constriction in the vocal tract (e.g., ventricular vocal folds, epilarynx) the maximum phonation time may increase, but with a negative effect on the larynx (Behrman, 2007). How, then, do you determine whether your aerodynamic measures were reached appropriately or by increasing phonatory effort? If you recognize a pressed, inappropriately loud, and/or effortful manner of phonation, and/or observe extraneous muscle activity in the neck, it is likely that your patient is using counterproductive strategies to extend his maximum phonation time (duration of /a/) and the duration of the /s/ and /z/ phonemes.

The vital capacity (VC) measure provides additional information to confirm or dismiss your suspicions regarding the adequacy of the patient's respiratory mechanism. Forced VC is obtained by having a patient take a maximum inhalation and then exhale all of the air into a handheld spirometer (dry spirometer). This measure quantifies VC in cubic centimeters (cc) of air. The measurements from a patient are compared to the normative data that accompany the device. The rule of thumb is that when a mean vital capacity measure is below 70% of the expected value, it is necessary to refer the patient for a pulmonary evaluation to rule out conditions such as asthma and chronic obstructive pulmonary disease (COPD) prior to the start of voice rehabilitation.

After you have completed both the mean vital capacity measure and the maximum phonation time for /a/, you can calculate the phonation quotient by dividing vital capacity by maximum phonation time (Raes & Clement, 1996). **Table 4-1** provides the normative data for vital capacity, maximum phonation time, and phonation quotient for young, healthy, adult, male and female individuals.

Mean flow rate during vowels and connected speech is related to **velopharyngeal competence** as well as glottal sufficiency and can have an effect on articulatory precision, voice quality, and intelligibility. If the flow is elevated, you will want to determine if it is due to velopharyngeal or laryngeal insufficiency. One way to make this distinction is to assess the voice quality. Increased nasal resonance is associated with velopharyngeal insufficiency.

Acoustic Analysis

Acoustic analysis has become widely used given the number of free programs readily available on the Web with algorithms that automatically calculate fundamental frequency, intensity, perturbation, voice range profiles, etc. However, the reliability of these automatic measures is affected by variations in equipment from clinic to clinic, the chosen protocol, the environment (e.g., ambient noise, distractions, presence of strong harmonics or subharmonics), aperiodicity in the signal, within-patient variation (within and between sessions), and test-retest variability. Further, subjective conditions may affect your acoustic results. If your patient is female, for instance, hormonal fluctuations during the premenstrual period may lead to temporary laryngeal swelling and an increase in the acidity and viscosity of the laryngeal mucus, thus influencing the findings (Abitbol, Abitbol, & Abitbol, 1999). For all patients, the reliability of the acoustic results may be

Table 4-1 Normative Data for Vital Capacity, Maximum Phonation Time for /a/, and Phonation Quotient

Norms	VC	MPT for /a/	PQ
Male	4800 ml	34.6 sec	269 ml/sec
	S.D. (600)*	S.D. (–11.4- +12.1)**	S.D. (88)***
Female	3500 ml	25.7 sec	233 ml/sec
	S.D. (600)*	S.D. (–6.5- +7.5)**	S.D. (82)***

*Ptacek & Sander, 1966.

**Hirano, Koike, & von Leden, 1968.

***Dobinson & Kendrick, 1993.

compromised by the time between the patient's last meal, hydration levels, caffeine intake, level of energy, and emotional state (Leong et al., 2012; Ma et al., 2006).

Unfortunately, the algorithms used to automatically calculate fundamental frequency, shimmer, and jitter are unreliable when fundamental frequency variability exceeds 6% per cycle (Titze & Lang, 1993), which is often the case when a vocal problem exists. Acoustic measurement programs calculate fundamental frequency by identifying zero-crossing or peak-picking, but when these features are not readily identifiable (due to excessive irregularity or noise in the signal due to excessive roughness or phonation breaks) the formula is not sufficiently robust to compensate for these irregularities. This may be the case, for example, when assessing the symptoms of spasmodic dysphonia. The strained-strangled voice quality typical of adductor spasmodic dysphonia frequently exceeds 6% per cycle. To check the validity of your results, you may compare your perceptual judgment with the data derived from the automatic acoustic measurement. When the objective data and your perceptual judgment do not match, it may be necessary to further analyze the voice sample using hand measurements, or to rely solely on perceptual assessment.

Fundamental frequency should be captured during running speech as well as sustained vowel phonation. Although F_0 has been shown to be repeatable, it does not expose the underlying, more obscure aspects of the voice disturbance. It does, however, supplement your perceptual observation of your patient's pitch and can be useful to document change over time and provide a tangible reinforcement for the patient of his progress over time (Behrman, 2005). The mean fundamental frequency for a typical adult male is between 85 and 155 Hz, and for a typical adult female range from 165 to 255 Hz (Fitch & Holbrook, 1970). However, age, gender, vocal intensity, intent, health, emotional state, and speech context affect these values.

It would not be unusual to find a higher than expected fundamental frequency in a patient with muscle tension dysphonia, whose larynx is elevated in the neck; a patient with a laryngeal web that decreases the length of the membranous portion of the vocal fold; or a patient with mutational falsetto resulting from hormonal effects, delayed maturation, psychological issues, habitual use, or personal choice. For these patients pitch typically lowers as an easier manner of phonation is implemented. Although mutational falsetto is more typically associated with pubescent males, it does occur in older adults and can lead to profound social and psychogenic consequences. Closely related to mutational falsetto in males is the juvenile, childlike voice exhibited by some adult females. This pattern may be conscious or unconscious and adopted to appear submissive and nonthreatening. A juvenile voice can be detrimental and undermine the individual's credibility as a competent, mature adult. In sharp contrast, **virilization**, which is most often seen in postmenopausal women, is an abnormal lowering of pitch due to an increase in the size and mass of the vocal folds that may be associated with high levels of androgenic hormones. Quantification of these deviations in pitch provides accountability for insurance companies, offers patients concrete data that monitors change over time, and is evidence that validates the patient's perceptual observations.

Measurements of jitter, shimmer, and harmonics-to-noise ratio provide additional information pertaining to the contribution of cycle-to-cycle variation, amplitude of variation, and noise in the signal. These measures vary based on fundamental frequency, the loudness of the signal, and the formula used to calculate the measure. Irregularity in vocal fold vibration associated with laryngeal pathology or even edema and stiffness or asynchrony in glottal closure may be reflected in the atypical perturbation measure. Again, these measures are useful when documentation is required by an insurance company in order to justify continued therapy because they represent concrete evidence of progress over time.

What Is a Diagnostic Hypothesis?

You make hypotheses every day. For instance, when you have been studying for hours and are having difficulty concentrating, you might hypothesize that if you take a nap your focus will improve. To test your hypothesis, you take a nap and when you return to your studies, if you are more alert and process the information more efficiently, you can accept your hypothesis. Diagnostic hypotheses allow you to apply your problem-solving skills to the development of an appropriate hierarchy of goals and procedures.

During the evaluation process, you identify the factors that precipitated, maintain, and/or exacerbate your patient's voice problem and formulate hypotheses based on these observations. If, for example, the patient reports that his spouse is hard of hearing, you might hypothesize that he uses excessive loudness and effort to communicate with her. In so doing, he uses excessive medial compression and stiffness of the vocal folds. In another case, if the patient works out and lifts weights, you might hypothesize that he is using strong laryngeal valving when he lifts instead of stabilizing the chest wall. Again, if he works as a bartender in a noisy club, you might hypothesize that he is using excessive expiratory drive to project his voice over noise.

In the *Recommendations: Voice Conservation* video, the clinician and patient discuss strategies that can be implemented to cope with ambient noise. Voice conservation is one of the early topics of conversation in therapy and can make a substantial difference in diminishing a common risk factor.

You use critical reasoning to rationalize what you hear and observe with your knowledge of appropriate coordination among the subsystems of respiration, phonation, resonance, and articulation. This information is central to developing a therapeutic plan that incorporates the physiological underpinnings of the voice problem into the procedures that you plan to use. As a clinician, you guide your patient as he modifies the manner by which he produces sound. Your understanding of vocal fold physiology and the laryngeal pathology will make your approach to assessment of change more accurate. You may remember that breathiness (perceptual rating) and increased flow (aerodynamic) are related to excessive air leaking through the glottis, possibly associated with bowing, unilateral vocal fold paralysis, an intrusive mass, posterior glottal chink, ankylosis of the cricoarytenoid joint, etc. (Colton, Casper, & Leonard, 2011; Ferrand, 2012). Similarly, if you note roughness (perceptual) and increased harmonic-to-noise ratio (acoustic), you might conjecture that the vocal folds are vibrating asymmetrically and/or asynchronously due to weighting and stiffness differences within or between them possibly due to the added weight from a unilateral vocal fold cyst or polyp. In another instance, if you observe a pressed manner of phonation (perceptual) you might theorize that the patient uses excessive medial compression and stiffness of the vocal folds, supraglottic squeeze, and excessive expiratory drive. If you hear abrupt voice onset, you might postulate that hyperadduction of the vocal folds and excessive expiratory drive occur prior to the onset of phonation.

What Is Diagnostic Voice Therapy?

As you move through the evaluation, you may begin **diagnostic therapy** (testing diagnostic hypotheses) and use the patient's repeated demonstration of your diagnostic voice tasks to determine the consistency or variability of his manner of phonation. If you observe that your patient uses frequent abrupt initiation of phonation, for example, you might hypothesize that he is using hyperadduction of the vocal folds and excessive subglottal pressure. Is he aware of any tightness or stiffness in the larynx associated with these behaviors? He may have so habituated these counterproductive behaviors that he no longer feels the effort he is using to make sound.

The process of diagnostic voice therapy begins with the patient's discrimination between and identification of easy versus effortful phonation. Does the patient accurately identify his own and your easy and effortful phonations of /mhm/? If not, how will he modify his phonatory effort? The patient's recognition and identification of effort contribute to your prognostic statement and the decision you make regarding therapeutic procedures. To facilitate this first step toward modification of effort, you, as the clinician, may present a pair of tokens and ask for identification of "same" or "different." You may exaggerate the difference between your productions of the /mhm/ tokens in order to sharpen the contrast. You may ask him to press his lips together tightly, say /mhm/ (feeling the tightness), release the lips, and repeat /mhm/ when the jaw and lips are released. If this proves ineffective, it may be useful to change the role of clinician and patient, whereby the patient is asked to produce tokens that he believes are very different from one another. You may follow his demonstration with a question that asks, "Which one of your tokens feels easier—less effortful?"

The frequent revelation that patients often experience when they feel the difference between the counterproductive effort they have used to "normalize voice quality" and the free and easy manner of phonation they experience during diagnostic therapy may provide an excellent starting point for modifying counterproductive behaviors. This first experience with an efficient manner of voice production after months or even years of effortful phonation provides a ray of hope that usually surprises patients. The patient's performance during these early modification exercises offers prognostic value as well. Whether your patient does or does not demonstrate identification and modification of effort, you have valuable information about his kinesthetic awareness and possible response to a sensory approach to treatment.

Based on your patient's accurate discrimination of easy versus effortful production, you may continue diagnostic therapy with a hypothesis that suggests that the vocal folds are hyperadducted to resist the excessive subglottal pressure. You can test your hypothesis with a back pressure exercise, such as /mhm/, with the expectation that the increase in supraglottal pressure will lead to a decrease in the transglottal pressure differential and decrease the excessive medial compression of the vocal folds. This technique provides an opportunity for your patient to reduce effort and for you to observe these changes as he decreases abrupt initiation of phonation and extraneous muscle activity in the head and neck.

Identification of effort is followed by modification. If the patient produces voice with abrupt initiation of phonation during a back pressure exercise, you might ask him to attend to the sensations in his throat as he repeats the /mhm/ exercise, hopefully, with less effort. You may suggest, "Do not push for sound." When he reduces effort (expiratory drive and medial compression of the vocal folds), he may become aphonic, look concerned, and say, "I feel like I'm doing nothing and no sound is coming out." It may be reassuring at this point to explain that the aphonia is due to the laryngeal pathology, and not something that he is doing "wrong." It may be difficult for the patient to give up the notion that voice at any cost is better than aphonia. Nevertheless, alteration of focus from the demand for sound to feeling a reduction in effort sets the stage for building your patient's kinesthetic awareness (Lessac, 1997).

Why Do I Consider All Aspects of Communication?

When a patient comes to you with a specific laryngeal diagnosis, you may not anticipate that he has other speech, language, hearing, or cognitive problems. Is the voice disorder a result of, or exacerbated by, another problem, such as a hearing loss, a submucous cleft of the palate, or a neurological disorder? It may seem obvious that changes in hearing, structure and function of the speech mechanism, cognition, language, articulation, fluency, and swallowing may have a negative effect on voice production. As a clinician, you need to screen these areas for factors that may coexist with or exacerbate the voice disorder. For instance, even a mild hearing loss may compromise the patient's perception of the inappropriate loudness of his voice. Structural changes, such as cleft palate, can lead to the use of counterproductive compensations, such as excessive expiratory drive and effortful phonation. A neurological disorder and associated dysphagia may be a result of decreased sensation in the laryngeal area, and this same decreased sensation may interfere with the patient's capacity to feel differences in the effort levels he uses when he produces sound. Furthermore, if your patient has cognitive deficits it may be difficult for him to follow directions and/or understand the purpose of your procedures. The patient may need additional demonstration and ongoing models of the intended goals as well as simple and concise verbal and written instructions for home use. It may be useful as well, to provide a recording of your voice explaining the steps of a recommended procedure to maximize independent, deliberate practice.

Diagnostic Impressions and Prognosis

Your **diagnostic impressions** are different from the diagnosis of the laryngeal pathology made by the otolaryngologist. You assess the overall severity of the dysphonia, describe the severity of the individual symptoms that characterize the dysphonia, gauge the patient's awareness of effort, judge the patient's response to stimulability testing, analyze the objective test results, use accurate empathy to probe the patient's narrative and emotional engagement during your assessment, and then incorporate that information with your knowledge of the physiology of normal and disrupted voice production. The integration of this information leads you to an understanding of the effect of this voice disorder on this specific patient and suggests a treatment path specific to his needs.

An essential extension of the diagnostic impression section is your prognostic statement. The prognosis forecasts your expectations regarding the patient's response to voice therapy. Prognostic statements may include expectations of return to clinically normal voice, significant improvement, or adequacy for activities of daily living. These prognostic statements exist along a continuum of achievement. It is possible, for example, that you hypothesize an excellent, good, fair, or poor potential for improvement. Your decision is based on several aspects of your initial evaluation. The laryngeal diagnosis, the chronicity of the problem, the patient's occupation and its ongoing demand on the voice, cognitive status, age, general health, severity of voice symptoms, response to diagnostic therapy, and verbal commitment to rehabilitation are key elements of the prognostic statement. This itemization is by no means all-inclusive, but does reflect many of the elements that you will consider when predicting outcome.

Summary

Assessment and formulation of diagnostic hypotheses are the first steps in the rehabilitation process. You conduct an assessment in order to determine the severity of the voice disorder, its impact on the patient's life, his awareness of effort and capacity to modify that manner of phonation, and how and where to begin the treatment process. The process of assessment is structured and facilitated by a Voice Evaluation Form, which provides the basic outline and categories of information that are necessary for the assessment, but the questions on the form are only the beginning. To perform an effective assessment and collect all the relevant information, you must be attentive to the patient's narrative in order to ask relevant follow-up questions and develop a multidimensional understanding of the patient and his problem. What are the unique characteristics of this patient and his voice disorder that you must consider? What are the patient's goals? How does the patient see his role in the treatment process? Are there other medical problems that interact with the voice disorder? What are the underlying physiological changes and counterproductive behaviors? What did your stimulability testing reveal about his kinesthetic awareness and modification of effort? You can use hypothesis development and testing as a framework for your assessment and treatment plan to address the whole patient in the rehabilitation process.

References

Abitbol, J., Abitbol, P., and Abitbol, B. (1999). Sex hormones and the female voice. *Journal of Voice, 13*(3), 424–446.

Angsuwarangsee, T., and Morrison, M. (2002). Extrinsic laryngeal muscular tension in patients with voice disorders. *Journal of Voice, 16*, 333–343.

Aronson, A.E., and Bless, D. (2009). *Clinical voice disorders: An interdisciplinary approach*. New York, NY: Thieme.

Barbara, D. (1968). *The art of listening*. Springfield, IL: Charles C. Thomas.

Bassich, C.J., and Ludlow, C.L. (1986). The use of perceptual methods by new clinicians for assessing voice quality. *Journal of Speech and Hearing Disorders, 51*(2), 125–333.

Belafsky, P.C., Postma, G.N., and Koufman, J.A. (2002). Validity and reliability of the reflux symptom index (RSI). *Journal of Voice, 16*(2), 274–277.

Behrman, A. (2005). Common practices of voice therapists in the evaluation of patients. *Journal of Voice, 19*(3), 454–469.

Behrman, A. (2007). *Speech and voice science*. San Diego, CA: Plural.

Carding, P., Carlson, E., Epstein, R., Mathieson, L., and Shewell, C. (2000). Formal perceptual evaluation of voice quality in the United Kingdom. *Logopedic Phoniatric Vocology, 25*, 133–138.

Colton, R., Casper, J.K., and Leonard, R. (2011). *Understanding voice problems: A physiological perspective for diagnosis and treatment* (4th ed.). Baltimore, MD: Lippincott Williams and Wilkins.

Dimon, T. (2011). *Your body, your voice: The key to natural singing and speaking*. Berkeley, CA: North Atlantic Books.

Dobinson, C.H., and Kendrick, A.H. (1993). Normal values and predictive equations for aerodynamic function in British Caucasian subjects. *Folia Phoniatrica (Basel), 45*(1), 14–24.

Ferrand, C.T. (2012). *Voice disorders: Scope of theory and practice*. Boston, MA: Pearson Higher Education.

Fitch, J.L., and Holbrook, A. (1970). Modal vocal fundamental frequency of young adults. *Archives of Otolaryngology*, 92, 379–382.

Franco, D., Martins, F., Andrea, M., Fragoso, I., Carrao, L., and Teles, J. (2014). Is the sagittal postural alignment different in normal and dysphonic adult speakers? *Journal of Voice*, 28(4), 523.e1–523.e8.

Gelfer, M.P., and Pazera, J.F. (2006). Maximum duration of sustained /s/ and /z/ and the s/z ratio with controlled intensity. *Journal of Voice*, 20(3), 369–379.

Gerratt, B.R., Kreiman, J., Antonanzas-Barroso, N., and Berke, G.S. (1993). Comparing internal and external standards in voice quality judgments. *Journal of Speech and Hearing Research*, 36(1), 14–20.

Hirano, M., Koike, Y., and von Leden, H. (1968). Maximum phonation time and air wastage during phonation: Clinical study. *Folia Phoniatrica*, 20, 185–201.

Hogikyan, N.D., and Sethuraman G. (1999). Validation of an instrument to measure voice-related quality of life (V-RQOL). *Journal of Voice*, 13(4), 557–569.

Kuhn, T.S. (1970). *The structure of the scientific revolution* (2nd ed., Vol. 2). Chicago, IL: University of Chicago.

Leong, K., Hawkshaw, M.J., Dentchev, D., Gupta, R., Lurie, D., and Sataloff, R.T. (2012). Reliability of objective voice measures of normal speaking voices. *Journal of Voice*, 27(2), 170–176.

Lessac, A. (1997). *The use and training of the human voice: A practical approach to speech and voice dynamics* (3rd ed.). Santa Monica, CA: McGraw-Hill.

Ma, E., Robertson, J., Radford, C., Vagne, S., El-Halabi, R., and Yiu, E. (2006). Reliability of speaking and maximum voice range measures in screening for dysphonia. *Journal of Voice*, 21(4), 397–406.

Martin, D.G. (1983). *Counseling and therapy skills*. Prospect Heights, IL: Waveland Press.

Prochaska, J.O. and DiClemente, C.C. (1984). *The transtheoretical approach: Crossing traditional boundaries of therapy*. Homewood, IL: Dorsey Professional Books.

Ptacek, P.H., and Sander, E.K. (1966). Age recognition from voice. *Journal of Speech and Hearing Research*, 9(2), 273–277.

Raes, J.P., and Clement, P.A. (1996). Aerodynamic measurements of voice production. *Acta Otorhinolaryngology*, 50(4), 293–298.

Rogers, C.R. (1951). *Client-centered therapy: Its current practice, implications, and theory*. Boston, MA: Houghton Mifflin.

Rosen, C.A., Lee, A.S., Osborne, J., Zullo, T., and Murry, T. (2004). Development and validation of the voice handicap index-10. *Laryngoscope*, 114(9), 1549–1556.

Schwarzer, R., & Jerusalem, M. (1995). Generalized self-efficacy scale. In J. Weinman, S. Wright, & M. Johnston, *Measures in health psychology: A user's portfolio. Causal and control beliefs* (pp. 35–37). Windsor, UK: NFER-NELSON.

Speyer, R., Bogaardt, H.C.A., Lima Passos, V., Roodenburg, N.P.H.D., Zumach, A., Heijnen, M.A.M., ... Brunings, J.W. (2010). Maximum phonation time: Variability and reliability. *Journal of Voice*, 24(3), 281–284.

Stone, R.E. (1983). Issues in clinical assessment of laryngeal function: Contra-indications for subscribing to maximum phonation time and optimum fundamental frequency. In D.M. Bless and J.H. Abbs (Eds.), *Vocal fold physiology: Contemporary research and clinical issues* (pp. 410–424). San Diego, CA: College Hill Press.

Titze, I.R., and Lang, H. (1993). Comparison of F_o extraction methods for high-precision voice perturbation measurements. *Journal of Speech and Hearing Research*, 36, 1177–1190.

Ventry, I.M., Schiavetti, N., and Denson, T.A. (1986). *Evaluating research in speech pathology and audiology*. New York, NY: Macmillan.

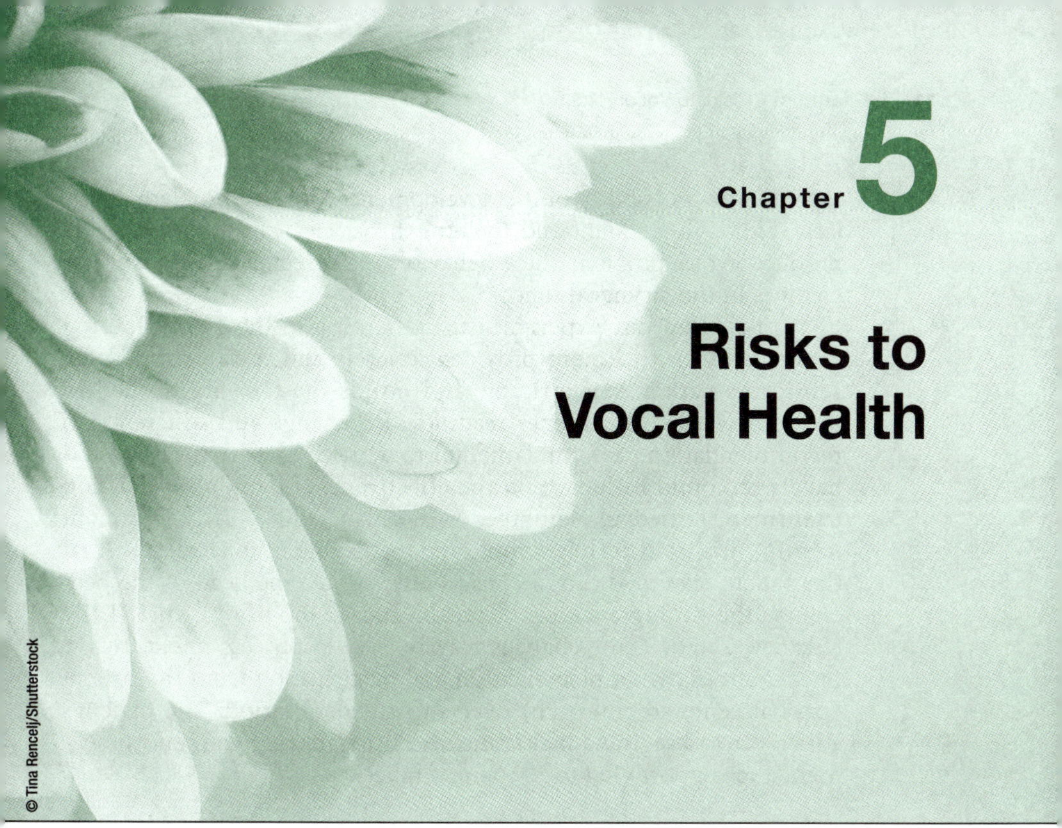

Chapter 5

Risks to Vocal Health

"You mentioned that it is difficult to read stories to your children. Does your throat ever feel tired?"

What Are Risks?

Anything that predisposes the larynx to a voice disorder may be considered a risk to vocal health and should be addressed in tandem with treatment that modifies the vibration of the vocal folds. A voice problem is not usually a result of one incident or one inappropriate vocal behavior, but habitual, repetitive, and effortful use of the voice over time. Speaking over noise for prolonged periods, for instance, does not in and of itself cause a laryngeal pathology, but it does represent a risk. Vocal fatigue, laryngeal stiffness, and excessive and prolonged compression of the vocal folds make the larynx more susceptible to and increase the probability of the development of a voice problem. Similarly, although frequent and forceful throat clearing do not directly produce a voice problem, these behaviors may precipitate or exacerbate changes in the laryngeal mucosa.

It has been our experience that attention to these contributing factors early in treatment provides concrete and rewarding results, reinforces patient self-efficacy, and builds the tenacity needed to move forward. The patient's readiness for change and adherence to recommendations are fundamental to a successful partnership and have a profound influence on the effectiveness of any plan of action (Behrman, Rutledge, Hembree, & Sheridan, 2008). Early treatment to minimize acid reflux symptoms, for example, may require that the patient take medication consistently, elevate the head of the bed, change the timing and size of meals, and/or modify his diet (Kelly & Lahey, 2009). These changes may be easy to process intellectually, but require active implementation and participation from the patient (patient-centered approach) over an extended period. The patient's adherence to a regimen may wane over time, making your encouragement and support vital to his perseverance.

Patient-Centered Rehabilitation Hypotheses

As you begin to organize your goals and procedures to reduce the impact of risk factors on the manner of phonation, you will need a hypothesis-driven framework to structure your follow-up questions, construct your hypotheses, and reconcile them with your clinical observations and your patient's report. The Voice Evaluation Form in Appendix 1 will guide you as you ask questions about the laryngeal diagnosis, surgery, medications, onset of the problem, alcohol use, etc. As you listen to the patient's description of the voice problem, surrounding factors, and ask follow-up questions to identify the significance of these factors—whether they are part of counterproductive compensations, unusual environmental circumstances, or medical complications—you will develop hypotheses that you will then test, accept, modify, or reject.

The process of transforming patient concerns and clinician observations into an organized framework that reduces the effect of risk factors is a complex one. You have many options from which to choose, and will be guided not only by what you observe as central to the patient's complaint but your awareness that no treatment plan or procedure will be effective with all patients. It is essential to tailor voice rehabilitation to meet the needs of the individual and the changes within the patient that occur over time. When you apply this concept to treatment, you rely on the patient's narrative and your perception of effortful versus easy voice production to gain insight into the effect of the risk on your patient's vocal health. The impact of the behavior, as well as environmental and/or medical risks, inform your recommendations regarding the modifications you believe will be beneficial.

When you begin therapy to reduce excessive loudness and make recommendations to alleviate contributing medical factors, it may be useful to refer to the transtheoretical model (TTM) and motivational interviewing (MI) to identify your patient's readiness for change. During the assessment and throughout treatment, you will reflect on this central aspect of therapy to enhance adherence. Readiness for change fluctuates both within the patient and within a particular phase of treatment. The patient may implement strategies easily in some areas before he will consider modifying his behavior in others. His attitude or behavior may suggest that he is in TTM stage 1 (precontemplation), and is unaware of the counterproductive factors that contribute to his voice problem, or he may be ready to consider stage 2 (contemplation) and work directly on these problems. Remember that you cannot convince anyone of anything. You can, however, discuss the patient's occupational demands, social life, and home environment to uncover previously unidentified opportunities for reducing counterproductive behaviors, and possibly identify discrepancies between his current mindset and the possibility of changing a behavior. A compliance lawyer, for instance, whose work requires constant talking during conference calls, presentations, and meetings for eight or nine hours per day, may be willing but feel unable to follow voice conservation recommendations (TTM stage 3, preparation) owing to the many responsibilities he has to his clients. Mutual problem solving may uncover possibilities for reducing his heavy vocal demand. He might become more of a listener with friends, avoid talking over noise, shift responsibility of play and reading aloud to the children to the spouse or older sibling, and limit social conversations on the telephone.

Tables 5-1 through 5-13 make this process more transparent by providing examples of hypotheses to reduce counterproductive behaviors (e.g., strategies commonly used by patients to enhance the voice), environmental challenges (e.g., noise, the need to project, environmental pollutants), and medical problems (e.g., asthma, surgery, respiratory disorders). These procedures and strategies act as a springboard to the problem-solving process as you and your patient decide how to manage these relentless and everyday stressors. Of course, all of these procedures should be developed in consultation with the patient to facilitate adherence. He may offer suggestions that will enhance the effectiveness of incorporating the procedure into his daily life. When you jointly discuss the process with your patient, not only will he better understand what he needs to do, but in all likelihood he will be more inclined to adhere to the recommendations.

The Intervention Process

The hypothesis-driven approach will serve you well as you organize the long- and short-term goals that represent your management plan. The rehabilitation hypotheses you develop will be associated with the underlying physiological changes that led to the development, maintenance, and exacerbation of the voice problem, as well as the counterproductive compensations the patient uses to cope with the voice disturbance. Your hypotheses take into account your observations of the patient's communicative strengths, temperament, and daily challenges (e.g., occupation, hearing-impaired spouse, young children). A **rehabilitation hypothesis** includes the identification of risk factors followed by a specific **therapeutic hypothesis**. This **intervention process** is demonstrated in **Box 5-1**.

Counterproductive Compensatory Behaviors

Excessive Laryngeal Valving

When an individual's voice deteriorates, he often instinctively clears his throat, coughs, or increases vocal intensity in a conscious or subliminal attempt to improve his voice. These behaviors may result in a temporary improvement in voicing, but this boost is ephemeral, creates more mucous production, increases dryness, and usually becomes entrenched and habituated. When you observe frequent throat clearing,

Box 5-1

Examples of Rehabilitation Hypotheses

Risk factor: Patient uses telephone extensively during work hours.

Therapeutic hypothesis: Delegation of phone duties to others will provide opportunities for **voice rest** and reduce effort during the workday.

Risk factor: Patient is a tennis athlete. He uses excessive laryngeal resistance during play (grunting).

Therapeutic hypothesis: Alternate strategy for chest wall stabilization during play will replace laryngeal valving.

Risk factor: Patient is a bartender and speaks over ambient noise for long periods.

Therapeutic hypothesis: Decrease of expiratory drive and extraneous muscle activity, especially in the larynx and neck (strap muscles), will facilitate more appropriate manner of production.

for instance, your goal is to discover whether it is related to a transient event, such as a cold, or if it is a habit. When throat clearing is habitual, it is necessary to facilitate your patient's awareness of the habit. Awareness is the first step to change. The counterproductive cycle for the management of mucus is illustrated in **Figure 5-1**.

Self-awareness takes place in several stages. The patient must recognize and acknowledge that frequent, effortful throat clearing is detrimental to vocal fold health, identify when the behavior occurs, and attempt to suppress the habituated impulse. Patients are often surprised that the behavior occurs as frequently as is identified during the session. A substitute behavior, such as a gentle hum, a sip of water, or a dry swallow when the urge first occurs or immediately after clearing one's throat addresses the underlying cause of the behavior (e.g., dryness, accumulation of mucus) during this initial stage of change and may facilitate cessation of the behavior. It may be of interest to your patient that frequent, aggressive throat clearing strips away the protective layer of mucus that covers the vocal folds. The dry vocal folds then create more mucus, and the patient finds himself in a self-perpetuating cycle of building and stripping mucus (King, 2006; Nadel, 2013). In **Table 5-1**, we link the clinician's observation of **excessive laryngeal valving** to a physiological hypothesis and procedure that address the counterproductive behavior. Your suggestions will consider the patient's readiness for change and the feasibility of easy integration of the procedure or strategy into his daily life.

Figure 5-1

Counterproductive Management of Mucus

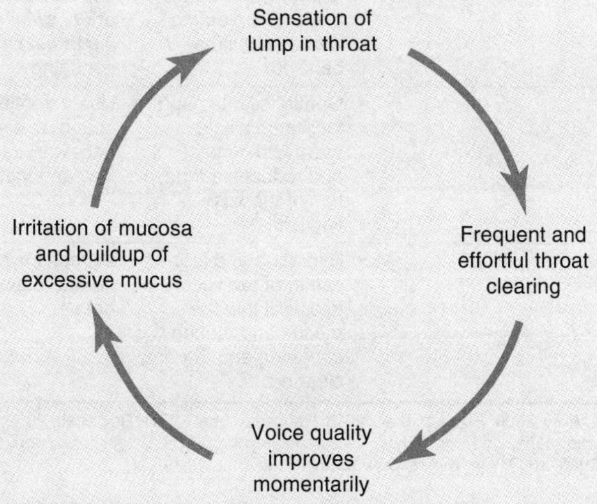

Table 5-1 Excessive Effortful Laryngeal Valving

Clinician's Perception and/or Patient's Report	Physiological Precipitating, Maintaining, and Exacerbating Factors	Hypothesis	Hypothesis Testing
• Patient inappropriately and excessively coughs or clears his throat during conversation.	• Patient uses excessive expiratory drive and medial compression of the vocal folds during coughing and throat clearing.	• Patient will reduce unnecessary coughing and throat clearing with awareness of its possible consequences.	• Discuss the effect of frequent, unnecessary coughing and throat clearing on the vocal folds. • Monitor frequency of throat clearing during the session. • Record frequency of throat clearing during the day (awareness of the activity will diminish its frequency). • Self-monitor and record successful suppression of the behaviors.
		• Patient will reduce unnecessary coughing and throat clearing if he has a substitute behavior.	• Discuss and practice options for gentle coughing and throat clearing. • Practice gentle /hmm/ (to dislodge mucus from folds). • Take small sips of water. • Use a dry or effortful swallow. • Suppress the cough and throat clearing.
		• Patient will reduce vocal fold stiffness following coughing and throat clearing with a substitute behavior.	• Produce a gentle /hmm/, take small sips of water, perform an effortful or dry swallow following throat clearing or coughing.
		• Gentle, silent cough facilitates a light vocal fold contact and reduces adduction of the false vocal folds.	• Use a gentle, silent cough as a substitute behavior (increase in airflow and minimal sound).
		• Hydration and lubrication of the vocal folds will thin the mucus and reduce coughing and throat clearing.	• Increase hydration and humidification of ambient air.

Data from: Deem & Miller, 2000; Pizolato et al., 2013; Rousseau et al., 2011; Roy et al., 2002; Solomon & DiMattia, 2000; Timmermans, De Bodt, Wuyts, & Van ede Heyning, 2004; Verdolini-Marston, Sandage, & Titze, 1994; Yiu & Chan, 2003; Yun, Kim, & Son, 2007.

Excessive and Inappropriate Loudness

One of the most common risks to vocal health is the habitual use of excessive effort and loudness during spontaneous speech. A significant decrease in strenuous voice use may be the patient's first step as he begins to gain control over his manner of phonation. The solution to excessive loudness may seem obvious and straightforward, but one's customary vocal intensity becomes habituated and eventually automatic, requiring first the development of awareness and then the implementation of procedures to establish and maintain a more cost-effective manner of phonation. Some patients may view their excessive vocal intensity not as a problem but as a personal asset and valued part of their personality. They may be reluctant to decrease the excessive expiratory drive that contributes to the effort they use. Others are genuinely surprised when you point out inappropriate loudness, but immediately adjust to a quieter, easier manner of phonation. Regardless of the patient's response to this counterproductive behavior, it is our responsibility to work with the patient to ensure longevity of the phonatory mechanism by providing information related to the consequences of excessive and prolonged effort and loudness.

Intervention to reduce habitual use of extreme loudness begins with the patient's acknowledgment of the behavior and the need to decrease the vocal intensity temporarily until he learns to increase loudness easily and efficiently. This adjustment appears straightforward, but when speakers become excited, vocal intensity naturally increases, usually without conscious awareness. Awareness develops over time and with more consistent implementation of strategies that offset this social response. **Table 5-2** offers some common clinician observations of excessive loudness and effort related to the physiological hypotheses and procedures that address this counterproductive behavior.

In the *Voice Conservation* video, the clinician reassures the patient that many of the voice conservation measures recommended early in the voice rehabilitation process are temporary and will be replaced by an efficient manner of phonation and adequate breath support that provide tools to cope with varying levels of vocal intensity.

Effortful Crying and Laughing

There may be times in a patient's life when psychological and emotional stress lead to prolonged periods of sobbing. If, for instance, the patient tells you that he recently lost a close relative and has had frequent episodes of uncontrollable sobbing, the clinician may provide information about the relationship between forceful sobbing and its effect on the laryngeal mucosa due to prolonged and strenuous crying.

Table 5-2 Excessive and Inappropriate Loudness

Clinician's Perception and/or Patient's Report	Physiological Precipitating, Maintaining, and Exacerbating Factors	Hypothesis	Hypothesis Testing
• Patient uses inappropriate, excessive effort and loudness during conversation.	• Patient is using excessive expiratory drive and medial compression of the vocal folds.	• Patient will produce voice with less effort if he decreases transglottal pressure drop, vocal fold stiffness, and medial compression of the vocal folds.	• Discuss benefits of using quiet, gentle phonation. • Implement confidential voice (speaking quietly without breathiness). • Decrease distance to listener (less need to project). • Enhance facial lighting (to facilitate lip reading).
• Patient reports that he "is a big talker."	• Prolonged talking with high expiratory drive leads to vocal fatigue.	• Vocal fatigue will decrease when the patient implements voice conservation.	• Identify ways to enhance awareness of loud talking. • Practice quiet talking in conversation to develop the *feel* of quiet speech. • Discuss feasibility of texting rather than talking on the telephone. • Engage family members and friends to monitor manner of phonation.
• During connected speech, the patient may use extraneous muscle activity: – furrow the brow – stiffen the jaw – purse the lips – engage the extrinsic laryngeal muscles – elevate the shoulders – stiffen the thorax	• Patient uses general, apparent, extraneous muscle activity in the head, neck and thorax.	• Manner of phonation will improve with decrease in extraneous muscle activity in the head, neck, and thorax.	• Jaw Release Exercises (see the *Introduction and Clinical Orientation* chapter). • Airway Reflex Exercise • Modify upper body posture with exercises that release shoulder and thoracic stiffness. • Release stiffness in tongue-root with gargling, yawning, sighing, protruding tongue while phonating, Masako, etc. • Incorporate exercise routines (e.g., yoga, Pilates, Feldenkrais, and Alexander technique).
		• Hydration and lubrication of the vocal folds will reduce high phonation pressure thresholds.	• Increase humidification of ambient air.

Data from Angsuwarangsee & Morrison, 2002; Behrman, Rutledge, Hembree, & Sheridan, 2008; Behrman & Sulica, 2003; Colton, Casper, & Leonard, 2011; Ferrand, 2012; Ferreira et al., 2010; Franco et al., 2014; Ilomaki, Laukkanen, Leppanen & Vilkman, 2008; Ishikawa & Thibeault, 2010; Pizolato et al., 2013; Rousseau et al., 2011; Roy et al., 2001; Roy et al., 2002; Timmermans, De Bodt, Wuyts, & Van de Heyning, 204; Yun, Kim, & Son, 2007.

Under these circumstances, the larynx closes tightly and the extrinsic laryngeal muscles stiffen to increase the medial compression of the vocal folds. This extraneous muscle activity may lead to vocal fatigue, tightness, pain, and eventually a lesion if the valving persists, even after the traumatic episode passes (Angsuwarangsee & Morrison, 2002). Given the highly charged nature of the patient's emotional situation, it is unlikely that he has considered the effect that prolonged crying might have on the larynx.

If the patient's grief becomes melancholia with reports of "crying all the time," a referral to a grief counselor or psychologist is certainly appropriate given that you are not expected to cope with problems that are outside of your scope of practice. If he is inconsolable, it may be appropriate to postpone therapy until the patient has come to terms with the emotional issues that interfere with the focus necessary to participate in the therapy process.

In contrast, intense laughter that is produced in a pressed, guttural, or inappropriately high-pitched manner may have a detrimental effect on the vocal folds, irritating and inflaming the mucosa. This effortful laughter can initiate fainting, asthma attacks, headaches, and arrhythmia. **Table 5-3** provides several hypotheses and strategies to modify these counterproductive behaviors.

It is normal and human to experience frustration, anxiety, and fear in response to a voice disorder. If the patient is a professional voice user, his concerns regarding employment are real ones. Your intuition and the patient's narrative guide you when these concerns warrant a referral for counseling services. Your delicacy and sensitivity should this problem arise will be crucial to the patient's willingness to follow your recommendation. The patient may be more open to the referral if it is couched within the framework of managing the voice problem. Perseverance and adherence to the voice rehabilitation process may hinge on resolution of co-occurring emotional, psychological stresses.

There may be times when your intuition, the patient's narrative, and/or his negative response to the therapeutic process suggest that a referral to a social worker, psychotherapist, or a counselor would be a more appropriate choice in the immediate circumstance than voice rehabilitation. It is not unusual to feel uncomfortable broaching this subject, especially if your patient has no prior experience with a psychologist and the idea is a foreign one. A referral of this kind is not appropriate until you feel relatively sure that you have pursued, tested, and modified all of the rehabilitation hypotheses relevant to this individual's voice problem, and that the patient's poor response to treatment will not change or improve under the present circumstances. Reassurance that the limited success in therapy does not represent a personal flaw in the patient, but may be a function of the current stresses in his life that should be addressed by the appropriate

Table 5-3 Effortful Crying and Laughing

Clinician's Perception and/or Patient's Report	Physiological Precipitating, Maintaining, and Exacerbating Factors	Hypothesis	Hypothesis Testing
• Patient is experiencing emotional turmoil and cries or laughs excessively or uncontrollably.	• Effortful crying and laughing may lead to phonotrauma.	• Decrease in laryngeal valving during crying and laughing will facilitate healing of vocal fold mucosa.	• Elicit options for gentle crying and laughing. • Demonstrate and practice efficient, effortless production. • Explore patient's receptiveness to counseling when appropriate.
• Patient suffers from acid reflux following episodes of crying and laughing.	• Effortful crying and laughing add pressure to the lower esophageal sphincter triggering reflux. The associated frequent coughing and throat clearing may irritate the vocal fold mucosa.	• Effective management of reflux will decrease episodes of throat clearing and coughing.	• Refer to gastroenterologist or otolaryngologist for assessment of reflux symptoms. • Follow procedures in Table 5-10.

Data from: Chamberlain, Garrod, & Birring, 2013; Chung, 2011; Morice, 2011; Murry & Rosen, 2000; Pizolato et al., 2013; Roy et al., 2001; Ryan, Vertigan, & Gibson, 2009; Sivasankar & Leydon, 2010; Vertigan & Gibson, 2011; Wiener et al., 1989; Yun, Kim, & Son, 2007.

professional; that you remain optimistic that the voice problem can be resolved; and that you will welcome the patient when he is ready to return to treatment are positive messages to convey. If your attitude remains nonjudgmental and reflects your positive regard for the patient, as well as an acknowledgment of how difficult it can be to change habituated motor patterns, you will communicate an expression of faith in his capacity to resolve the voice problem.

Extraneous Muscle Activity

At rest, the larynx is located anterior to the fourth, fifth, and sixth cervical vertebrae, but this position changes as the larynx rises during swallow, lowers with aging, and adjusts to head position and pitch modification. Stiffness in the surrounding musculature associated with forward, strained head and neck positions, tightening of the temporomandibular joint (TMJ), or **retroflection of the tongue base** decreases the freedom of laryngeal movement. Given that the larynx is suspended from the hyoid bone and held in place by the strap muscles, rigidity in the structures surrounding the larynx places pressure on the intrinsic musculature and affects pitch-changing efficiency. Unnecessary stiffness in the head, neck and thorax, clenching of the temporomandibular joint or stiffening the tongue base may indirectly interfere with effective voice production. When the thorax tightens or lifts and crowds the laryngeal collar, the balance of the passive (elastic) and active (muscular) respiratory forces is disrupted and may restrict the air flow and control necessary to produce voice. Release of these structures facilitates separate and independent movement of the jaw, tongue, and larynx and increases laryngeal control.

Reduction in extraneous muscle activity may be accomplished in several ways, including stretching and tactile and visual feedback. Stretches that are sustained for several seconds are most beneficial and are followed by a release in the hypercontracted structure following the sustained stretch. If, for instance, the patient holds a yawn or pre-yawn (initiation but not completion of the yawn) for a few seconds, release can be felt in the mouth, pharynx, and larynx, as the pharyngeal muscles dilate, allowing the larynx to lower to a rest position. Similarly, when laryngeal massage is used (tactile), the larynx may lower slightly. **Table 5-4** provides some potential sites of extraneous muscle activity followed by possible physiological factors, hypotheses for remediating the problem and, finally, procedures that test these hypotheses.

The following three videos—*Release of the Upper Body, Shoulder Release,* and *Sigh Therapy* videos demonstrate a patient with adductor spasmodic dysphonia releasing upper body stiffness. The release in extraneous muscle activity is reflected in the voice immediately following the exercises.

Environmental Challenges

Prolonged Talking Over Noise

Speakers in noisy environments (e.g., bars, clubs, restaurants, city streets, factories) often use excessive expiratory drive and loudness to compete with the ambient noise. This response to excessive loudness, known as the **Lombard effect**, is difficult to control because of the unconscious nature of the response, and the social demand to participate and be heard. The tendency may be exaggerated in situations involving large numbers of people engaged in many different types of activities. One common scenario involves different speakers fighting for the floor and talking over each other, such as working on the floor of the stock exchange, talking over noise at a party or restaurant, and pundits who argue on television. Still others, working as bartenders or waiters in noisy restaurants or bars, may be reluctant to forgo a lucrative job in order to conserve and protect the voice. Due to the financial and social implications of speaking more quietly in these situations, adherence to recommendations may be poor unless the patient determines that it is

Table 5-4 Extraneous Muscle Activity

Clinician's Perception and/or Patient's Report	Physiological Precipitating, Maintaining, and Exacerbating Factors	Hypothesis	Hypothesis Testing
• Patient uses excessive extrinsic laryngeal musculature during phonation.	• Patient elevates and stiffens the thorax crowding the laryngeal collar.	• Reduction in thoracic and extrinsic muscle stiffness will facilitate abdominal breathing.	• Identify and increase awareness of extraneous muscle activity. • Use visual feedback (mirror). • Employ tactile (hands-on) feedback. • Modify body position (e.g., fluid dance movement, stretches, Pilates ball). • Use of visualization (e.g., head floats up like balloon and spine pulls down like a string attached to the balloon).
• Patient exhibits extraneous muscle activity: jaw and tongue base stiffness, purses lips, furrows brow, clenches TMJ, and grinds teeth.	• Patient uses extraneous muscle activity during phonation.	• Decrease in extraneous muscle activity facilitates easier manner of voice production.	• Use visual and tactile feedback. • Identify and increase awareness of tightness inside the mouth. • Practice Jaw Release and Modified Jaw Release Exercises. • Perform Airway Reflex Exercise. • Allow tongue to protrude slightly and rest on the lower lip. • Masako Maneuver. • Produce /θa, θa, θa/ in a series (ascending to descending glissando). • Produce a gentle voiced gargle. • Yawn-sigh. • Perform voiceless and voiced lip and tongue trills and raspberries (Bronx cheer). • Laryngeal massage.

Data from: Angsuwarangsee & Morrison, 2002; Chapman, 2012; Ferreira et al., 2010; Koschkee & Rammage, 1997; Lessac, 1997.

in his interest to manage the problem in a way that mitigates the effect of ambient noise.

Several of the following procedures are similar to those in Table 5-2, but with attention to excessive loudness that is triggered by external stimulation. The first step identifies when and where this Lombard effect is activated in order to facilitate the patient's awareness of the problem. Only then can you work to identify ways to modify the behavior. Your patient may be a rich source of ideas for either manipulating the environment or his response to it because he is familiar with the situation and will implement only those suggestions that are feasible for his work and social life. Of course, all of these lifestyle changes are accompanied by therapy that builds effective voice production to meet the patient's needs. **Table 5-5** suggests several strategies that address this common problem.

Table 5-5 Prolonged Talking Over Noise

Clinician's Perception and/or Patient's Report	Physiological Precipitating, Maintaining, and Exacerbating Factors	Hypothesis	Hypothesis Testing
• Patient describes situations that demand talking over noise (e.g., restaurants, bars, factories, sporting events, city streets, subway platforms).	• The Lombard effect triggers excessive expiratory drive and medial compression of the vocal folds.	• Patient will decrease effortful manner of phonation by decreasing the medial compression of the vocal folds and decreasing the transglottal pressure drop.	• Identify situations that trigger the Lombard effect. • Strategies to recognize excessive vocal intensity (tactile-kinesthetic and auditory awareness). • Take opportunities to use confidential voice. • Use of amplification. • Reduce background noise (e.g., turn off or lower TV, music, radio). • Avoid noisy restaurants and sporting events. • Avoid talking on noisy streets, subways, when car windows are open. • Avoid using cell phone in noisy locations. • Reduce distance to listener. • Decrease distance to customer when taking orders. • Enhance facial lighting (to facilitate lip reading).
		• Thinning of the laryngeal secretions will reduce high phonation pressure thresholds.	• Increase hydration.

Data from: Colton, Casper, & Leonard, 2011; Ferrand, 2012; Ilomaki, Laukkanen, Leppanen, & Vilkman, 2008; McHenry & Carlson, 2004; Pick, Siegal, Fox, Garber, & Kearney, 1989; Roy et al., 2001; Roy et al., 2002; Sala et al., 2002; Shewmaker, Hapner, Gilman, Klein, and Johns III, 2010.

Classroom Teaching and Lecturing

As you probably know, the classroom teacher is at high risk for developing a voice disorder. Given the demand for prolonged voice use, projecting over noise (playground, cafeteria, and noisy classroom), frequent need for verbal discipline, and the vocal animation required to maintain students' attention, the teacher must have strategies to cope effectively with this challenging occupation.

A crucial aspect of your contribution involves identifying and exploring ways to implement strategies to cope with these challenging conditions. Although the classroom teacher may be peripherally aware of strategies to control the classroom environment, he may ignore them and rely solely on excessive vocal intensity to maintain discipline. This all too ubiquitous problem provides an excellent opportunity to use your partnership with the patient to find adequate solutions that are easily implemented. A strategy will be effective only when the patient feels that it fits his personality and that he is comfortable using it. **Table 5-6** addresses the problems of the classroom teacher with suggestions that pertain to manner of phonation and environmental obstacles.

In the *Discussion of Teaching Challenges* video, the singer/voice teacher acknowledges the importance of maintaining an awareness of the integration of flow and support while teaching. She agrees that using strategies to shift the burden of talking will facilitate the preservation of her voice.

Hearing Loss in Patient and/or Significant Others

We often see patients who have a voice problem and co-occurring hearing loss, or who are having difficulty interacting with people who are hard of hearing. This may be more common with your older patients, but it is not unusual for patients to have a parent, spouse, friend, or coworker with whom they have difficulty communicating owing to a hearing deficit. Too often, people attempt to cope with this challenging situation by increasing their vocal intensity, even shouting, which will actually exacerbate the problem for the hard-of-hearing listener and aggravate the patient's voice problem. The patient may have become so accustomed to shouting at the individual with the hearing loss, that he may not be aware that he is doing so. He may be convinced that the hard-of-hearing individual will not hear him if he speaks quietly, and does not realize that lip reading is facilitated by normal speed, articulation, and loudness.

It may not be immediately obvious that a hearing loss can actually enhance one's kinesthetic awareness given less reliance on sound for feedback. Nevertheless, we have worked with patients who become kinesthetically sensitive to voice use when they have a co-occurring

Table 5-6 Classroom Teaching and Lecturing

Clinician's Perception and/or Patient's Report	Physiological Precipitating, Maintaining, and Exacerbating Factors	Hypothesis	Hypothesis Testing
• The patient reports vocal fatigue, the necessity for longer recovery time, and persistent roughness related to a demanding teaching/ lecturing schedule.	• Sustained, loud, effortful phonation leads to vocal fatigue.	• Patient's persistent or recurring vocal fatigue will diminish with a decrease in vocal fold collision forces.	• Use of amplification. • Explore opportunities to maintain classroom discipline without shouting (e.g., speak quietly, clap, use a bell, whistle, blink lights, use reward system for quiet behavior). • Enhance communication (e.g., face the students when talking). • Decrease distance between teacher/ lecturer and students. • Divide class into small groups.
	• Prolonged vocal demand leads to vocal fatigue.	• Patient's persistent and/ or recurring vocal fatigue will diminish with voice conservation.	• Develop strategies to decrease vocal demand (e.g., involve teaching/lecturing assistants/student teachers, increase student presentations, use audiovisual aids, and increase independent, in-class desk work).
		• Hydration will thin laryngeal secretions and reduce high phonation pressure thresholds.	• Increase hydration.

Data from: Behrman, Rutledge, Hembree, & Sheridan, 2008; Colton, Casper, & Leonard, 2011; Ferrand, 2012; Jonsdottir, Laukkanen, & Siikki, 2003; McHenry & Carlson, 2004; Pizolato et al., 2013; Roy et al., 2001; Roy et al., 2002; Yun, Kim, & Son, 2007.

hearing loss. Your patient may already focus on kinesthetic feedback, and you can capitalize on this heightened awareness during therapy. **Table 5-7** contains a few hypotheses and procedures related to strategies that may facilitate planning, encourage adherence to treatment, and be effective when dealing with either of these situations.

Table 5-7 Hearing Loss in Patient or Significant Others

Clinician's Perception and/or Patient's Report	Physiological Precipitating, Maintaining, and Exacerbating Factors	Hypothesis	Hypothesis Testing
• Patient may suffer from a hearing loss.	• Hearing deficit interferes with communication exchange.	• Enhanced hearing acuity will facilitate vocal rehabilitation.	• Screen hearing acuity. • Refer for full audiometric evaluation and amplification, if necessary.
• Patient consistently misunderstands your message, uses excessive vocal intensity, and, when queried, denies a hearing loss.	• Sustained vocal fold hyperadduction persists when patient uses excessive expiratory drive.	• Manner of phonation will improve with a decrease in expiratory drive.	• Perform a hearing screening as part of the initial voice assessment. • Gently probe patient's readiness to investigate possible hearing loss with an audiologist. • Identify possible instances of miscommunication that might pertain to patient's hearing (e.g., spousal conflicts, need for repetition, increasing volume of television). • Refer for full audiometric evaluation and amplification, when necessary.
• Patient acknowledges a hearing loss, but despite audiologist's recommendation has not purchased a hearing aid.	• Same as above.	• Patient will reconsider use of amplification following appropriate counseling with audiologist and voice clinician.	• Explore options for insurance to pay for the hearing aid. • Discuss the benefits of new technology (smaller, in-the-ear aids). • Identify opportunities that will facilitate listener comprehension, such as lip reading, eye contact, close distance between talker and listener, and communicating in a well-lit environment. • Refer for full audiometric evaluation and amplification, when necessary.
• Patient purchased a hearing aid, but does not wear it due to difficulty with insertion, feedback from the aid, or discomfort.	• Same as above.	• Reevaluation with audiologist may resolve these problems.	• Refer patient back to audiologist to examine the hearing aid.

Table 5-7 Hearing Loss in Patient or Significant Others (*Continued*)

Clinician's Perception and/or Patient's Report	Physiological Precipitating, Maintaining, and Exacerbating Factors	Hypothesis	Hypothesis Testing
• Patient complains that the spouse or a relative, friend, or coworker has a hearing loss and does not wear a hearing aid.	• Patient's loud voice triggers excessive expiratory drive and medial compression of the vocal folds.	• Patient's persistent and/or recurring vocal fatigue will diminish with voice conservation.	• Develop awareness of vocal trauma associated with prolonged loud talking. • Explain the drawbacks of increasing vocal intensity. • Encourage the patient to maintain natural articulation, speed, and loudness to facilitate intelligibility when speaking to the individual who has a hearing loss. • Suggest that your patient enhance facial lighting to enhance lip reading. • Recommend that the speaker face the listener and decrease the distance to listener. • Encourage the spouse to purchase a hearing aid.

Data from: Colton, Casper, & Leonard, 2011; Roy et al., 2001.

Exercise

Your patient may unknowingly but habitually use excessive laryngeal valving (holding his breath) during exercise, and, because it is unrelated to speech, be unaware of its detrimental effect on his voice. The continued movement of air during exercise enhances the benefits of the exercise and protects the voice. Most exercise programs encourage continued breathing during all activities. Some exercise programs focus on inhalation during exertion and others on exhalation. Regardless of the philosophy, all encourage a continuous flow of air and discourage holding the breath during exertion.

If the patient holds his breath during exercise (e.g., during weight lifting), high levels of subglottal pressure and medial compression and stiffness of the vocal fold are generated, which may irritate the vocal fold mucosa or inflame an existing vocal fold lesion and prolong recovery time. A patient may notice a small dip in his strength during exercise when he stops laryngeal valving, but over time his strength will improve. Some approaches to minimizing this phonotrauma are presented in **Table 5-8**.

Table 5-8 Exercise

Clinician's Perception and/or Patient's Report	Physiological Precipitating, Maintaining, and Exacerbating Factors	Hypothesis	Hypothesis Testing
• Patient reports that he phonates during exercise (grunts during weight lifting). • Patient teaches an exercise class.	• Phonating during weight-bearing exercise leads to phonotrauma.	• Decrease laryngeal valving during exercise to minimize phonotrauma.	• Discuss strategies to reduce phonation during exercise. • Explore options to avoid excessive valving during weight lifting exercise, micturition, carrying groceries, or luggage, etc. • Advocate for patient use of amplification when teaching an exercise class.
		• Hydration will thin laryngeal secretions and reduce high phonation pressure thresholds.	• Increase hydration.

Data from: Pizolato et al., 2013; Verdolini, Titze, & Fennell, 1994; Yun, Kim, & Son, 2007.

The Vocal Athlete

The **vocal athlete** whose career requires negotiating broad ranges of loudness and pitch inflection in performance (singing or speaking), oration, announcing, and voice-overs for radio, film, and cartoons, and may have had extensive training to use his voice in his chosen profession, may not use his voice with the same ease during habitual conversation. In contrast, the individual who produces unusual character voices; the singer whose rough, creaky, pressed voice is what made him famous; and the television, movie, or radio actor whose voice is familiar to audiences but is produced inefficiently, often lack the appropriate techniques to meet these professional demands easily and effectively. These patients may or may not have had training with a voice teacher and may rely solely on intuition and emotional connection with the character or audience. In contrast, a patient may come to you having experienced no previous difficulty creating a character, singing an aria, or giving a speech to a large audience, but his voice is suddenly failing him. He may be worried that his professional career is at an end, express panic about an upcoming performance, and want his voice to improve immediately. He does not understand why the voice is failing now.

Commitment to voice therapy is seldom a concern with a professional voice user, but practicing with excessive enthusiasm, and the fear of losing both the identifying voice and the monetary rewards that come from that voice often lead to lack of adherence, or at the very least a difficult problem-solving circumstance. Treatment goals include production of the signature voice in a way that is easy and effortless, and require the patient to rely on changes in the vocal tract to create the sound he seeks. These goals may be different from the strategies that the vocal coach or singing teacher uses and may produce cognitive dissonance in the patient. You, as the clinician, will be faced with his anxiety, fragility, even denial of the problem when you attempt to counsel the patient at the beginning stages of the treatment process. **Table 5-9** provides a framework to address some of the stresses and schedule demands that the performer regularly encounters. These individuals may move through therapy more quickly than others because they usually have a developed kinesthetic vocal sensibility.

In the *Demonstration of Singing* video, the student clinician/singer complains of inadequate breath support, vocal fatigue, and a limited pitch range during singing. In this clip she demonstrates an excerpt from a song that is part of her repertoire. Note the extraneous muscle activity in her head and neck that, given the pleasantness of her singing voice, might be overlooked without careful scrutiny.

Medical Considerations

Acid Reflux: Laryngopharyngeal Reflux and Gastroesophageal Reflux Disease

Your knowledge of co-occurring medical problems that contribute to the voice problem gives you credibility. It is not unusual, for instance, for patients to receive a diagnosis of **gastroesophageal reflux disease (GERD)** and/or **laryngopharyngeal reflux (LPR)**, but deny the problem. You must have a clear understanding of the difference between GERD and LPR and the physiology of both, know what medication the patient is taking and its possible side effects, and be comfortable explaining appropriate diet and environmental modifications (Koufman, 2002). Again, it is the speech-language pathologist who most often discusses dietary and lifestyle modification with the patient, and encourages timely re-examinations with the otolaryngologist and/or gastroenterologist.

Table 5-9 The Vocal Athlete

Clinician's Perception and/or Patient's Report	Physiological Precipitating, Maintaining, and Exacerbating Factors	Hypothesis	Hypothesis Testing
• Patient's demonstration of character voices reveals pronounced phonatory effort.	• Forceful, strained phonation leads to vocal fatigue.	• Patient's vocal fatigue will diminish with a decrease in vocal fold collision forces.	• Provide information regarding the normal anatomy and physiology of voice production. • Discuss the benefits of using quiet, gentle phonation and implement confidential voice in conversation without breathiness.
• Patient exhibits extraneous muscle activity in the head, neck, and thorax when creating character voices.	• Patient narrows the supraglottal area and stiffens the jaw and tongue base to create the character voice.	• Interruption of excessive muscle contraction in the supraglottic space, jaw, and tongue base provides an opportunity to build kinesthetic awareness and muscle recovery time.	• Temporarily discontinue production of unusual voices (until direct therapy measures facilitate appropriate manner of phonation). • Explore scripts and stories that use a less demanding manner of phonation.
		• Dilation of the pharyngeal muscles and release of the jaw and tongue base facilitate more efficient expression of the character voice.	• Practice yawns, sighs, gargles, lip and tongue trills, Masako maneuver inverted megaphone (cup), straw phonation, laryngeal massage.
• Patient reads aloud (scripts, children's stories, poetry, etc.) with pressed phonation.	• Prolonged medial compression of the vocal folds and inadequate breath support lead to vocal fatigue, laryngeal stiffness, and abrupt initiation of voicing.	• Phonation neutral position (vocal folds are slightly abducted) facilitates reduction in adduction and more efficient oscillation of vocal folds.	• Use yawn-sigh, sigh phonation, lip/tongue trills, gentle-voiced gargle.

Table 5-9 The Vocal Athlete (*continued*)

Clinician's Perception and/or Patient's Report	Physiological Precipitating, Maintaining, and Exacerbating Factors	Hypothesis	Hypothesis Testing
• Patient is an actor/singer who performs regularly and complains of vocal fatigue following performances and prolonged warm-up time.	• Demanding performance schedule, travel, pre-performance eating, late night eating, frequent alcohol consumption, and general fatigue negatively affect stamina, endurance, pitch and loudness ranges, and phonatory control.	• Modification of diet, increase in hydration, avoidance of alcohol, more consistent sleep schedule will promote overall well-being.	• Increase hydration during airplane travel • Reduce alcohol consumption during a performance run. • Sleep 7 to 8 hours per night. • Schedule nap time before performances. • Allow at least 2.5 hours between eating and performance time. • Allow at least 3 hours between eating last meal and bedtime.
		• Hydration will thin laryngeal secretions and reduce high phonation pressure thresholds.	• Increase humidification of ambient air.

Data from: Abitbol, 2006; Angsuwarangsee & Morrison, 2002; Aronson & Bless, 2009; Behrman, Rutledge, Hembree, and Sheridan, 2008; Colton, Casper, & Leonard, 2011; Cooper, 1974; Ferrand, 2012; Ferreira et al., 2010; Ilomaki, Laukkanen, Leppanen, and Vilkman, 2008; Roy et al., 2001; Roy et al., 2002; Titze, Svec, & Popolo, 2003.

The gastroenterologist or otolaryngologist makes the diagnosis of GERD or LPR. Although treatment strategies remain controversial, it is generally agreed that (as with all voice therapy) a treatment regimen should be specifically tailored to the patient's complaints and symptoms. Medication, diet modification, and elevating the head of the bed can be effective management strategies. Given the chronicity and high incidence of LPR and GERD, it has become more common for the treating voice clinician to address and monitor these symptoms as part of the voice rehabilitation program.

Patients are often unaware of this problem and deny the possibility of chronic acid reflux even when laryngeal images illustrate inflammation and redness in the area of the arytenoid cartilages—even changes to the posterior larynx. Given that successful treatment of acid reflux symptoms depends on your patient's belief that he, in fact, has reflux, preliminary therapy may focus on developing awareness of symptoms. Early discussions may provide education and highlight frequently observed symptoms, the differences between GERD and LPR, and explore the possibility of keeping a food diary for a week to uncover a possible relationship between foods, smoking, size of meals, late-night eating, and the occurrence of reflux symptoms.

Although LPR, or silent reflux, may co-occur with GERD, its characteristics are quite distinctive. Chronic cough, morning roughness, worsening roughness, globus (sensation of lump in the throat most of the time), difficult or painful swallow, choking episodes, postnasal drip, excessive laryngeal mucus, frequent throat clearing, sore throat, shortness of breath, asthma, wheezing, halitosis, and dental disease represent the many symptoms that are associated with this problem. Typically, patients who suffer from silent reflux do not experience the heartburn or esophagitis that GERD sufferers do because the material that refluxes remains in the esophagus only for a short time—not sufficient to lead to inflammation.

The larynx and vocal tract are significantly more susceptible to irritation than the esophagus (Koufman & Stern, 2010). The symptoms of LPR occur generally during the daytime when the patient is upright, as opposed to GERD, which occurs primarily at night when the patient is lying down and the larynx is exposed to acid/pepsin for prolonged periods. Although many of your patients will not ask questions regarding the underlying patterns associated with reflux, the consequences of LPR and GERD are serious and can have a persistent, negative effect on your patient's general and laryngeal well being. In **Table 5-10** we suggest several hypotheses to address your clinical observations and the patient's complaints.

The clinician and student clinician in the *Management of Acid Reflux* video discuss diet modification and general guidelines to manage the patient's reported reflux problem. The clinician attempts to speak to the patient's individual needs and activities of daily living.

Prescription, Nonprescription, and Recreational Drugs

Your patient may complain of dryness in the oral cavity and throat (**xerostomia**) or take frequent sips of water during the session. He may be unaware of the origin of the problem or may indicate that he takes a medication that exacerbates the problem, or that he suffers from a medical condition that is associated with dryness (e.g., Sjögren's syndrome) (Tanner, Roy, Merrill, & Elstad, 2007). You can easily check oral lubrication with a tongue depressor placed inside the buccal area and on the surface of the tongue. If you note that the tongue depressor adheres to these areas, recommend an increase in hydration.

Table 5-10 Acid Reflux

Clinician's Perception and/or Patient's Report	Physiological Precipitating, Maintaining, and Exacerbating Factors	Hypothesis	Hypothesis Testing
• Patient complains of any one or more of the following: – Heartburn – Chest pain – Pain radiating to the ear – Lump in the throat – Choking episodes – Regurgitation – Sour taste in the mouth – Burping – Sneezing – Excessive mucus – Chronic throat clearing – Chronic cough – Voice that is rough in the morning and improves over the course of the day	• Reflux into the pharynx and larynx irritates the vocal fold mucosa.	• Reflux medication will control symptoms. • Identification and modification of the following factors may reduce reflux: – Diet – Fluid intake – Meal times – Portion size – Body mass index (BMI) – Smoking – Sleeping position	• Discuss symptoms of reflux. • Follow physician's recommendations. • Explore options to reduce intake of foods and beverages that trigger reflux episodes: – Caffeine (chocolate) – Fatty foods (e.g., cheese, nuts, fatty meat, fried foods) – Sugar/starch (e.g., cola, chocolate) – Acidic foods (e.g., tomato, orange, pineapple) – Alcohol – Carbonated drinks – Dense caloric foods (e.g., cola, cakes, candy) • Increase hydration. • Timing of meals: ~3 hours between eating and bedtime (including snacks) • Other: – Eat frequent small meals – Decrease BMI to 25 or less – Raise head of bed – Cessation of smoking – Acupuncture

Data from: Behrman, Rutledge, Hembree, & Sheridan, 2008; Bhattacharya & Siegmund, 2013; Cohen, Pitman, Noordzij, & Courey, 2012; Dettmar et al. 2011; Elam, Ishman, Dunbar, Clarke, & Gourin, 2010; Gibson & Vertigan, 2009; Hanson, & Jiang, 2000; Hicks, Ours, Abelson, Vaezi, & Richter, 2002; Leydon, Sivasankar, Falciglia, Atkins, & Fisher, 2009; Park et al., 2012; Verdolini et al., 2002; Zhang, Qin, & Guo, 2010; Yun, Kim, & Son, 2007.

Changes in lubrication are a common side effect of prescription and nonprescription drugs, and can change the mucosal lining of the larynx and interfere with the lubrication of the entire vocal tract. When the medications are provided by prescription, work with the physician to determine if the dryness is a possible side effect of the prescribed medication. If so, it may be possible to substitute a medication that will not affect the lubrication of the vocal tract. Oral and pharyngeal dryness may be further exacerbated if your patient inhales the substance, either by using an inhaler or smoking. If it is a recreational drug that affects the mucosa, it is necessary to discuss the possibility of reducing or stopping its use during therapy. The hypotheses in **Table 5-11** pertain to the possible sequelae of medication and recreational drugs.

Table 5-11 Prescription, Nonprescription, and Recreational Drugs

Clinician's Perception and/or Patient's Report	Physiological Precipitating, Maintaining, and Exacerbating Factors	Hypothesis	Hypothesis Testing
• Patient is taking prescription medication.	• Prescription drugs can irritate the vocal fold mucosa, diminish hydration, and negatively affect cognition.	• An alternate medication may have fewer side effects, and enhance hydration without affecting cognitive status.	• Discuss the medication side effects with physician.
• Patient is using over-the-counter medications and/or recreational drugs.	• Nonprescription drugs can irritate the vocal fold mucosa, diminish hydration, and/or change cognitive status.	• Review and modification of use of nonpharmaceutical drugs (e.g., over-the-counter medications, herbal, or recreational), may foster homeostasis and improve hydration.	• Explore ways to reduce or eliminate the use of non-pharmaceutical drugs (if appropriate).
• Patient reports excessive alcohol consumption.	• Alcohol dries and irritates the vocal fold mucosa, and changes cognitive status.	• Reduction of alcohol consumption will facilitate lubrication of the vocal tract and improve cognition.	• Elicit options to reduce or eliminate alcohol consumption. • Refer patient for appropriate counseling program (if appropriate). • Refer patient to AA (if appropriate).
• Patient smokes cigarettes.	• Smoking irritates and dries the nasal, pharyngeal, laryngeal, and tracheal membranous lining.	• Reduction or cessation of smoking promotes adequate hydration of the vocal tract.	• Explore options to reduce or eliminate smoking. • Refer to American Cancer Society or similar program for advice and strategies (if appropriate). • Refer to physician for medical treatments to facilitate cessation of smoking (if appropriate).

Data from: Guimaraes & Abberton, 2005; Mathieson, 2001; Muscat & Wynder, 1992; Titze & Verdolini-Abbott, 2012.

Respiratory Disturbances

The power source for phonation is breath flow, and the respiratory problems that sometimes co-occur with a voice problem may interfere with your patient's progress if not appropriately addressed during treatment. A patient with emphysema, asthma, severe allergies, chronic obstructive pulmonary disease (COPD), or paradoxical vocal fold motion may experience dyspnea (shortness of breath) and air hunger. He may produce fewer syllables per breath group than is customary for his age and gender and run out of breath before the end of the phrase. The work required to sustain phonation may produce extraneous muscle activity in the head, neck, and thorax, as well as laryngeal and supralaryngeal constriction, and lead to vocal fatigue (Angsuwarangsee & Morrison, 2002).

It is generally the case that a physician will treat a patient who presents any of these respiratory difficulties. There are, however, effective voice rehabilitation strategies that will ameliorate the symptoms and maximize the coordination between the respiratory and phonatory subsystems. If your patient does not take his medication regularly or continues to smoke, you will need to reinforce the physician's recommendations and explore the patient's reasons for nonadherence to the physician's recommendations. In **Table 5-12**, we suggest several hypotheses that pertain to the consequences of a respiratory problem. These hypotheses and procedures focus on decreasing the effort used during inspiration and expiration, increasing breath control, and coordinating the voice production subsystems.

Preoperative Voice Therapy

Some laryngeal lesions may require surgery, some may resolve with voice rehabilitation alone, and some require a combination of both. A patient with a polyp at the midmembranous portion of the vocal fold, for example, is often referred for **preoperative voice therapy**, or for a trial period of voice therapy to ascertain whether the polyp will resolve without a surgical procedure. It is possible (although not probable) that the polyp will completely resorb with preoperative voice therapy focused solely on lifestyle change if it is a result of a sudden, acute laryngeal event. Even partial resolution (shrinking in size, reduction of inflammation and swelling), will make surgery more straightforward. Furthermore, it is essential that your patient understands voice conservation, the significance of acid reflux, and the process of wound healing, and begins to integrate an appropriate coordination among the vocal subsystems in order to avoid a recurrence of the polyp following surgery. During this preoperative time, you can include exercises to capitalize on a semi-occluded vocal tract with resonant voice therapy,

Table 5-12 Respiratory Disturbances

Clinician's Perception and/or Patient's Report	Physiological Precipitating, Maintaining, and Exacerbating Factors	Hypothesis	Hypothesis Testing
• Patient's medical history includes the following: – Emphysema – Asthma – COPD – Allergies – Paradoxical vocal fold motion	• Limited expiratory drive leads to increased expiratory effort and, possibly, pressed phonation.	• Balance of expiratory drive with vocal fold adduction facilitates flow phonation.	• Increase reliance on diaphragmatic-abdominal breathing. • Release thoracic stiffness. • Modify posture. • Use abdominal breath control.
	• Allergies and respiratory disease may increase lung compliance and decrease elastic recoil of the lungs.	• Use of abdominal breath control facilitates coordination between respiration and phonation.	• Use abdominal breath control.
• Patient's medical history includes negative response to air pollution and airborne irritants.	• Allergies irritate the nasal, laryngeal, and tracheal membranous lining.	• Avoidance of known allergens to prevent irritation of the nasal, laryngeal, and tracheal membranous lining.	• Discuss ways to avoid known allergens (e.g., pet dander, seasonal plants, molds, foods, detergents, chemicals, smoke, perfume).
• Patient intermittently holds his breath during conversation.	• Paradoxical vocal fold motion obstructs the airway by closing the glottis during inhalation.	• Easy, uninterrupted breathing facilitates flow phonation.	• Release thoracic stiffness. • Stretch the torso. • Free shoulders during inhalation. • Increase reliance on diaphragmatic-abdominal breathing. • Yawn-sigh. • Develop awareness of physical symptoms that forewarn of impending attack. • Refer to physician for pharmacological treatment if GERD is identified as a trigger.

Data from: Colton, Casper, & Leonard, 2011; Ferrand, 2012; Franco et al., 2014; Lowell, Barkmeier-Kraemer, Hoit, & Story, 2008; Zemlin, 1998.

straw phonation, and lip and tongue trills. When surgery is required, these exercises establish a more efficient manner of phonation prior to surgery, and provide the springboard for treatment and an easier transition into postoperative therapy.

The recommendation for and duration of complete or modified voice rest before or after laryngeal surgery differs among voice care professionals. Voice rest offers the mucosa time to recover, but it can result in muscle atrophy. It is a particularly complex decision for the professional voice user, who requires highly controlled movements of the larynx, and the elderly patient who has already lost muscle mass due to aging (Sandage, 2013). Complete voice rest for these individuals may result in more than the typical loss of muscle tone and strength. A protracted period of rehabilitation may be required for these individuals to rebuild strength, tone, and flexibility.

Preoperative meetings are held in order to alleviate the anxiety that your patient feels as he prepares for surgery. It may be his first experience with a surgical procedure; it may be that your patient is a professional voice user and is especially frightened about an invasion of his larynx; or, it may be that the outcome of a previous surgical procedure was suboptimal. A systematic description of what can be expected during the procedure may go a long way to help the patient cognitively and psychologically justify the event and decrease the dread and trepidation that surround any surgical procedure. The patient's heightened state of anxiety may facilitate his adherence to your recommendations to use confidential voice, reduce vocal demand, and follow a consistent and deliberate practice schedule with the exercises you develop together, or he may believe that the surgery will meet all of his needs and that he can ignore your recommendations.

Postoperative Voice Therapy

The time immediately following laryngeal surgery is a stressful one for your patient. A sense of relief may be followed by the frustration associated with complete voice rest, the nuisance of continued voice therapy, and the nagging worry that the voice may never fully recover. Although these emotions are common, they may interfere with your patient's adherence to both the otolaryngologist's and your recommendations. As Portone-Maira and Johns III (2013) suggest, some patients are so frustrated by the anticipated length of the rehabilitation process that they fail to come to their scheduled sessions. It can be many months before a patient returns, and then only because he is again experiencing a problem with the voice. At this point, the problem faced by you and the otolaryngologist becomes a more complicated one because the time when therapy provides a major contribution to the healing process of the surgical scar may have passed.

Although there are varying opinions as to the duration of complete voice rest following laryngeal surgery, the patient is generally asked to refrain from speaking for anywhere from two to four days to one week (Branski, Verdolini, & Sandulache, 2006). When a physician orders complete voice rest, he intends for the patient to remain silent for the period that he designates as beneficial for the initial phase of wound healing in order to avoid flap dehiscence (rupturing of the wound along the suture). General wound healing is described as a dynamic process that has three main stages with common characteristics (Branski, 2013; Clark, 1998). Immediately following surgery, the structures are inflamed. Shortly thereafter, new tissue starts to grow to fill the wound, and then the mucosal tissue forms a scar (Clark, 1998). Management during these phases may be linked to the specific phase. During the acute management phase (post surgery to 2 weeks), the scar tissue forms (Branski, 2013; Portone-Maira & Johns III, 2013), and most often complete voice rest is the treatment of choice during this time. However, the debate continues as to whether complete cessation of voice or an easy, gentle, quiet manner of phonation (relative voice rest) is most efficacious for recovery (Branski, Verdolini, Sandulache, Rosen, & Hebda, 2006; Ishikawa & Thibeault, 2010).

The otolaryngologist who recommends voice therapy after laryngeal surgery usually asks the patient to wait one to two weeks after surgery before initiating the voice therapy process. The initial phase of postoperative voice treatment continues a protocol started during the preoperative meetings, and includes quiet, confidential voice and voice conservation. During this phase, work begins to restore vocal strength and flexibility in a systematic and cautious manner. Phonation is limited to a few minutes per hour (2 to 5 minutes), and confidential voice without breathiness is encouraged. Gradually and carefully, the duration and loudness of phonation may be increased, but these increments must be geared to your perception of the postsurgical roughness and breathiness associated with residual edema, the patient's successful integration of ease during the exercises provided, and the otolaryngologist's recommendations (Friedman, Johnson, Novaleski, & Rousseau, 2013). A 60-year-old acting coach, for instance, who offers frequent master classes and socializes with friends in noisy restaurants, must return to these highly demanding speaking situations gradually and with caution. Your partnership with the patient at this time is critical for his successful transition from

Table 5-13 Laryngeal Surgery

Clinician's Perception and/or Patient's Report	Physiological Precipitating, Maintaining, and Exacerbating Factors	Hypothesis	Hypothesis Testing
• Patient reports recent surgery or medical treatment.	• Laryngeal surgery or vocal pathology irritate the nasal, pharyngeal, laryngeal, and tracheal membranous lining (type and duration of voice rest is determined by the treating surgeon).	• Total voice rest will facilitate wound healing during the acute phase of management.	• Describe total voice rest. • Discuss possible problems associated with whispering. • Explore alternative communication strategies (e.g., writing, texting).
		• Modified voice rest will facilitate healing of vocal fold mucosa.	• Describe partial voice rest. • Explore process of limited voice use and gradual return to loudness.

Data from: Behrman & Sulica, 2003; Branski, Verdolini & Sandulache, 2006; Hansen & Thibeault, 2006; Ishikawa & Thibeault, 2010; Portone-Maira & Johns III, 2013; Rousseau et al., 2011; Salter, 1996; Sandage, 2013.

complete voice rest to modified voice rest to unrestricted voice production. In **Table 5-13** we present some hypotheses and procedures to facilitate recovery from laryngeal surgery.

Dialogue: Management of Risk Factors

The following dialogue with a patient represents a portion of a voice evaluation. Her symptoms and complaints were addressed first with lifestyle changes and then with intervention to modify her manner of phonation. Although this case provides an opportunity to address several aspects of change, it is impossible for one patient to demonstrate all the symptoms that require attention. During **Dialogue 5-1**, the clinician's attention shifts between the patient's report, the patient's manner of phonation, and the provision of an appropriate clinical voice model. The clinician's internal monologue is italicized.

Dialogue 5-1
Mother of Three Sons

Ms. E is a 34-year-old homemaker and mother of three sons (ages 3, 5, and 7 years). Although she employs a nanny, she spends quite a lot of time reading and playing with her children. She has an active social life, frequents noisy restaurants, eats late dinners, travels, and has extensive phone conversations with friends. She called and insisted that I squeeze her in for an evaluation the next day because she was so concerned that her persistent voice problem was preventing her from reading to her children, coping with her mother's hearing loss, and socializing with her friends. Although my day was full, I worked her into my schedule during my break for lunch.

She arrived 20 minutes early for the assessment and engaged the receptionist in a long conversation with questions about her voice during her wait, including "Do you think therapy will help my voice? How long will it take? Does it work?"

Excerpt from the Voice Evaluation

I began with an open-ended question, "Tell me about the problem you've been having with your voice."

As if the floodgates had opened, Ms. E blurted out, "I have been evaluated by four different otolaryngologists (twice by one of them), and I got four different diagnoses: cyst, nodule, polyp, and finally polypoid lesion. The last one also said I have acid reflux, and that I should take some medication, but I haven't filled the prescription because I don't feel any acid [clearing her throat]. I've taken Z-Pak several times and it has always helped my voice, but the ENT wouldn't prescribe it this time. He said I need voice therapy. Do you think he would give it to me if you give him a call?"

For a moment, I was at a loss as to what to address first. As she described her visit with her physician, I noted a moderate dysphonia characterized by inappropriate loudness, frequent abrupt initiations of phonation, moderate roughness, pressed phonation, and stridency. She exhibited excessive expiratory drive, and apparent generalized extraneous muscle activity in the head, neck, and thorax. I felt that if I didn't dissipate her anxiety and apprehension right away, it would be almost impossible to build a positive relationship. "Why don't you tell me a little about how and when your voice problem started, and we can see if the two of us can find some alternatives to medication that will make your throat feel better."

Ms. E snapped, "I just want a Z-Pak. I have spoken the same way all of my life. I don't think that talking is the problem."

Despite her insistent tone, I explained that it would not be appropriate for me to recommend any medication because I am not a physician.

Ms. E huffily countered, "Well, I guess I'll just have to call him again myself [clearing her throat]. I know it [Z-Pak] works."

Noting her pronounced phonatory effort, increasing stridency, and stiffened torso, I queried, "You mentioned that it is getting difficult to read stories to your children. Does your throat ever feel tired?"

Ms. E barked, "I don't know. Sometimes it sounds hoarse after I read and sometimes it just gives out."

Trying to focus her on feeling the sensations in her throat rather than the sound of her voice, I modeled an easy manner of phonation. I hoped that she might unconsciously match my model, almost through osmosis. "What I mean is, when it gives out on you, does it feel uncomfortable or like it is worn out?"

As if reflecting on the experience of reading to her children, Ms. E said pensively, "I don't really know. It always feels sore. Is that what you mean?"

Seeing an opening to engage her, and continuing to model easy phonation, "When you push your voice and you do it for a long time, it probably gets tired. Your vocal folds may become irritated so you feel like you have a sore throat. Is it very loud in your home?"

She retorted, "Oh! Of course, I have young kids. The music is always blasting, the TV is always loud, and the kids are always yelling, so I feel like I have to scream to be heard. I come from a family of loud talkers."

Noting two phonation breaks and probing to ascertain self-management, "Have you tried anything on your own to cope with the noise and sore throat?"

"Well," *Ms. E said in an exasperated tone [clearing her throat]*, "I've had to cut back on the storytelling. And I just don't know what to do about the noise... that's kids."

I saw the agitation on her face and noted the increasing effort she used to explain herself. "That can be frustrating. It might be helpful if you read to the children in a quiet place and with a quiet voice."

Rolling her eyes, Ms. E retorted, "I'm not sure they would listen. But, it's not just the storytelling. They won't listen to me if I talk quietly."

Taking a chance, and with genuine curiosity, I queried, "Are they listening when you yell at them?" *I had captured her attention.*

Looking at me for the first time, Ms. E laughed and with a pronounced decrease in vocal effort, she sighed, "Well... no."

I recognized the positive change in her manner of phonation, and saw an opening to engage her in problem solving. "Do you think it makes sense to use quiet talking and see how they respond?"

Chuckling skeptically, "I don't think it will work, but I suppose so. I'm at the end of my rope, so I guess I'll try it. But how will that help the thing on my vocal folds?"

Her vocal intensity had diminished even more. Her question gave me the opportunity to suggest changes in her routine, and I described counterproductive compensation. I continued to model easy phonation, "When you speak in an easier, quiet voice, your vocal folds vibrate gently and you avoid the potential for hurting your throat. When you yell, you squeeze your vocal folds together tightly and build up a lot of air pressure below them. Your vocal folds blow very far apart and then really slam together [I clap my hands loudly]. When you do this often enough the vocal fold tissue becomes irritated, inflamed, and you may develop something on your vocal folds."

Ms. E took this information in and asked, "Do you think that's what happened to me?"

She appeared receptive to learning more about her voice problem and I continued, "The kind of lesion you have on your vocal folds usually comes from using a lot of effort when you talk, especially when you talk over noise or use character voices."

Incredulously, "Are you saying I can never speak loudly or read to the kids?"

Noting her rising volume and pitch, "Absolutely not. But, you're asking an important question. I'm saying that for the time being, until we've found a more effective way for you to talk over noise, and until your vocal folds recover, using an easier, more confidential style of speaking will avoid more damage. But this is only temporary. Eventually, you should be able to use your voice in any way you choose, and the way you make sound will be more effective."

Thoughtfully, "My mom is a real problem. She won't admit that she can't hear, and I'm always pushing my voice when I talk to her. She comes over a lot to play with the kids, and I love having her around, but the other day my voice just broke."

I observed that she was speaking more quietly. "What kinds of things have you tried to do to deal with your mom's hearing loss?"

Icily, with some irritation, Ms. E replied scornfully, "Well, I try my best [clearing her throat]. I talk as loudly as I can."

She had misunderstood my question. "Is there something you could do to save your voice and have her hear you at the same time?"

"Hmm... like what?"

Continuing in a confidential voice, "Well, if you make eye contact, so she can see your lips, and if you exaggerate your speech a little, you may not need to talk as loudly."

"Oh, I never thought of that. You mean that we should be close to each other, face-to-face, because I'm always trying to talk to her from another room, and she never answers me. It is so frustrating."

"Yes, exactly."

With a sigh of resignation, "Should I talk less?"

She is beginning to understand the connection between effort and her voice and has reduced her loudness. "Yes, that's a good idea temporarily because if you talk less you save your voice, especially if you have been talking over noise for a long time."

Now that she had some awareness of the extra effort she was using to make sound, it was time to find out if she strained her voice in other ways. "I noticed that you have been clearing your throat during our talk. Do you do this very often?"

With surprise and concern [clearing her throat], Ms. E said, "I stopped smoking, cold turkey, two months ago. I had a bad smoker's cough, and I was afraid that I was getting lung cancer, so I stopped. Thank goodness my cough is better, but I still need to clear my throat and I still cough occasionally. It feels like I have something down there all the time."

Her commitment to the cessation of smoking was a good prognostic indicator (i.e., self-efficacy). I described the changes that can occur after smoking and explained how the lungs and sinuses sometimes secrete excessive mucus to clean out the lungs. She seemed relieved. I also suggested that she see her physician if the symptoms didn't abate in another month. I knew that she had three children that she likes to read to and asked, "Do you talk in character voices or make funny sounds when you read?"

Ms. E smiled proudly, "I am great at reading to the kids. I have three boys, they love the 'Three Billy Goats Gruff' story, and I love to read it. I talk like each of the billy goats, they copy me, and then we all laugh. Is this bad for my voice?"

I was pleased that she was asking questions about potential harm to her throat and replied in a confidential voice, "Well, it all depends on how you do it. It's kind of like what we talked about earlier with loudness. For now it is probably a good idea to avoided making those sounds until you develop a more effective way to produce them."

Ms. E furrowed her brow. Speaking in pressed phonation and with significant roughness, "I do it like this, 'I will gobble you up!'"

I could almost feel the tightness in her throat. Before I could speak, Ms. E said, "Wow! I can feel it getting sore already. Does this mean that I can't read to my boys?"

I detected three things simultaneously: the effort she used, her awareness of the effort, and her fear that she would have to stop reading to her kids. What should I address first? "I am impressed that you were so quickly aware of the soreness in your throat. If you are aware of what you feel in your throat it will be easier to change how you produce your voice."

"Oh?"

Her concern was clear, and I knew that we needed to figure out a way to make reading stories easier on her voice. Hoping to engage her in finding a solution to this problem, "How old are your boys?"

Ms. E, smiling, "The oldest is 7, the middle one is 5, and the little one is 3. Oh! I know, maybe they could do the voices. They might really like that."

I changed the focus to explore her problem with acid reflux. I attempted to engage her in problem solving. "You mentioned that you have been diagnosed with acid reflux."

With a roll of her eyes and in a prickly tone, "Yes, the last ENT said my throat looks red in the back, and that I have acid reflux. [She produced the laryngeal images from her examination and pointed to the arytenoid cartilages.] I am sure he was wrong. I don't have any heartburn."

I had heard this many times before. The advertisements on TV for anti-reflux medication have volcanoes with lava. I continued to use confidential voice. "It's not uncommon for people to be unaware of their reflux. It's called 'silent reflux.' With silent reflux, you don't burp and you don't experience heartburn, but you can cough, need to clear your throat often, and have a sore throat, which we have talked about. These symptoms aren't just related to smoking, but could be associated with silent reflux or allergies. Did your doctor prescribe any medication?"

Ms. E replied sheepishly, "He did, but I didn't fill the prescription because I didn't think I had reflux. Should I fill the prescription now?"

To encourage adherence to her physician's recommendations and wanting to know what he had suggested, I said, "It's probably a good idea to follow his recommendation. You and I can talk about your diet and lifestyle to see if they are contributing to the problem. Did he ask you about your diet?"

"He just said, 'Cut back on coffee, alcohol, and spicy or fatty foods.'"

"Did you follow his suggestions?"

Lowering her eyes and exhaling, Ms. E replied, "No, I didn't realize that it was important. I thought it was kind of a silly thing to do."

Over the last several conversational turns, I had noticed her increasing willingness to engage in mutual problem solving. I took this opportunity to explore lifestyle strategies that would ameliorate her symptoms of reflux. "Why don't we talk about some changes that you can make right away that may decrease your need to clear your throat and the soreness that you talked about. Do you eat late at night?"

"Yes, I love to cook but we also go out a lot. The kids eat around 5:30, but my husband gets home around 7:30 or 8:00. We relax with a glass of wine and then have dinner around 8:30 or 9:00."

Continuing to model a confidential voice, "What time do you usually go to bed?"

Ms. E responded pleasantly, "My husband leaves for work early in the morning, so we go to bed around 10:30."

I recognized that changing this pattern could be difficult because it is a special time for her and her husband, and I knew that allowing at least three hours between eating and lying down is one of the easiest ways to reduce acid reflux. "Hmm, let me show you a little bit about how reflux happens. [I drew a stick figure of a person with a stomach, esophagus, larynx, and mouth and held the picture vertically.] When you sit up while you are eating, your stomach fills up part way and gravity helps to hold the food in your stomach. [I point to the lower esophageal sphincter.] This is the hiatal sphincter. It closes tightly and helps hold the food in your stomach. You've probably heard of a hiatal hernia."

Ms. E nods.

"When the sphincter is weak, stomach acid and food can leak into the esophagus. When you lay down [I turn the picture sideways], the hiatal sphincter is below the level of the stomach contents and this makes the sphincter work even harder. If we can keep the stomach contents below the sphincter, it is more difficult for the stomach contents to reflux. There are a couple of ways to help the sphincter close more tightly. You can raise the head of the bed so that the sphincter is higher, eat smaller meals so that the stomach is partly empty, and have at least three hours between when you eat and when you go to bed."

"I had no idea. Can I have that picture?"

I noted that she was receptive to the information and continued, "One of the easiest ways to reduce the reflux is raising the head of the bed. You can buy lofting cups at any home decorating store, put thick books under the top legs of the bed, build a riser, or use a special pillow called an 'anti-reflux pillow.' It is shaped like a long triangle and goes all the way down to your bottom so that the sphincter is raised." *[Pointing to the soft spot between my ribs.]*

Ms. E was listening intently and did not seem to have any questions.

I continued quietly, "Do you think you could eat earlier or go to bed later? When we eat, the acid levels in our stomach decrease for about an hour because of the food in our stomach. After one hour, the acid levels increase and remain elevated for at least two hours. So it is best if you can wait to go to bed for at least three hours after you eat."

Thoughtfully, "I don't think that I can eat earlier; my husband gets home late. I probably could elevate the head of the bed or eat smaller meals. Maybe I could have a bite with the kids and then eat a smaller meal when he gets home."

She had just become a partner in finding solutions to her voice problem.

I hadn't asked her yet about any possible allergies, which could potentially cause the sore throat and excessive mucus. "Do you have allergies?"

Ms. E answered, "No, not that I am aware of."

To explore the question more thoroughly, "So you don't have any itchy or watery eyes, sneezing, or notice any changes in the spring and fall?"

"No, my husband and kids have allergies to cats and spring pollen, but I seem to be okay."

Although we had talked about the Z-Pak, I had not inquired about other medications. I wanted to make sure that we did not overlook other medical issues. "Are you currently taking any medication?"

"Well, I'm on birth control pills and I've taken the Z-Pak for my throat."

Knowing that the medications she mentioned do not usually have a negative effect on the voice, "Anything else?"

"Maybe I will go get that prescription filled for reflux."

"That's probably a good idea."

I asked one last open-ended question. "Is there anything else I should know?"

We finished the session by scheduling an appointment for the following week. I provided a written list of the recommendations we discussed during the evaluation. I wondered if she would return, given her high level of ambivalence about whether voice therapy would help her.

Therapy Session 1

Ms. E returned the following week and we continued our discussion of voice conservation, talked about hydration, diet modification, and carryover of the suggestions made during the evaluation.

Ms. E had avoided producing unusual character voices as she read to her boys (letting them play the characters), and had started making eye contact and speaking more quietly when talking with her mother. She had difficulty using a quieter voice with her kids, stating, "I lost my confidential voice" when they were acting out. She said that she had been clearing her throat less frequently and seemed to have less mucus. During her description of the changes she had made she maintained a conversational level of vocal intensity.

Her success with diet modification was variable. She had bought lofting cups for the head of her bed, but had not yet installed them. Ms. E claimed that her evenings with her husband were too important to her to change, and she was unwilling to eat before he came home. She did, however, reduce the amount of caffeine, spicy foods, and alcohol in her diet. She thought that her throat felt less "sore" and that it "seems less tired."

Summary

During the time between your assessment and the first therapy session, you will have time to digest and filter not only the information provided by the patient but your observations regarding the manner of phonation, the severity of the voice problem, posture, and coordination between the vocal subsystems. How do you decide what is most salient in the counterproductive characteristics you have identified during the voice evaluation? Where in the subsystems is it most beneficial and straightforward to begin? The patient's history and your observations provide the material for the decisions the two of you make as you develop and test your hypotheses. The modifications that the patient is willing to make at the beginning of treatment to manage the risk factors that have been identified will remain relevant and be revisited and modified as the therapeutic process unfolds. In this chapter, we suggested hypotheses and procedures to support your patients' efforts to modify their effortful, compensatory behaviors, environmental stressors, and the medical, emotional, and occupational challenges they encounter daily. As we continue, we will use a hypothesis-driven and patient-centered framework to facilitate control and coordination of the vocal subsystems.

References

Abitbol, J. (2006). *Odyssey of the voice.* San Diego, CA: Plural.

Angsuwarangsee, T., and Morrison, M. (2002). Extrinsic laryngeal muscular tension in patients with voice disorders. *Journal of Voice, 16,* 333–343.

Aronson, A.E., and Bless, D. (2009). *Clinical voice disorders: An interdisciplinary approach*. New York, NY: Thieme.

Behrman, A., Rutledge, J., Hembree, A., and Sheridan, S. (2008). Vocal hygiene education, voice production therapy, and the role of patient adherence: A treatment effectiveness study in women with phonotrauma. *Journal of Speech, Language and Hearing Research*, 51(2), 350–366.

Behrman, A., and Sulica, L. (2003). Voice rest after microlaryngoscopy: Current opinion and practice. *Laryngoscope*, *113*(12), 2182–2186.

Bhattacharya, P., and Siegmund, T. (2013). A computational study of systemic hydration in vocal fold collision. *Computer Methods in Biomechanical Biomedical Engineering*, *17*(16), 1835–1852.

Branski, R.C. (2013). Perioperative voice recovery: A wound-healing perspective. *Perspectives on Voice and Voice Disorders*, 23(2), 42–46.

Branski, R.C., Verdolini, K., Sandulache, V., Rosen, C.A., and Hebda, P.A. (2006). Vocal fold wound healing: A review for clinicians. *Journal of Voice*, 20(3), 432–442.

Chamberlain, S., Garrod, R., and Birring, S.S. (2013). Cough suppression therapy: Does it work? *Pulmonary PharmacologicalTherapy*, 26(5), 524–527.

Chapman, J. (2012). *Singing and teaching singing: A holistic approach to classical voice* (2nd ed.). San Diego, CA: Plural.

Chung, K.F. (2011). Chronic "cough hypersensitivity syndrome": A more precise label for chronic cough. *Pulmonary Pharmacology Therapy*, 24(3), 267–271.

Clark, M. (1998). Removing the "estimates and guesses" from practice—evidence based tissue viability. *Journal of Tissue Viability*, 8(2), 3–5.

Cohen, S.M., Pitman, M.J., Noordzij, J.P., and Courey, M. (2012). Management of dysphonic patients by otolaryngologists. *Otolaryngology-Head and Neck Surgery*, *147*(2), 289–294.

Colton, R., Casper, J.K., and Leonard, R. (2011). *Understanding voice problems: A physiological perspective for diagnosis and treatment* (4th ed.). Baltimore, MD: Lippincott Williams and Wilkins.

Cooper, M. (1974). *Modern techniques of vocal rehabilitation*. Springfield, IL: Charles C. Thomas.

Deem, J.F., and Miller, L. (2000). *Manual of voice therapy* (2nd ed.). Austin, TX: Pro-Ed.

Dettmar, P.W., Castell, D.O., Heading, R.C., Dettmar, P.W., Ell, S., Fagan, M.J., ... Watson, M. (2011). Review article: Reflux and its consequences—The laryngeal, pulmonary and oesophageal manifestations. *Alimentary Pharmacology & Therapeutics*, 33, 1–71.

Elam, J.C., Ishman, S.L., Dunbar, K.B., Clarke, J.O., and Gourin, C.G. (2010). The relationship between depressive symptoms and voice handicap index scores in laryngopharyngeal reflux. *Laryngoscope*, *120*(9), 1900–1903.

Ferrand, C.T. (2012). *Voice disorders: Scope of theory and practice*. Boston, MA: Pearson Higher Education.

Ferreira, L.P., de Oliveira Latorre, M.R., Pinto Giannini, S.P., de Assis Moura Ghirardi, A.C., de Fraga Karmann, D., Silva, E.E., and Figueira, S. (2010). Influence of abusive vocal habits, hydration, mastication, and sleep in the occurrence of vocal symptoms in teachers. *Journal of Voice*, 24(1), 86–92.

Franco, D., Martins, F., Andrea, M., Fragoso, I., Carrao, L., and Teles, J. (2014). Is the sagittal postural alignment different in normal and dysphonic adult speakers? *Journal of Voice*, 28(4), 523.e1–523.e8.

Friedman, J.G., Johnson, J.P., Novaleski, C.K., and Rousseau, B. (2013). Peri-operative voice recovery: Adherence to treatment, quality of life, and patient personality. *Perspectives on Voice and Voice Disorders*, 23(2), 61–66.

Gibson, P.G., and Vertigan, A.E. (2009). Speech pathology for chronic cough: A new approach. *Pulmonary Pharmacological Therapy*, 22(2), 159–162.

Guimaraes, I., and Abberton, E. (2005). Health and voice quality in smokers: An exploratory investigation. *Logopedics Phoniatrics Vocology*, 30, 185–191.

Hansen, J.K., and Thibeault, S.L. (2006). Current understanding and review of the literature: Vocal fold scarring. *Journal of Voice*, 20(1), 110–120.

Hanson, D.G., and Jiang, J.J. (2000). Diagnosis and management of chronic laryngitis associated with reflux. *The American Journal of Medicine*, 108(4A), 112S–119S.

Hicks, D.M., Ours, T.M., Abelson, T.I., Vaezi, M.F., and Richter, J.E. (2002). The prevalence of hypopharynx findings associated with gastroesophageal reflux in normal volunteers. *Journal of Voice*, 16(4), 564–579.

Ilomaki, I., Laukkanen, A.M., Leppanen, K., and Vilkman, E. (2008). Effects of voice training and voice hygiene education on acoustic and perceptual speech parameters and self-reported vocal well-being in female teachers. *Logopedics Phoniatrics Vocology*, 33, 83–92.

Ishikawa, K., and Thibeault, S. (2010). Voice rest versus exercise: A review of the literature. *Journal of Voice*, 24(4), 379–387.

Jonsdottir, V., Laukkanen, A.M., and Siikki, I. (2003). Changes in teachers' voice quality during a working day with and without electronic sound amplification. *Folia Phoniatrica Logopedics*, 55, 267–280.

Kelly, J.H., and Lahey, K.P. (2009). Gastroesophageal reflux disease and voice disorders. In M.P. Fried and A. Ferlito (Eds.), *The larynx* (3rd ed., pp. 27–36). San Diego, CA: Plural.

King, M. (2006). Physiology of mucus clearance. *Pediatric Respiratory Reviews*, 7, S212–S214.

Koschkee, D.L., and Rammage, L. (1997). *Voice care in the medical setting*. San Diego, CA: Singular.

Koufman, J.A. (2002). Laryngopharyngeal reflux is different from classic gastroesophageal reflux disease. *Journal of Ear, Nose, and Throat*, 81, 7–9.

Koufman, J.A., and Stern, J. (2010). *Dropping acid: The reflux diet cookbook and cure*. Elmwood Park, NJ: TLLC. G and H Soho.

Lessac, A. (1997). *The use and training of the human voice: A practical approach to speech and voice dynamics* (3rd ed.). Santa Monica, CA: McGraw-Hill.

Leydon, C., Sivasankar, M., Falciglia, D.L., Atkins, C., and Fisher, K.V. (2009). Vocal fold surface hydration: A review. *Journal of Voice*, 23(6), 658–665.

Lowell, S.Y., Barkmeier-Kraemer, J.M., Hoit, J.D., and Story, B.H. (2008). Respiratory and laryngeal function during spontaneous speaking in teachers with voice disorders. *Journal of Speech, Language and Hearing Research*, 51(2), 333–349.

Mathieson, L. (2001). *Greene and Mathieson's the voice and its disorders* (6th ed.). London, UK: Whurr.

McHenry, M.A., and Carlson, H.K. (2004). The vocal health of auctioneers. *Logopedic Phoniatrica Vocology, 29*(1), 41–47.

Morice, A.H. (2011). Postnasal drip syndrome: A symptom to be sniffed at? *Pulmonary Pharmacology Therapy, 17*, 343–345.

Murry, T., and Rosen, C.A. (2000). Phonotrauma associated with crying. *Journal of Voice, 14*(4), 575–580.

Muscat, J.E., and Wynder, E.L. (1992). Tobacco, alcohol, asbestos, and occupational risk factors for laryngeal cancer. *Cancer, 69*(9), 2244–2251.

Nadel, J.A. (2013). Mucous hypersecretion and relationship to cough. *Pulmonary Pharmacology Therapy, 26*(5), 510–513.

Park, J.O., Shim, M.R., Hwang, Y.S., Cho, K.J., Joo, Y.H., Cho, J.H., Sun, D.I. (2012). Combination of voice therapy and antireflux therapy rapidly recovers voice-related symptoms in laryngopharyngeal reflux patients. *Otolaryngology—Head and Neck Surgery, 146*, 92–97.

Pick, H.L., Siegal, G.M., Fox, P.W., Garber, S.R., and Kearney, J.K. (1989). Inhibiting the Lombard effect. *Journal of the Acoustical Society of America, 85*, 894–900.

Pizolato, R.A., Rehder, M.I., Meneghim, M.C., Ambrosano, G.M., Mialhe, F.L., and Pereira, A.C. (2013). Impact on quality of life in teachers after educational actions for prevention of voice disorders: A longitudinal study. *Health and Quality of Life Outcomes, 27*, 11–28.

Portone-Maira, C., and Johns, M.M., III. (2013). Perioperative voice recovery and the vocal folds: Perspectives from the voice care team. *Perspectives on Voice and Voice Disorders, 23*(2), 53–60.

Rousseau, B., Cohen., S.M., Zeller, A.S., Scearce, L., Tritter, A.G., and Garrett, C.G. (2011). Compliance and quality of life in patients on prescribed voice rest. *Otolaryngology—Head and Neck Surgery, 144*(1), 104–107.

Roy, N., Gray, S.D., Simon, M., Dove, H., Corbin-Lewis, K., and Stemple, J.C. (2001). An evaluation of the effects of two treatment approaches for teachers with voice disorders: A prospective randomized clinical trial. *Journal of Speech, Language and Hearing Research, 44*(2), 286–296.

Roy, N., Weinrich, B., Gray, S.D., Tanner, K., Walker-Toledo, S., Dove, H., Corbin-Lewis, K., and Stemple, J. (2002). Voice amplification vs. vocal hygiene instruction for teachers with voice disorders: A treatment outcomes study. *Journal of Speech and Hearing Research, 45*, 625–638.

Ryan, N.M., Vertigan, A.E., and Gibson, P.G. (2009). Chronic cough and laryngeal dysfunction improve with specific treatment of cough and paradoxical vocal fold movement. *Cough, 5*, 4–11.

Sala, E., Airo, E., Olkinuora, P., Simberg, S., Ström, U., Laine, A., . . . Suonpää, J. (2002). Vocal loading among day care center teachers. *Logopedics Phoniatrica Vocology, 27*(1), 21–28.

Salter, R.B. (1996). History of rest and motion and the scientific basis for early continuous passive motion. *Hand Clinics, 12*, 1–11.

Sandage, M.J. (2013). Perioperative voice recovery: An exercise physiology perspective. *Perspectives on Voice and Voice Disorders*, 23(2), 47–52.

Shewmaker, M.B., Hapner, E.R., Gilman, M., Klein, A.M., and Johns, M.M., III. (2010). Analysis of voice change during cellular phone use: A blinded controlled study. *Journal of Voice*, 24(3), 308–313.

Sivasankar, M., and Leydon, C. (2010). The role of hydration in vocal fold physiology. *Current Opinions in Otolaryngology Head and Neck Surgery*, 18(3), 171–175.

Solomon, N.P., and DiMattia, M.S. (2000). Effects of a vocally fatiguing task and systemic hydration on phonation threshold pressure. *Journal of Voice*, 14(3), 341–362.

Tanner, K., Roy, N., Merrill, R.M., and Elstad, M. (2007). The effects of three nebulized osmotic agents in the dry larynx. *Journal of Speech, Language, Hearing Research*, 50(3), 635–646.

Timmermans, B., De Bodt, M., Wuyts, F., and Van de Heyning, P. (2004). Voice quality change in future professional voice users after 9 months of voice training. *European Archives of Otorhinolaryngology*, 261(1), 1–5.

Titze, I.R., Svec, J.G., and Popolo, P.S. (2003). Vocal dose measures: Quantifying accumulated vibration exposure in vocal fold tissues. *Journal of Speech, Language and Hearing Research*, 46(4), 919–932.

Titze, I.R., and Verdolini-Abbott, K.V. (2012). *Vocology: The science and practice of voice rehabilitation*. Salt Lake City, UT: The National Center for Voice and Speech.

Verdolini, K., Min, Y., Titze, I.R., Lemke, J., Brown, K., van Mersbergen, M., . . . Fisher, K. (2002). Biological mechanisms underlying voice changes due to dehydration. *Journal of Speech, Language and Hearing Research*, 45, 268–281.

Verdolini, K., Titze, I.R., and Fennell, A. (1994). Dependence of phonatory effort on hydration. *Journal of Speech and Hearing Research*, 37(5), 1001–1007.

Verdolini-Marston, K., Sandage, M., and Titze, I.R. (1994). Effect of hydration treatment on laryngeal nodules and polyps, and related measures. *Journal of Voice*, 8, 30–47.

Vertigan, A.E., and Gibson, P.G. (2011). The role of speech pathology in the management of patients with chronic refractory cough. *Lung*, 190(1), 35–40.

Wiener, G.J., Koufman, J.A., Wu, W.C., Cooper, J.B., Richter, J.E., and Castell, D.O. (1989). Chronic hoarseness secondary to gastroesophageal reflux disease: Documentation with 24-h ambulatory pH monitoring. *American Journal of Gastroenterology*, 12, 1503–1508.

Yiu, E.M., and Chan, R.M. (2003). Effect of hydration and vocal rest on the vocal fatigue in amateur karaoke singers. *Journal of Voice*, 17(2), 216–227.

Yun, Y-S., Kim, M-B., and Son, Y-I. (2007). The effect of vocal hygiene education for patients with vocal polyp. *Otolaryngology—Head and Neck Surgery*, 137, 569–575.

Zemlin, W.R. (1998). *Speech and hearing science: Anatomy and physiology* (4th ed.). Needham Heights, MA: Allyn and Bacon.

Zhang, C.X., Qin, Y.M., and Guo, B.R. (2010). Clinical study on treatment of gastroesophageal reflux by acupuncture. *Clinical Journal of Integrative Medicine*, 16(4), 278–303.

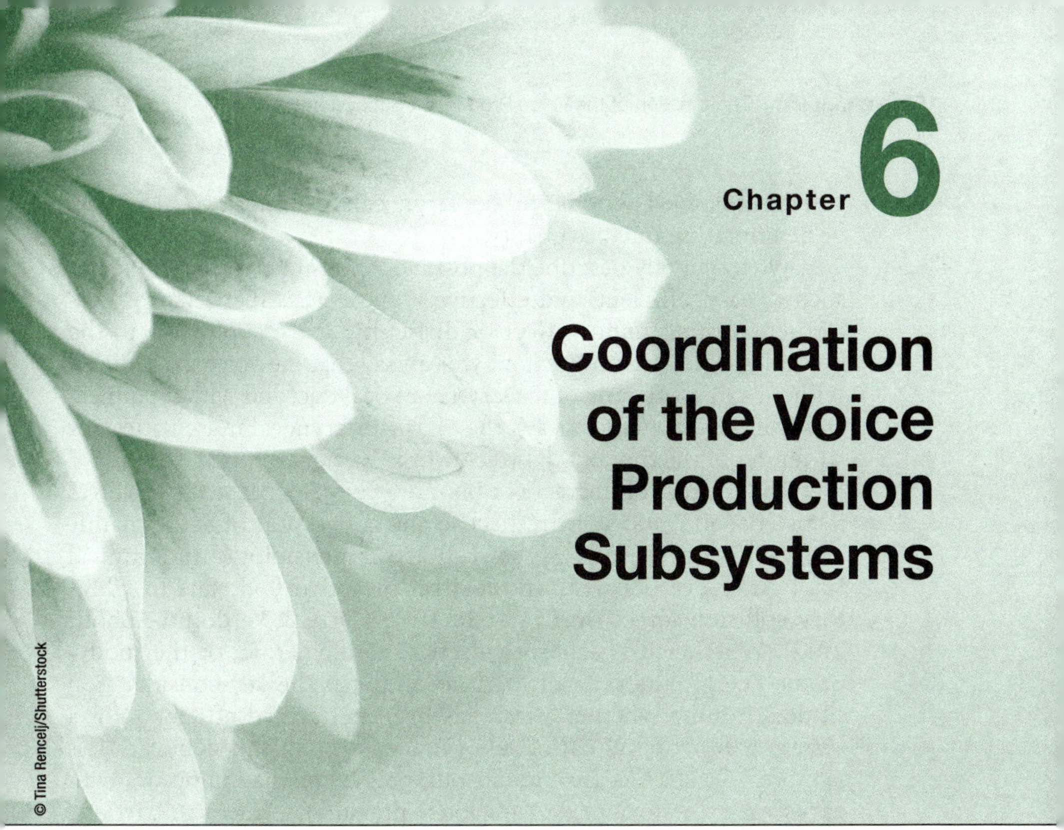

Chapter 6

Coordination of the Voice Production Subsystems

"Do not think the sound first!
Avoid listening in order to judge your vocal sounds!
Turn off the outer ear and turn on the inner 'feel!'" (Lessac, 1997, p. 19)

How Does Your Patient Achieve Vocal Longevity?

As voice clinicians, we strive for a similar outcome for all our patients: a voice that will withstand the vocal challenges that the patient will meet throughout his lifetime. The vocal stamina and durability implicit in this concept are a result of an optimum coordination among the respiration, phonation, resonation, and articulation subsystems of voice production. When such a balance exists among the vocal subsystems, the speaker is then capable of producing a voice that meets his needs in a variety of emotional, occupational, and recreational circumstances, and for prolonged periods without laryngeal discomfort, vocal fatigue, or deterioration in voice quality.

We frequently describe the positive aspects of a voice with terms such as easy, efficient, and effective. *Easy* suggests that a task is performed without undue effort or difficulty. If we apply ease to the physiology of voice production, we can say that the voice is produced without extra stiffening of the larynx or vocal tract and without unnecessary engagement of the jaw, the extrinsic laryngeal musculature, or stiffening of the thorax. The voice works without effort.

The concept of *efficiency* is a bit more complex because it involves a cost–benefit ratio with respect to the conversion of aerodynamic energy to acoustic energy, as well as the physiologic and clinical implications of the wear and tear on the vocal folds due to vibratory collision forces over one's lifetime (Titze & Verdolini-Abbott, 2012). Whether it is acoustic, electric, aerodynamic, or thermodynamic energy, the ratio of input to output is the key consideration in determining whether a task has been performed efficiently or a system is functioning efficiently (Titze, 1994). In this context, "less is more." Or is it? As Titze points out, pressed phonation occurs with excessive expiratory drive (subglottal pressure), inadequate airflow, and extreme glottal constriction. A pressed phonation may be aerodynamically and acoustically efficient, but the derived acoustic gain may come at a high cost to the larynx due to the excessive medial compression of the vocal folds.

Together, ease and efficiency underscore the clinical importance of appropriate coordination among the subsystems. When we describe an efficient manner of phonation, we consider whether a balance exists among expiratory drive, the chosen level of vocal intensity, the target pitch, the specific voice quality, and the vibratory mode of the vocal folds (Titze, 1994). When we add subglottal pressure to increase loudness efficiently, a simultaneous adjustment takes place in the medial compression of the vocal folds and abdominal control so that expiratory drive does not overwhelm the elasticity of the vocal folds. Without the concomitant adjustments at the vocal tract (back pressure, inertance) and laryngeal levels as well as the skill necessary to manage the respiratory forces when increasing or decreasing loudness and fundamental frequency, the speaker places an undue stress on the vocal folds. Two of the most frequently observed vocal problems occur when limited airflow leads to a pressed manner of phonation or when a counterproductive, excessive expiratory drive is used to maintain phonation. Under these circumstances the presence of a laryngeal lesion will interfere with vocal fold vibration due to vocal fold asymmetry and the associated asynchrony of vibration.

In order to increase fundamental frequency the vocal folds lengthen and stiffen, which requires a matching increase in breath control.

A balance among the length and stiffness of the vocal folds and expiratory drive is crucial to maintain efficient phonation during connected speech. In singing, if a soprano were to negotiate an ascending/descending scale without the necessary and concomitant adjustments in subglottal pressure and breath control, she might experience a break in the passaggio as she transitions from the chest to the **head voice**, and again as she lowers the fundamental frequency from the head to the **chest voice**. It is not unusual for young singers to push the system in this way and complain of a break in the passaggio, vocal fatigue, and laryngeal discomfort related to the delicate challenge of balancing subglottal pressure and dynamic changes in fundamental frequency.

Even more elusive are the underlying components of an *effective* voice. We use this term to describe a voice that meets all of one's vocal demands, whether it is sustaining expected levels of vocal intensity in a large theatre; quietly telling a fairytale to a child before bedtime; shouting for a taxi that is out of physical reach; singing an aria, rock song, or heavy metal; teaching a second grade class for a five-hour stretch; performing beat-box on Forty-Second Street; ad infinitum. The effective voice negotiates, seduces, intimidates, consoles, befriends, or disciplines, irks, manipulates, teases, questions, and humiliates. If we were to watch a film in a foreign language without subtitles, we might rely on what we see and hear to extract the actors' meaning. If the actors use their voices effectively, the story may unfold even without the subtitles.

Is it possible to produce a voice effectively in the absence of ease and efficiency? Probably so. Nevertheless, if the speaker sacrifices ease and efficiency for effectiveness, the consequences of that phonatory choice may be limited vocal stamina and endurance (vocal longevity). The rock or heavy metal singer, for instance, who effectively engages an audience with the dramatic intensity of his vocal style, may pay a heavy laryngeal price for the effect that he creates on stage if he achieves that effect with hyperadduction of the vocal folds. Further, the teaching profession is one with a high incidence of voice-related problems. The teacher who disciplines his class with his voice may do so effectively. His students may respond to the shouting, yelling, and stridency of his voice quality with compliance and cooperation, but the long-term vocal consequences may reduce his enjoyment of teaching and shorten his teaching career. Over a long period, excessive vocal fold collision forces may lead to phonotrauma, permanent change to the vocal fold tissue, and a change in voice quality.

Many of your patients will say, "I want my voice to *sound* better," while you, as a savvy clinician, know that kinesthetic awareness is a more effective guide when coordination among the vocal subsystems goes awry. This subtle paradigmatic shift is necessary because, unless and until your patient begins to feel the difference between ease and effort, it will be difficult for him to make other kinesthetic adjustments. Sensory feedback becomes more central as you facilitate appropriate coordination of the subsystems, eliminating the counter-productive compensations associated with excessive expiratory drive, hyperadduction of the vocal folds, and increased stiffness in the vocal tract. It is likely that an insistence on the importance of sound will sabotage those goals. Longevity, stamina, and strength evolve as your patient learns to use kinesthetic awareness rather than his ear to regulate phonation.

The patient in the *Education: Effort Versus Ease* video is a singer who teaches singing and uses her voice to explain and demonstrate **vocalise** to her adolescent students. Her awareness and modification of effort during the back pressure exercises and long teaching days are crucial to the longevity of her career.

Sensory Feedback and Manner of Phonation

Sensory feedback pertaining to voice production may be more difficult for patients to evaluate than feedback from other motor activities (van Leer & Connor, 2010) such as golf, tennis, aerobatic flying, and even knitting. The acquisition and refinement of a motor skill may be measured by the speed and accuracy of the trajectory of a ball, the smoothness of the maneuvers a pilot executes, or the evenness of stitches in a knitted sweater. During the process of voice rehabilitation, on the other hand, the speaker is asked to shift from the habitual reliance on auditory monitoring to the subtle, tactile, and kinesthetic cues from the vibrating air column and air flowing through the mouth. This shift from listening to feeling sensations is made because the auditory assessment of sound is misleading given that a clear sound can be produced with effort. *Auditory feedback is not trustworthy.* Consequently, the process of modifying voice production requires deliberate attention and self-assessment in order to minimize effort and facilitate ease and coordination.

Although it is often the case that our work indirectly facilitates the resolution of a vocal fold lesion, voice therapy does not directly address this goal. Our primary goal is the optimal coordination among the respiratory, phonatory, resonation, and articulatory subsystems of voice production for a given task. It is obvious that voice problems associated with effortful use of the laryngeal mechanism (muscle tension dysphonia, nodules, polyps, vocal hemorrhage, varices, and edema) respond well to a treatment process focused on optimum coordination of the subsystems. It may not be as obvious when the laryngeal diagnosis is associated with a neurological or oncological etiology that the manner of phonation continues to be relevant to possible worsening of the voice symptoms. The counterproductive, compensatory behaviors (effort) that patients implement to cope with vocal changes from neurological disorders disrupt the coordination among the subsystems and usually lead to more effort, which exacerbates the voice disorder. Regardless of the etiology of the voice problem, your plan to modify and reduce harmful behaviors and to reduce the negative impact of an existing lesion or neurological problem always includes the development of rehabilitation hypotheses and treatment hierarchies.

Physiological Empathy

You may remember from our discussion of patient-centered therapy that Rogers (1951) emphasizes the importance of accurate empathy in order to appreciate the patient's perspective of his problem. In the context of voice rehabilitation, we use **physiological empathy** as well as accurate empathy—that is, the clinician's kinesthetic awareness of the patient's manner of phonation and his kinesthetic sensitivity to the sensations of ease with which the clinician produces the model. Of course, physiological empathy can be one-sided—you are aware of the effort the patient uses as he produces voice, but he does not feel it. At the beginning of therapy your patient may have a limited awareness of the effort he uses to make sound because of a predisposition to listening to the voice. Your initial goal then is to engage and enhance sensory awareness and his capacity to discriminate between an effortful and an easier manner of phonation. It may take time to prepare him to use physiological empathy in order to take advantage of your models as you facilitate ease and efficiency of phonation. When the patient responds positively to an approach that includes physiological empathy, he uses sensory rather than auditory feedback to discriminate between ease and effort. It is almost as though the process of osmosis allows your patient to absorb your appropriate model of phonation.

Development of the Management Plan

The Intervention Process

A consideration of the relationship among disrupted physiological patterns, counterproductive compensations, and vocal symptoms will serve you well as you organize the long- and short-term goals that are part of your management plan. Your rehabilitation hypotheses, then, will emerge from the factors that may have led to the development, maintenance, and exacerbation of the voice problem. We have described some of the most common voice characteristics of dysphonia and suspected

Box 6-1

Rehabilitation Hypotheses

Observation: Patient habitually uses effortful phonation.

Expected underlying physiology: Patient uses excessive expiratory drive and hyperadducts the vocal folds (excessive medial compression) during phonation.

Therapeutic hypothesis: Patient's enhanced awareness of ease versus effort facilitates a more appropriate manner of phonation.

Observation: Patient habitually uses abrupt onset of phonation.

Expected underlying physiology: Patient adducts the vocal folds *prior* to phonation.

Therapeutic hypothesis: Coordinated release of the airstream with initiation of phonation facilitates easy onset of phonation.

Observation: Patient habitually uses a pressed manner of phonation.

Expected underlying physiology: Patient uses limited air flow and excessive medial compression of the vocal folds during phonation.

Therapeutic hypothesis: Increased back pressure and inertance capitalize on the resonating properties of the vocal tract.

underlying physiological changes that accompanied those symptoms. In **Box 6-1** we link the underlying physiology to a management plan that includes rehabilitation hypotheses, goals, and procedures.

The patient's viewpoint and the patient–clinician partnership are especially meaningful during the planning phase of treatment. For that reason, the long- and short-term goals that you plan with your patient will take into account not only an estimate of the best performance that can be expected within a given period of time, but the patient's narrative regarding his preferred learning style, readiness for change, previous therapy experience (if any), and your perception of his self-efficacy. **Table 6-1** proposes several possible long- and short-term goals to guide you as you develop your treatment plan.

The *Description of Effort: Lack of Resonance* video reveals the patient's awareness that she does not capitalize on the resonating characteristics of the vocal tract. Her awareness of the importance of resonance is a favorable prognostic indicator.

Framework for Deliberate Practice

During the early stages of therapy, it is desirable to keep the vocal tract relatively stable in order to optimize patient discrimination of appropriate manner of phonation and to minimize the cognitive load. Attention to the sensations of the new motor pattern requires full and deliberate concentration on the fine details of the motor control

Table 6-1 Guidelines for a Management Plan

Hypothesis	Long-Term Goals	Short-Term Goals	Session Goals	Session Procedures
• Patient's enhanced awareness of ease versus effort facilitates more appropriate manner of phonation	• To establish consistent differentiation of ease versus effort	• To refine discrimination and identification of excessive loudness and chronic throat clearing	• To develop alternatives to detrimental vocal behaviors	• Voice conservation recommendations (decrease amount of speaking, increase listening; decrease laryngeal stiffness by sip-swallowing water—especially following throat clearing and coughing) • Verbal reasoning (describe the purpose of procedure and format, turn-taking style, prompts, preferred manner of phonation) (see Dialogue 6-1) • Identify preferred manner of phonation (use speech samples beginning with repetition of the clinician's simple utterances within a turn-taking format) (see Dialogue 6-1) • Identify ease of phonation (use basic back pressure exercise in turn-taking format with clinician model, followed by feedback and reinforcement or modification of patient production. Initial utterances should be short and provide a relatively high back pressure) (see Dialogue 6-1)

(continues)

Table 6-1 Guidelines for a Management Plan (*continued*)

Hypothesis	Long-Term Goals	Short-Term Goals	Session Goals	Session Procedures
		• To develop a generalized motor schema for easy, efficient, and effective manner of phonation	• To reinforce physiologic memory of appropriate manner of production • Enhance recall and recognition schema (specify criterion—90%)	• Self Assessment (Intermittent queries of patient self-discrimination and awareness of ease of production and awareness of sensory feedback) (see Dialogue 6-1)
• Decrease in excessive expiratory drive, vocal fold stiffness, and medial compression facilitates more appropriate manner of phonation	• To improve coordination of voice production subsystems for professional and personal use	• To decrease expiratory drive • To decrease medial compression of the vocal folds • To decrease extraneous muscle activity in head, neck, and thorax	• To decrease expiratory drive • To decrease medial compression of the vocal folds • To increase back pressure • To decrease extraneous muscle activity in head, neck, and thorax	• Confidential voice during conversation • Yawn-sigh • Voiceless or voiced gargle • Airway Reflex Exercise • Voiceless or voiced tongue and lip trills • Raspberries
• Dynamic control of the expiratory drive facilitates appropriate coordination of the vocal subsystems and more appropriate manner of phonation	• To coordinate expiratory drive with varying levels of vocal intensity and utterance length	• To establish adequate control of expiratory drive to cope with varying levels of vocal intensity	• To develop awareness, strength, and then stamina for a given task • To develop adequate breath control to cope with varying levels of vocal intensity • To establish appropriate intonation patterns as patient develops an efficient manner of phonation	• Basic breathing exercises (Box 6-13) • Phrases, utterances of increasing length • Ladder (loudness) exercise (Box 6-15) • Ascending and descending scales • Incorporate intonation patterns for emotions such as happiness, sadness, fear, etc.

necessary for voice production (Ericsson, Krampe, & Tesch-Romer, 1993). The careful and deliberate repetition of a more efficient motor pattern builds a stronger imprint of the new motor memory trace and increases the patient's awareness of the distance between the intended target and the actual production.

Although blocked practice builds consistency within a prescribed context, it does not provide the variation in practice that is required to meet the demand that generalization places on the speaker. **Learning theory** suggests that greater transfer and flexibility occur when the patient engages in random practice, which increases the cognitive load during the motor acquisition process. Consequently, when ease of production becomes consistent within a structured context, it is time to take advantage of the benefits of *random practice* and facilitate transfer of the skill. Random practice facilitates self-recognition and modification of errors to improve retention and generalization of a new motor skill. You may vary initial phonemes in words or phrases, mix voiced and voiceless sounds, and increase utterance length and linguistic complexity in order to augment the cognitive load as it becomes evident that the patient is ready to manage greater complexity. When you insert a delay, ask for novel responses, or require self-evaluation, cognitive load and complexity increase. Combined random and blocked practice schedules facilitate the acquisition and consolidation of the targeted motor pattern (Wong, Whitehill, Ma, & Masters, 2013).

Deliberate practice requires careful focus on the small details of voice production and experimentation with manner of phonation as the patient achieves the most effective way to produce the new motor pattern (Ericsson et al., 1993). Deliberate practice leads to mastery of a motor skill through repeated, thoughtful performance and repetition under different conditions, with a critical review of one's performance. Deliberate practice is active. In contrast, practice that takes place when distractions interfere with complete concentration (e.g., while driving, walking down the street, watching TV) produces either little positive result, or worse, the habituation of an ineffective, inappropriate, counterproductive behavior.

How do we establish an environment within which the patient is more likely to use deliberate practice? Your support in this endeavor begins with the information you provide regarding the process of deliberate practice and your encouragement to practice only when full concentration and attention are possible. During the early stages of therapy, the level of attention necessary for deliberate practice is quite high. As stronger memory traces and a more robust generalized motor program become integrated the patient generalizes these skills to more challenging environments. Consequently, the practice schedule and procedures will be adapted to meet the patient's developing skill level.

A general guideline for home practice is that frequent, short practice periods (i.e., 30 seconds to a minute at a time) that are interspersed (i.e., 6, 12, or 18 times) throughout the day are usually more effective than single, half-hour practice sessions. Frequent reminders to focus deliberately on the production of the voice, in conjunction with the period of spontaneous improvement that usually follows a practice session, facilitate carryover, especially when practices take place in different settings throughout the day. Patients usually like the short practice periods because they are easy to incorporate into a daily routine and require limited periods of the intensive, deliberate control of voice production. A watch or phone set to beep on the hour can serve as a reminder to perform a deliberate practice.

At the beginning of a session, we generally ask the patient to describe his daily practice routine in order to support his efforts, and if practice has been irregular, to develop strategies that enhance adherence. He may report that he practiced regularly but had difficulty maintaining deliberate attention and did not have success very often. You might shape your responses with motivational interviewing (MI) as a model, and remind him that the habituated effort he uses to produce sound takes time to change. Alternatively, he might report that he practiced regularly and had good success, but you observe effort during the session (e.g., increased apparent general extraneous muscle activity, abrupt initiations of phonation, and excessive loudness). This suggests that the patient may need support to discriminate between ease and effort, and encouragement to maintain the high level of concentration necessary for this highly focused practice. Again, you might use the MI framework (i.e., reflective listening, problem recognition) to develop greater accuracy in his assessment of effort. On the other hand, he may report that he practiced regularly and had some success maintaining his deliberate focus on the sensations in his vocal tract, which you observe during the session (e.g., you observe decreased apparent general extraneous muscle activity, the absence of abrupt initiations, and quiet phonation on the trials). It may be time to increase the cognitive load.

The patient with adductor spasmodic dysphonia in the *Discussion of Home Practice* video discusses his adherence to the clinician's suggestions from the previous session. The patient has followed through with the recommendations and reports some success.

Resonance: Back Pressure and Inertance

When we enhance resonance, we capitalize on the shape and configuration of the vocal tract to make vocal fold vibration more efficient, to project the voice without effort, and to increase stamina and vocal longevity. Resonance was described by Lessac (1997) as the **Y-Buzz** and was expanded and enhanced by Titze (1983, 1988, 1994), Titze and Story (1997), Verdolini (1998, 2000a), and Titze and Verdolini-Abbott

(2012) to include back pressure and inertance. Lessac emphasizes the use of tactile (vibratory) cues in the front of the hard palate, the gum ridge, and nasal septum to maximize resonance. **Resonant voice** is "the ideal mix of laryngeal adduction (somewhere between breathy and pressed) [phonation neutral position] and ample reinforcement of vocal fold vibration by the vocal tract" (Titze, 2001, p. 519). *Clinically*, resonant voice is enhanced by deliberately attending to the vibrations in the vocal tract. Resonance is more easily experienced on nasal rather than open sounds (i.e., vowels). It is obvious that the nasal phonemes facilitate a heightened sensation in the nasal cavity as a result of the amplified acoustic energy in the cavity. Your hierarchy of therapy can be modified by varying the phonemic structure of an utterance to increase or decrease the strength of these vibratory sensations. Titze and Verdolini-Abbott (2012) point out that acoustic energy moves away from the source (the vocal folds) "along the entire airway system" (p. 287). An efficient conversion of energy spreads strong vibrations throughout the air column above and below the vocal folds, but an inefficient conversion concentrates small vibrations around the vocal folds.

The hypotheses you develop as part of the voice rehabilitation process are based on your observations of the patient's patterns of vocal behavior and your knowledge of the underlying physiology of voice production. When you observe abrupt onset of phonation, you hypothesize that the patient is using excessive medial compression of the vocal folds and subglottal pressure, and that a decrease in expiratory drive will increase the probability of an effective coordination of the subsystems and an easier manner of phonation. You might test your hypothesis by asking the patient to do the Puffy Cheeks Exercise (Chapman, 2012) or the Airway Reflex Exercise because you know these techniques create a high supraglottal pressure (back pressure). The increase in back pressure facilitates a decrease in the difference between the pressure above and the pressure below the vocal folds (transglottal pressure drop), thereby decreasing medial compression of the vocal folds. The patient executes the procedure with deliberate attention to the sensations in the vocal tract and then produces a phrase that begins with a vowel-initiated word (e.g., "I am on my way"). You note a remarkable shift from the previous abrupt to a gentler onset of phonation with the initiation of "I." Based on this behavioral change, you accept your hypothesis. Additional semi-occluded procedures are linked with hypothesis development in **Box 6-2**.

During an early session (even during the assessment), the clinician might introduce a back pressure exercise to decrease expiratory drive and medial compression and stiffness of the vocal folds and facilitate awareness of nasal resonance. The basic hierarchy for this back pressure exercise begins when the clinician models /mhm/ once, the patient

Box 6-2

Selected Semi-Occluded Procedure

Hypotheses and Short-Term Goal	**Procedure**
• Patient's conscious awareness of ease versus effort will facilitate more appropriate manner of phonation. • Nasal phonemes facilitate increased awareness of the vibrations in the head (the resonance on nasal sounds is strong in the anterior face and is enhanced because nasals can be prolonged). • The voiceless phoneme /h/ partially abducts the vocal folds and facilitates easy initiation of phonation. • The patient uses physiological empathy and kinesthetic feedback to imitate the clinician's model.	Within a turn-taking format, the clinician models easy, resonant manner of phonation. Clinician: "/mhm/" Patient: "/mhm/" Clinician: "/mhm/" Patient: "/mhm/" Clinician: "/hu/" Patient: "/hu/"

responds /mhm/, the clinician repeats and the patient responds /mhm/ again. This format allows for *immediate* imitation of the clinician's model, provides kinesthetic support, and maximizes physiological empathy.

In **Dialogue 6-1**, the clinician uses a combination of three philosophical and theoretical frameworks to facilitate change: a client-centered approach, an education model, and physiologically based rationales for the procedures. The clinician explores the patient's self-knowledge, and includes the patient as a partner responsible for the changes that take place with growing self-awareness and kinesthetic sensitivity. The clinician provides a model and notes the patient's ease of production but does not give immediate feedback, allowing the patient to recognize the need for deliberate attention to the sensations.

Dialogue 6-1
Modification of Vocal Fold Vibration

Ms. F returned for her first therapy session following the assessment and a week of practice with a back pressure exercise and confidential voice. She expressed concern and uncertainty regarding the accuracy of her manner of phonation during the procedures.

Using a quiet, resonant voice while providing information about voice production, I reviewed, "During the evaluation we talked about how squeezing the vocal folds together for long periods may lead to the vocal fatigue you have described to me."

Ms. F stiffened her jaw and produced voice with abrupt initiations and moderate roughness, "Yes, I have been trying to talk more easily and quietly and my throat is a little less sore, but I still lose my voice by midday."

I was aware of her mixed feelings of success and frustration and thought that working directly on her voice might provide encouragement. Continuing the resonant voice model, "Yes, it's frustrating when your voice is not dependable. But talking quietly and deliberately attending to the sensations in your nose and lips is a big change for you. Well done! I know it is frustrating when things don't change as quickly as you would like. So I thought we might try a procedure that will make your more aware of the sensations in your nose and lips and may make you more comfortable using your voice in this gentler, quieter way. We will do this exercise as if we are having a conversation. I'll say /mhm/ and you will answer me, /mhm/. I'll do it again and you will answer me again. Then, I'll say, /hu/ and you will answer me with /hu/. I want you to deliberately attend to the sensations in your nose and lips and do the /mhm/ and /hu/ as gently and easily as you can. *Do not push for voice* during the exercise. If you get voice without effort that's fine, but what we're working toward is your deliberate attention to the feelings of ease, not sound. That means it should *feel* so easy that it's as if you are doing nothing. So let's start."

The procedure is practiced in a series of three groups of turn-taking sequences. The clinician maintains an easy manner of phonation during each token to provide a physiological model that the patient imitates. During this initial turn-taking procedure, the clinician notes the patient's response to the physiological model, observes the manner of phonation and any extraneous muscle activity, determines whether the patient modifies the effortful tokens, but provides no feedback. The patient has an opportunity then to determine independently whether she produced the tokens more easily.

Clinician: "/mhm/." *This model and subsequent models are produced with ease and resonance.*

Ms. F: "/mhm/," *produced with abrupt onset on both syllables and extraneous muscle activity in the head, neck, and shoulders.*

Clinician: "/mhm/."

Ms. F: "/mhm/," *produced with the same high effort levels.*

Clinician: "/hu/."

Ms. F: "/hu/," *again with effort.*

Clinician: "/mhm/," *with a gentle, floating gesture.*

Ms. F: "/mhm/," *produced with abrupt onset on both syllables, but less extraneous muscle activity.*

Clinician: "/mhm/."

Ms. F: "/mhm/," *maintaining less effort.*

Clinician: "/hu/," *pairing the /mhm/ with a gentle extension of the arm to suggest ease.*

Ms. F: "/hu/," *produced with abrupt vowel onset and no extraneous muscle activity in her head and neck.*

Clinician: "/mhm/."

Ms. F: "/mhm/," *same as previous token.*

Clinician: "/mhm/."

Ms. F: "/mhm/," *same as previous one.*

Clinician: "/hu/."

Ms. F: "/hu/," *produced with abrupt vowel onset and no extraneous muscle activity.*

I perceived instability in her phonatory output, but a subtle decrease in effort as we continued the procedure. I also observed a slight decrease in the apparent, general extraneous muscle activity in her neck and I asked, "What did you feel?"

Ms. F looked confused, "What do you mean?"

She asked her question with excessive vocal intensity and moderate extraneous muscle activity. I wanted to direct her attention to the sensations in her vocal tract and see if her effort levels would decrease. I gestured to the area of the mask, "I mean, what did you feel in the front of your face?"

With an expression of curiosity and a slight drop in loudness, Ms. F repeated, "/mhm/ . . . I feel . . . buzzing."

Her repetition of /mhm/ and her statement suggested that she had not initially focused on feeling during the /mhm/ turn-taking procedure. I was impressed that she had attended to the vibrations on this additional trial. It is not easy to focus on sensation, and it probably felt awkward to her. I wanted to see if she could be more precise in her description, "Good. Did your /mhm/ feel as easy as mine or did you feel like you were pushing for sound?"

Her eyes opened widely and Ms. F smiled. Her effort decreased somewhat, "I'm not sure. What do you mean by pushing?"

Continuing to model an easy voice, "Do you feel like your voice is just flowing, or are you demanding sound?"

With a look of curiosity and a reduction in the extraneous muscle activity Ms. F said, "I'm not sure. Can we do it again?"

In a quiet, resonant voice, I modeled, "/mhm/."

With greatly reduced effort and a gentle onset and no extraneous muscle activity, Ms. F produced, "/mhm/" . . . I feel . . . buzzing, but I don't think mine was as gentle as yours. Was I pushing?"

Pleased that she was deliberately focusing on the sensations in her nose and lips, "You are right, you used some effort, but not as much as on the previous ones."

"It is really difficult to focus on feeling. I'm such an aural person. Can we try it again?"

I wanted to support her insight and attention to the sensations in her nose and lips, "I know it is very hard when you make such a big shift from listening to feeling, but just attend to whether it feels easy or you need to push to get sound."

With practice, ease of phonation stabilizes and becomes more consistent. The procedures are continued in the same turn-taking manner presented, and the clinician continues to model a quiet, resonant voice on each trial. The clinician continues to give intermittent feedback to the patient and solicit descriptions regarding what the patient feels during the tokens.

Sample Hierarchy of Back Pressure Exercises

The nasal sounds provide an inroad to building your patient's kinesthetic sensitivity, and are therefore effective during these introductory back pressure exercises. When you create a **hierarchy** of procedures based on back pressure, they may progress from /mhm/, /mhm/ with /hu/, to /mhm/, /mhm/ with phrases that begin with the /m/ phoneme in order to heighten the vibrations experienced in the lips and the face—what is referred to by singers as "the mask." The /m/ and /n/ phonemes are traditionally used early in the process. Nasals can be sustained and provide the most powerful vibratory sensations in the lips, in the hard palate, the gum ridge, and the bridge of the nose, making it easy to attend to the nasal resonance. Bear in mind, however, that our phonemic repertoire varies across a wide spectrum of sounds, with /m/ and /n/ representing only two of them. The nasal consonants, while a part of that repertoire, do not provide an appropriate model for the timbre (color tone) of the voice and vowel production across the non-nasal sounds. In addition, the extreme forward placement and vibratory sensation created by the nasals might bring some hypernasality to the voice (Lessac, 1997).

The following procedures combine the /mhm/ with a variety of /m/-initiated phrases to capitalize on the nasal resonance and a semi-occluded vocal tract, which reduces the collision forces between the vocal folds. This technique is best performed in a turn-taking manner similar to that illustrated in the previous dialogue in order to develop physiological empathy between you and the patient, which encourages attention to the sensations in the vocal tract. The clinician models a phrase, such as "more and more," and the patient responds, "more and more." Your clinical model of easy phonation makes this possible. We generally perform these phrases over a series of several turn-taking sequences before asking the patient for feedback regarding his manner of phonation. When you ask, "What did you feel?" "Were yours as easy as mine?" "Did you let the vocal folds do what they want to do?" "Did you feel like you were pushing to make sound or demanding sound on the /mhm/?" you are directing the patient's conscious awareness to the kinesthetic aspect of the exercise, and reinforcing his self-efficacy. The patient's analysis, the **congruence** of his self-assessment, and your appraisal of his manner of phonation will determine the next step. A reminder that the deliberate attention and ease with which the /mhm/ is produced should be carried over to the phrases that ensue is useful to clarify the goal of the exercise as you move into connected speech.

When the /mhm/ has become highly stabilized through practice, it can be used to set the vocal tract up for easy, efficient phonation during connected speech (phrases), and cue the patient to attend to the sensations in the facial mask. As you work with your patient, you can create additional phrases to supplement the ones provided in **Box 6-3**. If the patient's name begins with /m/, for instance, you can incorporate his name into the practice sentences. The /mhm/ is the sound we use when we listen and agree with someone during a conversation; it is an easy sound to work into a conversation as a "sneak" practice and within which to attend to resonance as he begins the process of transfer.

The sample phrases in Box 6-3 incorporate the nasal phonemes with the /mhm/ token, which sets up the vocal tract for easy phonation and reminds the patient to deliberately focus on the sensations in the facial mask. Each example can be used multiple times. Although these procedures take place within a structured context, the changes made as you modify articulatory placement (nasal to glide to vowel) provide a beginning in the process of random practice and generalization.

Box 6-3

Sample Phrases Incorporating Nasal Phonemes

Hypotheses and Short-Term Goal	Procedure
• The /mhm/ sets the larynx up for an appropriate manner of phonation during connected speech. • Nasal phonemes (i.e., /m/, /n/) provide high back pressure and sensation of resonance in the mask. • The patient will attend to the vibratory sensations created by the nasal phonemes and identify their location in the vocal tract.	The turn-taking format provides an opportunity for the patient to repeat the utterance and use physiological empathy to match the clinician's ease of phonation on phrases with multiple nasal sounds (e.g., "more and more," "many, many men," "Mamie and Naomi," "maybe on Monday," "Mama made marmalade," "moon over Miami," "Mona married Nathan," "me and Bobby Magee," "no, no Nannette," "never say never," "ninety-nine knives," "never on Monday"). Clinician: "/mhm/, /mhm/," *<easy breath>* "More and more." Patient: "/mhm/, /mhm/," *<easy breath>* "More and more." Clinician: "/mhm/, /mhm/," *<easy breath>* "Many, many men." Patient: "/mhm/, /mhm/," *<easy breath>* "Many, many men." Clinician: "/mhm/, /mhm/," *<easy breath>* "No, no Nannette." Patient: "/mhm/, /mhm/," *<easy breath>* "No, no Nannette."

Nota bene: Easy breath is a cue for the patient to remember to breathe before producing the phrase. Before the procedure, the patient is cued to focus on the vibrations in the mask.

The clinician and patient in videos *Back Pressure Hierarchy, Back Pressure + /m/Phrases, Back Pressure + /j/ Phrases,* and *Back Pressure + Vowel Phrases* participate in these exercises progressing from /m/, to /j/, and finally vowel-initiated phrases. As the complexity of the exercise increases, the patient uses her kinesthetic awareness to produce the vowel-initiated phrases with gentle onset and flow phonation.

When we follow two /mhm/ tokens with a phrase (e.g., /mhm/, /mhm/, "more and more"), the cognitive load increases because the patient must consciously self-monitor not only the kinesthetic information from the back pressure (/mhm/, /mhm/) set-up, but across the entire utterance. Patients often inquire as to the need for breath management during this procedure. Given the minimal subglottal pressure needed at this quiet level of phonation, the breath that is available is sufficient to produce the /mhm/, /mhm/ portion of the utterance. The patient then takes an easy breath for the phrase that follows. We find it useful, as a way of building an awareness of "easy, natural breath," to discourage either an excessive intake of air or initiation of the phrase without an inhalation. We ask the patient to pay attention to the body, allowing it time to decide when it needs to take the breath. The rib cage will naturally spring into action and expand when the system is ready for the next breath. The coordination between respiration and phonation is disrupted when the inhalation occurs before the system returns to resting expiratory level (REL).

The shift from the turn-taking format in the clinical setting to practice at home often leads to "rushing" through an exercise, rather than focusing on the sensations in the nose and oral cavity, allowing the body to dictate when it is ready for the next breath. Home practice may be difficult in the absence of the clinician's model and the turn-taking format which serve to slow the process. This motor insecurity can be disquieting during the process of the acquisition and stabilization of a new motor pattern. The patient may communicate frustration regarding self-assessment of the appropriateness and efficiency of the practice trials. His uncertainty reflects his difficulty directing attention appropriately and trusting the sensations in his body.

We increase the cognitive load during this semi-occluded series by inserting a delay, either prior to the production of a short phrase (i.e., "/mhm/, /mhm/" <pause> "more and more"), or following the clinician's model of the entire utterance (i.e., clinician's model, "/mhm/, /mhm/, more and more" <pause> patient's response). The insertion of a short pause increases the cognitive load by asking the patient to retain the sensory attributes of the clinician's model for a short period before he produces the utterance. During the pause, the patient has time to establish deliberate attention to the sensations in his vocal tract, rehearse (repeat) the phrase, and silently modify the manner of phonation of the utterance to come, thus solidifying the motor traces that require habituation.

The next level of complexity in this hierarchy integrates the /j/ phoneme into phrases, providing a change in placement as we move from the most forward place in the head with the nasal sounds toward the level of the vocal folds, with the glide serving as a transition placement between these extremes. We use the glide to enhance the kinesthetic awareness of flow as the tongue blade lifts to the boundary between the hard and soft palate to produce the /j/ sound. This technique, described by Lessac (1997) as the *Y-Buzz*, or "call" technique, creates an easy, fluid, and resonant tone that is projected without unnecessary constriction in the vocal tract or hyperadduction of the vocal folds. The term *call* derives from the train conductor's call to passengers when boarding the train, "All aboard." A sensation of a relaxed half-yawn, slight protrusion of the lips, and the tongue tip resting gently behind the lower teeth accompanies the production of the /j/ to create an inverted megaphone shape that provides an open pharynx and vibratory sensations along the hard palate and alveolar ridge (Lessac, 1997; Titze & Verdolini-Abbott, 2012).

You can begin this series using the /mhm/, /mhm/ setup followed by phrases that begin with the /j/ phoneme. This series of semi-occluded tokens with the /j/ phoneme may be performed in a similar turn-taking format to the utterances that incorporate the nasal phonemes. Remember to maintain deliberate attention as you produce a comfortable pitch and model the fluid manner of phonation associated with the glide. The breath will come easily and spontaneously as it floats along with this continuing sound. The voice should flow with the breath. Visualization may be useful during this phase of establishing the feeling of flow and buzz that may, initially, be elusive. If you picture a pond (the breath) and a lily pad (the word) floating on the top of the water, you can imagine the buoyancy and suspension of the pad as it floats, never piercing the surface of the pond—just riding along the surface of the water. In this way, the voice floats atop the breath—rides along with it, never pressing or pushing the sound.

Continue to direct the patient's attention to the sensations (buzz) on the alveolar ridge and the hard palate, provide intermittent feedback, and query the patient regarding kinesthetic awareness. Given that the /j/ phoneme is a *glide*, the **proprioceptive feedback** will differ from the *nasal* phonemes used in the previous series. The glide contributes to a fluid, flowing phonation and oral resonance that prevents nasalization of the vowel and abrupt initiation. Sample /j/-initiated phrases are presented in **Box 6-4**.

As we increase complexity by decreasing back pressure in the vocal tract, the third series of phrases combines the back pressure setup with vowel-initiated phrases. The vowel is the most challenging phoneme

Box 6-4

Sample Phrases Incorporating the /j/ Glide

Hypotheses and Short-Term Goal	Procedure
• The /mhm/ sets up the larynx for an appropriate manner of phonation during connected speech. • The glide /j/ heightens the awareness of vibrations along the hard palate and on the alveolar ridge. • The patient will identify the difference in kinesthetic feedback between the nasal and glide phonemes.	The clinician uses a turn-taking format to encourage physiological empathy and integration of ease while repeating sample phrases (e.g., "yummy, yummy, yummy," "yummy, yummy yams," "yonder in Wyoming," "yes and no," "you and me," "yummy, yummy avocado," "yellow and orange," "yummy, yummy apples"). Clinician: "/mhm/, /mhm/," *<easy breath>* "Yummy, yummy, yummy." Patient: "/mhm/, /mhm/," *<easy breath>* "Yummy, yummy, yummy." Clinician: "/mhm/, /mhm/," *<easy breath>* "Yummy, yummy yams." Patient: "/mhm/, /mhm/," *<easy breath>* "Yummy, yummy yams."

Nota bene: The patient attends to the elevated tongue blade, tongue tip resting behind the lower teeth. He may feel the air stream as it flows across the boundary that separates the hard and soft palate.

to produce with ease, and it is not possible to feel the same forward placement or resonance experienced with the nasals or glide with an open sound that has minimal back pressure. During these tokens, the patient *thinks* the glide on to the vowel to facilitate a feeling of flow and fluidity that facilitates easy, gentle onset of the vowel. The phrases in **Box 6-5** may be practiced in the same turn-taking format. You may gradually extend the length of the utterance. Again, the activity is created to produce memory traces and build stability into the productions.

As your patient progresses to a semi-structured format, you may introduce variation to the procedure and increase the cognitive load by asking questions that can be answered with overlearned information such as family names, addresses, or phone numbers. In this initial phase, the topics should be neutral and require little reasoning or original thought because the question-answer format itself increases the cognitive load and the difficulty of maintaining attention to the sensory feedback. We continue to precede phrases with the /mhm/ to set the larynx up for efficient phonation and encourage the patient to attend to the vibratory feedback from the resonating chamber.

As you make a transition from semi-structured to spontaneous speech, the incorporation of prosody increases the cognitive demand. It is not uncommon for patients to adjust pace and/or use monopitch or monoloud patterns and unusual pauses or prosody while attempting

Box 6-5

Sample Phrases Incorporating Vowel-Initiated Words

Hypotheses and Short-Term Goal	Procedure
• The /mhm/ sets the larynx up for an appropriate manner of phonation during connected speech. • The open vocal tract during production of vowels diminishes back pressure significantly. • The patient will think the glide onto the vowel in order to establish flow and easy onset of phonation.	Within the turn-taking structure, the patient imitates the clinician's manner of phonation while echoing phrases incorporating vowel-initiated words (e.g., "on and on," "over and over," "apples and oranges," "apricots and apples," "I eat apricot ice cream," "I appreciate the Aegean," "over the Atlantic Ocean," "I always enjoy artichokes," "I enjoy almonds and olives"). Clinician: "/mhm/, /mhm/," *<easy breath> <think /j/>* "On and on." Patient: "/mhm/, /mhm/," *<easy breath> <think /j/>* "On and on." Clinician: "/mhm/, /mhm/," *<easy breath> <think /j/>* "Over and over." Patient: "/mhm/, /mhm/," *<easy breath> <think /j/>* "Over and over."

Nota bene: The patient is encouraged to attend to the vibrations of the /mhm/ and to note if the onset of the vowel is smooth or begins abruptly as he *thinks* the glide onto the vowel. The vibrations experienced on the vowels are not as strong as those felt on the nasals and glides.

to acquire and stabilize new motor patterns. You can integrate prosody into your procedure by adding an emotional context to your phrases (e.g., happy, sad, frightened), various accents (e.g., British, western, southern), or a communicative goal (e.g., to seduce, to explain, to threaten) to the description of an object.

The hierarchy of complexity increases when the patient demonstrates an easy manner of phonation across the spectrum of phonemes you have chosen. You then move from a structured to a semi-structured format, adding linguistic complexity, while still incorporating back pressure to prepare the larynx for easy phonation. Until this point, the patient simply has repeated phrases from the clinician's model. Now the patient is responsible not only for monitoring the manner of phonation, but creating the phrase himself as well as incorporating resonance. Given that it is impossible to think about content and technique simultaneously, you will continue to use the /mhm/ in this series to provide a physiologic set up *prior* to production of a phrase. Your effective model of the procedure remains critical to the patient's capacity to integrate the newly acquired motor patterns created by the semi-occluded vocal tract.

Semi-structured Format

In the following turn-taking interaction, an object is chosen for description and placed on the table between the clinician and patient. The clinician begins by producing /mhm/ twice, followed by a phrase that describes the object (e.g., "/mhm, mhm/, the pencil is made of wood"). The patient continues in the same vein, but must produce a different phrase from the one chosen by the therapist (e.g., "/mhm, mhm/, it needs to be sharpened"). The exchanges continue over five or six turn-taking sequences during which the patient focuses on integrating the feeling of vibration and flow developed in the previous, structured back pressure exercises as he creates each new description and strengthens his memory trace for the generalized motor program.

Although the following series in **Box 6-6** represents a very early stage of incorporating flow and kinesthetic awareness of vocal tract vibration in connected speech, and breath control would be minimal in this circumstance, you and your patient maintain a deliberate awareness of and a connection to the breath. It is at these times (when we introduce spontaneous speech) that any imbalance between

Box 6-6

Sample Semi-Structured Exercise (Description of an Object)

Hypotheses and Short-Term Goal	**Procedure**
• The /mhm/ sets the larynx up for an appropriate manner of phonation during connected speech. • To facilitate carryover of an appropriate manner of phonation during a semi-structured format with utterances of increasing complexity. • To consolidate the memory trace of resonant voice in a semi-structured context.	Within a turn-taking format, the clinician demonstrates an easy, resonant voice on all models. The patient then creates a new description of the object while using physiological empathy to imitate the clinician's manner of phonation. Clinician: "/mhm/, /mhm/," *<easy breath>* "The pencil is yellow." Patient: "/mhm/, /mhm/," *<easy breath>* "It has an eraser." Clinician: "/mhm/, /mhm/," *<easy breath>* "The pencil is sharp." Patient: "/mhm/, /mhm/," *<easy breath>* "The eraser is new." Clinician: "/mhm/, /mhm/," *<easy breath>* "The wood is smooth." Patient: "/mhm/, /mhm/," *<easy breath>* "The point is sharp."

Nota bene: During this series be sure to monitor integration of breath with phonation.

respiration and phonation would become evident. The structure of the procedure provides an opportunity for the patient to maintain an awareness of coordination between inhalation and exhalation during phonation, which will become more relevant as complexity increases and you transition to longer and more complex utterances.

As the exercise continues, it becomes increasingly difficult to create new descriptions, which places a greater cognitive demand on the patient's attention and makes the integration of flow and ease even more challenging and complex. Some inconsistency in manner of phonation is expected because the patient needs time to integrate your model and the increased cognitive load, which may negatively affect his deliberate attention to the targets.

If you observe that the patient has reached a level where vibratory awareness, ease, and flow are incorporated within this level of complexity, it is time to remove the /mhm/ as a preparatory set-up and engage in a simple conversation—perhaps using the question-answer format to restrict the length of the responses required from the patient (**Box 6-7**). A simple, straightforward conversation over five to six turns serves as another step toward generalization of the flow

Box 6-7

Sample Semi-Structured Exercise (Everyday Activities)

Hypothesis and Short-Term Goals	Procedure
• Random practice facilitates consolidation and transfer of motor patterns. • To increase the cognitive load by increasing linguistic demands. • To facilitate carryover of ease and efficiency during spontaneous speech.	Continuing the turn-taking format within a short conversation, the clinician asks simple questions while modeling an easy, resonant manner of phonation. The patient is encouraged to use physiological empathy to promote carryover. Clinician: "Have you purchased a bed-wedge yet?" Patient: "Yes, but I haven't used it." Clinician: "Is there something stopping you?" Patient: "I'm afraid it will be uncomfortable." Clinician: "It can take some time to acclimate to it." Patient: "Maybe I'll try it tonight." If the patient has difficulty integrating an appropriate manner of phonation, the "/mhm/, /mhm/" can be inserted prior to each response.

Nota bene: Renew the patient's focus on the sensation of the flow under the hard palate and the alveolar ridge.

and ease you hope your patient will eventually use automatically. The hierarchy of complexity continues to increase as you create procedures that pertain to topics corresponding to your patient's interests, occupation, and lifestyle. It is useful to incorporate the linguistic and prosodic features most often used in the patient's daily life with the techniques developed over the course of treatment. Actors bring their scripts to sessions, lawyers bring their opening statements to the court, and telemarketers rehearse their selling routines—all with the purpose of making these newly acquired motor patterns their own. The patient continues to consciously focus on the tactile-kinesthetic feedback in order to maximize stability of the motor pattern and continue to build the generalized motor program. Further, the semi-structured context provides the opportunity not only to integrate the technique you hope to solidify, but a context within which you can obtain information relevant to the therapeutic program (e.g., "Are you taking your anti-reflux medication?") (see Box 6-7).

Modification of Hypothesis

Semi-occlusion of the vocal tract provides the physiological foundation for the sample hierarchy of procedures described in the previous sections. The various stages of the process may be accomplished in a straightforward manner or may be complicated by the patient's difficulty understanding the procedures, connecting with the concept of physiological empathy, deliberately focusing on the resonant feedback, or even limited awareness of the sensations in the vocal tract that facilitate a more appropriate placement for the voice. Furthermore, the severity of a laryngeal pathology may preclude phonation on any of the back pressure exercises that are followed by a phrase. When the patient's response to the procedures does not support your hypothesis, it is necessary to modify or reject that hypothesis. Certainly, there are many possible ways to modify an effortful pattern of production. We have chosen several responses (Dialogues 6-2 and 6-3) in order to illustrate the process of critical reasoning within hypothesis testing and modification.

Facilitation of Awareness of Vibratory Sensations

During the early stages of therapy with a patient who focuses on listening to his voice rather than feeling the effort he uses to produce voice, you develop hypotheses that will, in a direct and perhaps concrete manner, facilitate a shift in the patient's attention from listening to feeling.

This seemingly small shift in the patient's awareness actually represents a paradigmatic shift from an auditory to a kinesthetic focus. Your patient may have sought therapy because of the way his voice sounds. The customary speaker may find it "weird" to attend to the sensations in the vocal tract. On the other hand, a singer is most often accustomed to attending to these sensations during singing, but not necessarily during speech, and might make the transition more easily. Straw phonation, lip and tongue trills, and the airway reflex exercise are useful procedures to quickly achieve this goal. The session excerpt presented in **Dialogue 6-2** illustrates the difficulty that can be encountered when attempting to facilitate this paradigmatic shift.

Dialogue 6-2
Hypothesis Modification in Real Time: Facilitation of Awareness of Vibratory Sensations

Mr. G demonstrates a moderate dysphonia characterized by moderate roughness, mild stridency and breathiness, frequent abrupt initiations, limited loudness range, and apparent, general extraneous muscle activity in the head, neck, and thorax. According to the otolaryngologist, he has a small, unilateral vocal fold nodule on his right vocal fold. He participated in a voice evaluation and several therapy sessions that focused on creating a semi-occluded vocal tract. Following the assessment and each therapy session, he was encouraged to do home practice with /mhm/ and attend to the sensations in the nose and lips. The following excerpt is part of his first voice therapy session following the evaluation. The clinician reviews the instructions for the back pressure exercise and asks Mr. G to copy the clinician's model of an easy manner of production, while attending to the sensations in the lips, nose, and mouth.

The following hypothesis guides the procedure: deliberate attention to the sensations in the vocal tract following increased back pressure and inertance will decrease the medial compression of the vocal folds to optimize coordination among the subsystems and facilitate a more appropriate manner of phonation.

Modeling a quiet, resonant voice on each trial, I began the sequence of back pressure exercises, "I want you to consciously focus on the sensations in your lips and nose and say /mhm/."

Mr. G: "/mhm/," *with an abrupt initiation of phonation on both syllables and apparent extraneous muscle activity in the head, neck, and thorax.*

Nota bene: The clinician assesses each production, but does not necessarily give feedback on each token.

Clinician: "/mhm/."

Mr. G: "/mhm/," *similar effortful phonation.*

Clinician: "/mhm/."

Mr. G: "/mhm/," *again with effort.*

Clinician: "/hu/."

Mr. G: "/hu/," *with abrupt onset on both syllables and extraneous muscle activity in the face, neck, and shoulders.*

I repeat the sequence four more times and the effort levels do not diminish over the four turns. I want to know if he is aware of the effort and the abrupt onsets. In an attempt to focus his attention on the sensations in the vocal tract, I say, "What do you feel?"

Mr. G uses a rough, strident, pressed voice, "It sounded bad."

Recognizing the high effort levels and wanting to direct his attention to the sensation in his vocal tract, I confirmed his assessment and asked, "Yes, your voice is rough, but how did it feel?"

Mr. G did not modify the high level of effort when he responded, "I don't understand what you mean by feel."

Attempting to clarify, "Did you focus on the vibrations in your lips and nose? Did it feel easy? Did you push to get voice or did you just let it happen?"

Continuing with high effort levels and abrupt initiations, Mr. G said, "Of course I was pushing. It is the only way I can get my voice out."

I noticed a big increase in the effort he was using to make voice and realized that he did not understand the purpose of the exercise, "I know it seems awkward to change the focus from hearing to feeling, but this is an effective way to reduce the effort in your throat and allow your vocal folds to vibrate more efficiently. Does your throat get tired?"

With continued effort, Mr. G admits, "It is pretty good in the morning, but it gets tired around 1:00."

I consider that we have been working to establish deliberate attention to the resonating cavity for two sessions and are having limited success, so I shift to a new hypothesis: higher back pressure and inertance created by straw phonation will facilitate a decrease in the medial compression of the vocal folds and a more appropriate manner of phonation. Giving the patient a straw, "We are going to increase the pressure above your vocal folds and take it away from your throat in another way. I want you to produce sound through the straw, like this." (Demonstration of easy /u/ phonation through the straw.)

With a reduction in effort, Mr. G produces easy phonation through the straw.

Nodding, "What did you feel?"

Continued mild reduction in effort, Mr. G states, "It sounded weird."

Refocusing him to the kinesthetic feedback, "Yes, it is strange. It is similar to the sound of a steam ship horn in the fog. How did it feel?"

Drawing his eyebrows together, frowning, Mr. G phonates through the straw again, "I felt a buzz through the straw."

"Great! Did you feel a buzz anyplace else? The next time you try it, see if you feel vibration in your fingers as you hold the straw, almost as if the voice is coming from outside of your head."

Smiling, Mr. G lifts his eyebrows and phonates /u/ through the straw again, "Wow, I feel a buzz in my lips and a little bit in my fingers. How did I do that?"

"The vibrations have been there all along. You were just unaware of them. When we focus our awareness on feeling, we notice it. Try it again and deliberately focus on the feelings in your lips."

Mr. G phonates through the straw, "Wow, I really felt them that time."

Capitalizing on his incipient, kinesthetic awareness, "Great! Now, play with that buzzing and see if you can make the vibrations bigger and smaller. You can change the pitch, tighten or loosen your lips, and get louder or quieter. Just play with the sound for a few minutes."

Mr. G shrugs and phonates through the straw again with various loudness and pitch changes.

Pursuing the proprioceptive focus, "What did you feel?"

Dropping his gaze, Mr. G seems to reflect on the production, "I felt vibrations in my lips and tongue. It is weird, but they seem to get bigger when I soften my lips."

Thrilled that the patient found this on his own, "Yes, when you let go and do not tighten your lips, tongue, or jaw, the air is freer to move and the vibrations are stronger. I know that it is counterintuitive, but less is more. Now let's try it again and continue to focus on the vibrations."

Chuckling, looking somewhat bemused, and then dropping his gaze as though he is focusing inward on the sensations, Mr. G phonates through the straw.

Noting the easy, continuous, resonance from the vibrations, "What did you feel?"

Mr. G lowers his eyes as though he is recalling the sensations and using reduced expiratory drive, "It feels funny. I feel vibrations in my lips, nose, and top of my mouth. Is that right? Should they be there all the time?"

"Yes, you just need to deliberately focus to feel them." *Going to the next step,* "When you just answered me, you used an easy, resonant voice. Now, let's pair the straw phonation with /mhm/. I want you to phonate through the straw and then remove the straw and say /mhm/ using the same easy level, feeling the continued vibrations, like this." *I demonstrate phonating /u/ through the straw by removing the straw, and then producing /mhm/ in a quiet, resonant voice.*

Slowly putting the straw in his mouth, Mr. G phonates through the straw, and then produces /mhm/ with ease.

Perceiving the continuation of the resonance in both the straw phonation and /mhm/, I ask, "What did you feel?"

With a curious smile, Mr. G says, "I feel vibrations in my lips, nose, and top of my mouth on both."

Noticing resonance in his speech, "That is great! Let's do some more."

Nota bene: The clinician repeatedly cued the patient to deliberately attend to the sensations in the vocal tract during this procedure.

All of the following **semi-occluded maneuvers** create high back pressure and generate inertance. Often, when these maneuvers are introduced independently or immediately prior to the /mhm/ they lead to an enhanced sensation of resonance. The speaker experiences the positive effects of the semi-occluded vocal tract as a notable decrease in effort and a more resonant voice quality.

Early in the rehabilitation process, the patient may be uncertain as to where he should expect to experience the vibratory sensations that occur with increased back pressure and inertance. He may wonder whether there is a "correct" place in the vocal tract to feel them because they seem ephemeral. During straw phonation, he may be aware of vibration in the lips or in the fingers while he holds the straw. The nasal sounds (/m/ and /n/) facilitate awareness of vibration in the lips, nose, or hard palate, but with other consonants and vowels the vibratory feedback may be minimal or absent. The procedures listed in **Box 6-8** can be used to facilitate attention to the resonance in the nose and lips.

The inclusion of nonspeech, back pressure, and inertance exercises facilitates awareness of resonant voice production. You may find it helpful to alternate between the maneuvers, because each one encourages tactile-kinesthetic awareness in slightly different locations to facilitate resonance. A patient may find some maneuvers to be more effective than others at enhancing resonance. These semi-occluded procedures also release stiffness in specific structures (lips, tongue, jaw) and encourage freedom of movement throughout the vocal tract to set the system up for easy vibration. If the patient has difficulty feeling vibrations, it may be because he is stiffening his lips, tongue, jaw, and shoulders. As he releases these structures the vibrations may

Box 6-8

Selected Voiced Semi-occluded Maneuvers

Hypotheses and Short-Term Goals	Procedures
• The high back pressure generated by these procedures is especially effective in reducing medial compression of the vocal folds and supralaryngeal stiffness. • The high back pressure generated by these procedures facilitates an increased awareness of the vibrations in the head (lips, tongue, hard palate, larynx) and encourages an easy manner of phonation. • To enhance discrimination between ease and effort. • The patient will rely on kinesthetic feedback to attend to vibration in the lips, tongue, hard palate, pharynx, larynx, and upper thorax.	The clinician models the following procedures: phonation through a straw, voiced Puffy Cheek Exercise, lip kazoo, voiced raspberries, voiced lip and tongue trills, voiced gargle.

Nota bene: These procedures have no linguistic significance. They set up the system for an easy manner of phonation and should be followed by connected speech.

Box 6-9

Decrease Extraneous Muscle Activity

Hypotheses and Short-Term Goal	Procedures
• Extraneous muscle activity in the head, neck, and thorax negatively affects voice production. • Awareness of muscle stiffness is a necessary precursor to implementing strategies that effect change. • Contrasting stiffness with release facilitates recognition of ease versus effort. • The patient will discriminate between stiffness and the freedom to act during procedures that facilitate heightened kinesthetic feedback.	The patient performs the following procedures and then describes what he feels: • Clench and release the hands • Compress and release the lips • Clench and release the jaw • Press tongue tip against the roof of the mouth and release • Extend the tongue as far as possible and produce /heI/, /hi/, /haI/, /ho/, /hu/ • Perform the Masako swallowing technique (swallow with tongue protruded)

Nota bene: These exercises may release long-standing stiffness in the vocal tract.

become more palpable and widespread throughout his vocal tract. The exercises listed in **Box 6-9** contrast a consciously stiffened posture with a more released one to develop sensory awareness.

High Transglottal Pressure Drop and Intermittent Aphonia

Phonotrauma occurs when a high transglottal pressure drop and excessive medial compression of the vocal folds result in abrupt initiation of phonation. With persistent hyperadduction of the vocal folds and its resulting trauma, intermittent aphonia is not unusual. If a lesion develops, adding weight to the vocal fold cover, initiation of phonation will require a matching increase in subglottal pressure. If the subglottal pressure is reduced (by decreasing excessive expiratory drive and loudness), the transglottal pressure drop may no longer exceed the 3 to 4 cm H_2O necessary to initiate phonation, and the voice may become aphonic. Aphonic productions are disconcerting and may be even frightening to some patients, and intermittent aphonia may be the symptom that prompts your patient to seek voice treatment. Typically, a new patient will be extremely uncomfortable if you suggest that he permit his voice to be aphonic during a **back pressure** exercise. His automatic response will be to stiffen the vocal folds and push his voice. But if he continues to push the system beyond its capability, if he continues to *demand* sound, the existing lesion will probably worsen. Inflammation may increase, swelling may increase, and the excessive medial compression he uses to produce voice may exacerbate the overall voice problem.

The patient will be unaware of the delicate balance between expiratory drive and medial compression of the vocal folds. When you ask him to decrease vocal intensity (expiratory drive) and focus on the sensations in the vocal tract, he will, almost certainly, become aphonic and his anxiety will be activated. It takes high levels of self-control and self-efficacy to follow the clinician's instructions and to allow the tokens to be aphonic. You can support self-control and self-efficacy by explaining that the goal of these procedures is to reduce effort and allow the larynx to release. The clinical reasoning and hypothesis development and revision used in this situation is explored in **Box 6-10**.

Box 6-10

High Transglottal Pressure Drop and Intermittent Aphonia

Your patient demonstrates a moderate-to-severe dysphonia characterized by severe roughness and stridency, mild breathiness, frequent abrupt initiations, limited pitch and loudness range, and apparent, general extraneous muscle activity in his head, neck, and thorax. He reports having frequent episodes of aphonia in the early morning and in the evening for the past three weeks. He says, "It's a lot of work to talk now." According to the otolaryngologist, he has bilateral vocal fold nodules, inflammation, and edema.

Therapeutic Hypothesis	Testing the Hypothesis	Outcome
A decrease in excessive expiratory drive, vocal fold stiffness, and medial compression facilitates a more appropriate manner of phonation.	You ask the patient to copy your easy model of /mhm/, /mhm/, /hu/, and attend to the sensations in his nose and lips. The /mhm/, /mhm/ increases back pressure and decreases the transglottal pressure drop. The /hu/ decreases the medial compression of the vocal folds.	During the first trial, he initiates /mhm/ abruptly and louder than expected. His production of /hu/ begins appropriately, but the vowel is aphonic. The second and third trials of /mhm/ remain effortful and the /hu/ continues to be aphonic.

Physiological Rationale

Why would this happen? The loud production of the /mhm/ with the abrupt onset of phonation suggests that there is excessive vocal fold resistance and buildup of subglottal air pressure that results in a high transglottal pressure drop (abrupt onset) with large excursions of the vocal folds, which result in loud phonation.

The aphonic vowel during the production of /hu/ suggests that the decreased medial compression triggered by the voiceless consonant resulted in a decrease in the transglottal pressure drop. The transglottal pressure drop on the /hu/ was below that needed to initiate vibration of the vocal folds. Consequently, the /u/ was aphonic.

You realize that at this point in the process while swelling or inflammation exists, aphonia is probably the only possible outcome when the transglottal pressure drop decreases. You know that the way to reduce swelling and inflammation is to decrease the excessive collision forces, and so you proceed. Given your fund of knowledge of normal and disordered voice production, you modify your hypothesis to include the following rationale.

(*continues*)

Box 6-10 (*continued*)

Modified Therapeutic Hypothesis	Testing the Hypothesis	Outcome
Patient will become aphonic if he decreases the transglottal pressure drop, vocal fold stiffness, and medial compression of the vocal folds.	You continue in a turn-taking format with the /mhm, mhm, hu/ exercise. You ask the patient to allow the larynx to do what it wants to do, and explain that the larynx may not make sound on each syllable when he reduces effort. Most patients are uncomfortable with this at first. You ask him to note the air passing through the nose and lips. Reassure him that the vocal folds are still moving and that mild exercise reduces swelling (intermittent aphonia is common when there is vocal fold swelling and inflammation).	During the following trials, /mhm/ is aphonic. His production of /hu/ begins appropriately, but the vowel is aphonic. The patient appears to be uncomfortable.

The patient in **Dialogue 6-3** is having difficulty accepting that aphonia during the back pressure exercise represents a beneficial modification, and that this new, easier manner of phonation will facilitate a reduction in the swelling of the vocal folds that was reported by the otolaryngologist. The patient is intent on making phonation on each trial and is uncomfortable with the tokens that are aphonic. Your acknowledgment that it takes time for the system to modify an old habit provides encouragement during this early phase of the process.

Dialogue 6-3
High Transglottal Pressure Drop and Intermittent Aphonia

The following dialogue is an excerpt from an early session with Mr. H who demonstrates the moderate-to-severe dysphonia described in Box 6-10. He reports periods of aphonia during the afternoon and then some improvement in the voice later in the evening. He is concerned that he will lose his job if his voice does not improve. Although Mr. H is easily frustrated, he reports that he is eager to make progress. We pick up in the middle of the third session. . .

Attempting to direct Mr. H's focus to the sensory feedback from easy manner of phonation and an easy, resonant voice, "Let's try the /mhm/, /mhm/, /hu/ again. I want you to do less. Don't demand voice. Allow your throat to do what it wants. It may feel like you are doing nothing, but that's what we want."

With similar high levels of effort, Mr. H participates in the turn-taking format again and we complete three turns.

I ask, "How did those feel?"

Mr. H responds, "I don't know. My voice kept stopping."

"I felt that one of your /mhm/ tokens was quite easy, but the other two seemed effortful. Did you feel any differences between them?"

Almost in a truculent tone and with increased effort and stridency, Mr. H grunted, "Yes, the second one was easier, but I didn't get sound on that one."

Acknowledging his frustration and recognizing that he might be contemplating change, but not be ready for change, "I think I understand what you mean. It can be very awkward when you don't hear anything because that is how you have always judged your voice. I'm asking you to change your focus to feeling when you're so used to listening to your voice."

Definitely in a truculent tone, Mr. H barked, "Well, you get sound when we do it together, so why don't I?"

He is committed to auditory feedback and doesn't trust the kinesthetic shift. Remaining unflappable, I take a slightly different approach and provide some information, "I think it's because your vocal folds are a bit irritated, and in order to make sound you have to push to make them vibrate. When you don't push for sound, the vocal folds move, but do not necessarily touch all the time and sometimes you don't get sound. Mild exercise is good to reduce swelling, and this easy manner of production represents mild exercise. When you don't close the vocal folds so tightly, the inflammation has a chance to subside, which is what we want."

Mr. H paused for a long time, and then in an incredulous tone he asked, "So you're saying it's better if I don't get sound?"

His confusion was apparent. Was he merely resistant to the idea of focusing on the vocal sensations, was he unable to feel the kinesthetic differences, or was it something else? "No, I'm saying that 'sound' isn't the target, one way or the other. If you get sound without effort that's fine, but if you have to push and use effort in order to make sound we're on the wrong track. The focus is on how it *feels*, not how it *sounds*. You may feel the gentle flow of air through your nose."

Mr. H looked skeptical and massaged his stiff neck, "I keep getting to the place where if I just go a little further I will get sound, and I can't stop myself from doing that because I should be able to get sound."

Checking to see if I understand his meaning, "It sounds like you think you are doing something wrong if you don't get sound. Is that true?"

Mr. H sighed, "Well, if I did it better, I would get sound."

Recognizing his frustration, "It is really frustrating to have this kind of voice problem. I know that it is awkward when you don't hear your voice, but allowing your throat to do only as much as it can is how you reduce the irritation. When you allow that to happen your voice may break. This exercise isn't about *doing*; it's about *feeling* the difference between ease and effort."

Mr. H nods reluctantly.

"Let's try another one to see if you can dial down the effort. I don't care about sound." *I model an easy, resonant /mhm/, and he follows with an easy production that is aphonic.* "Wow! That was great. I would like you to do another one just like that. Everything was balanced and easy. Keep dialing down the effort."

Mr. H nods and we do three more tokens. Two of them are effortless and aphonic.

Reduction of Medial Compression of the Vocal Folds

The hypothesis development and modification described in **Box 6-11** reflects the clinical reasoning and formulation of an additional alternative to addressing the behaviors associated with excessive expiratory drive, vocal fold stiffness and medial compression, and a high transglottal pressure drop. The goal of the procedures is to facilitate a gentle onset of phonation by incorporating a voiceless phoneme at the

Box 6-11

Reduction of Medial Compression of the Vocal Folds

Your patient has a severe dysphonia characterized by severe roughness and stridency, moderate breathiness, frequent abrupt initiations, limited loudness range, and apparent, general extraneous muscle activity in the head, neck, and thorax. He reports frequent episodes of aphonia throughout the day over the past six months and difficulty with prolonged speaking. He avoids speaking on the telephone whenever possible and complains of a mild ache in his throat following these conversations. According to the otolaryngologist, he has large, well-defined, bilateral vocal fold nodules.

You demonstrate an easy production of /mhm/, /mhm/, /hu/ with a slight downward inflection. When the procedure is performed in the turn-taking format the patient produces the /mhm/ tokens with abrupt onsets, but the /hu/ is produced with gentle airflow on the /h/ and an easy initiation of the vowel. Your knowledge of the physiology of normal voice production and the perceptual consequences of inefficient manner of phonation remind you that voiceless sounds in the initial position are made with slightly abducted vocal folds, permitting air to pass through the glottis without vibration. You hypothesize that the patient will produce voice with less effort if he decreases adduction of the vocal folds and stiffness in the vocal tract. When you note considerable reduction in abrupt onset and an increase in easy onset of phonation, you accept your hypothesis. It is appropriate to explore other /h/-initiated syllables followed by a vowel to see if a similar reduction in effort is noted. The next phase introduces short phrases that begin with the aspirated sound (e.g., "Who are you?" "How are you?" "Where are you?"), followed by short phrases that combine voiced and voiceless phonemes. You can introduce many intermediate tasks by simply modeling the procedure rather than discussing each procedure in detail.

Therapeutic Hypothesis	Testing the Hypothesis	Outcome
A decrease in medial compression of the vocal folds will facilitate a more appropriate manner of phonation.	You ask the patient to copy your easy model of /hu/ and attend to the sensation of the air flowing across the tongue and through the lips. The /hu/ decreases the medial compression of the vocal folds.	During the first trial of /hu/ the vowel is initiated smoothly. The second and third trials are similar to the first.

Physiological Rationale

Why would this happen? The easy onset of the vowel during production of /hu/ suggests that the decreased medial compression of the vocal folds triggered by the aspirated sound leads to a decrease in the transglottal pressure drop. The lowered transglottal pressure drop is appropriate for quiet phonation. You accept your hypothesis and expand it to include other voiceless fricatives (e.g., /h/, /s/, /f/, /θ/).

Box 6-12

Selected Voiceless Semi-Occluded Maneuvers

Hypothesis and Short-Term Goal	Procedures
• The high back pressure generated by these procedures is especially effective in reducing supralaryngeal stiffness. • To enhance discrimination between ease and effort.	The clinician models the following procedures: blowing through a hollow stir-straw, Airway Reflex Exercise, voiceless Puffy Cheek Exercise, voiceless raspberries, voiceless lip and tongue trills, voiceless gargles.

Nota bene: These maneuvers have no linguistic significance. They can be practiced hourly to consolidate a more efficient motor pattern.

Chapman, 2012; Titze, 1994

beginning of a word or phrase. We remain attentive to the patient's responses in order to modify the hypothesis when necessary, and reorganize the procedure to enhance kinesthetic awareness (feeling versus listening).

All of the following maneuvers in **Box 6-12** are voiceless, produced with partially abducted vocal folds and a semi-occluded vocal tract. The resulting high back pressure can be used to set up the vocal tract for easy phonation on other voice procedures in therapy. They serve as an excellent warm-up prior to auditions, singing lessons, rehearsals, and performances. These maneuvers may be alternated with their voiced cognates when laryngeal control has improved.

Breath Control

To Intervene or Not to Intervene—That Is the Question

Given the complexity and intricate interplay between the inspiratory and expiratory musculature, it is no surprise that the physiology and application of breath control has received a great deal of attention in the speaking literature. Opinions vary as to whether clinicians should or should not address breathing as part of their voice rehabilitation program. Some believe that breathing is spontaneous, natural, and part of an automatic process that requires no special attention, and others propose that the unique demands made on the respiration system—changing linguistic environments and rapid and irregular shifts in rhythm, stress, and intonation—warrant training.

Within the context of voice rehabilitation and the coordination between respiration and phonation, the common counterproductive strategies used by patients to cope with negative changes and imbalances often manifest as excessive expiratory drive (subglottal pressure) or pressed phonation (insufficient airflow). If we take into account the demands made on the respiratory system by high elastic recoil forces during the initial phases of exhalation, as well as the consequences of an inappropriate manner of phonation (poor coordination among the subsystems), formal attention to the efficient coordination between respiration and phonation is frequently an implicit part of the rehabilitation process.

In the *Jaw Stiffness and Breath Control* video, the patient complains that she has always struggled with maintaining adequate breath support. She recognizes stiffness in her jaw that has a negative effect on her singing voice.

Development of Breath Control

If your voice therapy program includes the development of appropriate abdominal control, the physiological rationales for your chosen procedures must be considered. Under typical circumstances, for example, quiet breathing takes place without conscious awareness of the continuous flow from inspiration to expiration and back again. We often ask patients to breathe through the nose during structured breathing exercises in order to slow the inhalation phase and warm, filter, and moisten the air as it passes through the cilia in the nasal cavity. This pattern of inhalation is not practical during spontaneous conversation or singing, of course, when we take quick breaths through the mouth or both the nose and the mouth in order to fill the lungs rapidly, but breathing through the nose is useful in order to establish a more relaxed, efficient respiratory pattern (Chapman, 2012).

The following series of basic breathing exercises releases extraneous muscle activity in the upper airway and engages the abdominal muscles to coordinate breath flow with the voice. These introductory procedures establish a connection to a lower abdominal-diaphragmatic breathing pattern. Your patient may find an easier inhalation and greater release if you begin the exercises in **Box 6-13** by lying on the floor to observe the natural rise and fall of the abdomen.

The clinician in the *Basic Breathing Exercises: Transgender Voice Group* video guides the participants in the transgender voice group through three breathing exercises that facilitate the abdominal support necessary to project the voice efficiently.

The singer/voice teacher in the *Basic Breathing Exercises: The Singer* video uses these breathing exercises to warm-up before teaching her students and before her performances.

Box 6-13

Basic Warm-up Breathing Exercises

Hypotheses and Short-Term Goal	Procedures
• Checking action (activation of the muscles of inhalation) is necessary to manage excessive relaxation pressure. • Engagement of the muscles of exhalation permits efficient management of a prolonged exhalation phase. • The patient will increase the exhalation phase in steps from 10, to 15, to 20 seconds. • The patient will attend to the active engagement of the abdominal musculature as he exhales slowly.	1. Take an easy breath through the nose (remember, breathing through the nose warms, moistens, and filters the air), release the jaw, and exhale on an easy sigh (think voiceless /a/). Your throat should feel open (similar to a yawn) as you exhale. There should be no turbulent sound during the expiration phase. Repeat this step three times. 2. Take an easy breath through the nose and exhale on the /s/ phoneme until you are comfortably out of air. The /s/ provides a resistance at the teeth that extends the exhalation phase. Actively focus on feeling the connection with the abdomen that the resistance at the teeth facilitates. This is the first step in feeling control and coordination. Repeat this step three times. 3. Take an easy breath through the nose, bring the lips forward into an /u/ phoneme, and exhale slowly (and silently) for 20 seconds. You will focus on feeling how the abdominal muscles resist the impulse to collapse. You are now using your expiratory muscles to control your rate of exhalation. Repeat this step three times. These breathing exercises should be practiced twice daily.

Over time, ease and duration of the sustained breath will increase. You can pair these exercises with speech in order to carry over the awareness of ease and flow into conversation. Initially, serial speech (e.g., counting, days of the week, and months of the year) provides a straightforward, introductory exercise during which the patient integrates abdominal control.

Nota bene: If the patient has difficulty decreasing excessive expiratory drive during Step 3, it is useful to hold a tissue at its upper edge in front of the face during exhalation with the intent of keeping the tissue as still as possible. The visual feedback provided by the tissue facilitates the implementation of checking action and the abdominal control necessary to slow the expiratory phase.

You may have a patient who speaks in vocal fry or whose voice fades into vocal fry toward the end of an utterance. This phenomenon may be motivated culturally or socially and has been observed more frequently in female speakers (Abdelli-Beruh, Wolk, & Slavin, 2014). **Vocal fry (pulse register)** is associated with limited airflow. In **Box 6-14**, a three-step procedure demonstrates the process of initiating and sustaining the respiratory energy necessary to support modal phonation during prolonged utterances.

Box 6-14

Breath Control During Extend Utterances

Hypothesis and Short-Term Goal	Procedures
• Smooth transition between the implementation of checking action and the engagement of the expiratory musculature facilitates efficient prolongation of extended utterances. • The patient will monitor easy expansion of the abdomen and rib cage during inhalation and a slow, steady flow of air during production of utterances that increase in length and complexity. • The engagement of the muscles of exhalation becomes relevant as the individual approaches resting lung volume.	The following exercise is performed most effectively in a standing position. 1. Inhale through the nose, feeling an easy expansion of the abdomen and rib cage. 2. Imagine you will count to 10, but count only to 5, using a flowing, sustained voicing similar to intoning. Maintain a slightly lifted eye-gaze during phonation to enhance the feeling of the voice floating on the breath and carrying over a long distance. 3. Continue the exercise by adding a number until you reach 10 (count to 6, imagine counting to 11; count to 7, imagine counting to 12, and so on.).

Nota bene: Remind the patient to exhale following each series before initiating the next breath in order to avoid tightening in the thorax.

Breath Control and Loudness Inflection

The elusive and somewhat abstract nature of kinesthetic feedback, and the challenges associated with acquisition and consolidation of new motor patterns, may lead to a misinterpretation of sensory information. In his effort to reduce abrupt initiation of phonation the patient may simply reduce vocal intensity rather than attend to the sensations of coordination among the subsystems in order to achieve a more efficient vibratory pattern of phonation. He may become unduly careful and maintain a quiet phonation, continuing to listen rather than rely on the more effective kinesthetic feedback. Furthermore, the quiet phonation may be accompanied by limited expiratory drive, which often leads to pressed phonation. Modification of loudness with flow phonation, on the other hand, facilitates efficiency of vocal fold oscillation and reinforces a balance among the subsystems of voice production.

If loudness variation is not included as an inherent part of the therapeutic process, the patient may become fearful of and reluctant to implement loudness inflection. As you begin to incorporate loudness variation into your procedures, the coordination among the vocal subsystems becomes more complex. **Loudness control** requires a balance between subglottal air pressure and vocal fold resistance. Changes in loudness depend on the requirements of the voice task. If a conversational level of loudness is the target, for example, only ~7–8 cm H_2O are necessary. If ambient noise in a restaurant or a noisy street requires an increase in vocal intensity, possibly for an extended period, the subglottal pressure and glottal resistance will increase in tandem to permit sustained vocal volume without placing stress on the larynx. During the turn-taking format in **Dialogue 6-4**, the patient is encouraged to attend to the sensations in the vocal tract and make small adjustments in loudness inflection.

Dialogue 6-4
Breath Control and Loudness Inflection

When the patient consistently produces the back pressure exercise /mhm/ plus a short phrase, easily and efficiently, it is time to introduce loudness variation into the process.

During the first step the patient produces the /mhm/, /mhm/ followed by a short phrase at a level of loudness that is easy and effortless. The goal during this step is to feel resonance during production of the phrase.

With an easy model, "Now we will start working on loudness flexibility. I want you to copy my model and maintain the same ease on the production of the phrase 'Maybe on Monday' as you do on the /mhm/, /mhm/. Focus carefully on feeling the sensations in your nose, lips, and mouth."

Mr. I, using a resonant, conversational level of loudness, "/mhm/, /mhm/. Maybe on Monday."

"Was the phrase as effortless as the /mhm/, /mhm/?"

In an easy, resonant voice Mr. I said, "Yes, they both felt the same, and I could feel the vibrations in my nose."

"Great. I want you to say the /mhm/, /mhm/ the same way and reduce the loudness of the phrase by half, like this [conversational loudness] /mhm/, /mhm/, [half loudness] Maybe on Monday."

In conversational loudness, Mr. I produced "/mhm/, /mhm/," *and then in an easy, quiet voice*, "Maybe on Monday."

"How was that?"

With ease and a questioning inflection Mr. I stated, "It was weird. I had trouble thinking about the loudness and attending to the vibrations and flow. I think it was okay."

"Okay, now I want you to double the loudness on the phrase like this [conversational loudness] /mhm/, /mhm/, [twice the loudness] Maybe on Monday."

At the same conversational level, Mr. I produced, "/mhm/, /mhm/" *and in a louder voice,* "Maybe on Monday."

"That was really good. You kept the /mhm/ quiet and made the phrase louder. What did you feel on the phrase?"

We continue to alternate between *slightly* quieter and louder phrases, because at this juncture of the process the demands made on the subsystems should be small ones to facilitate control.

Nota bene: Due to the high nasal resonance, the vocal intensity of the /mhm/ will not increase substantially. The setup /mhm/ is used to facilitate easy production of the following phrase. It may be counterintuitive, but the quieter productions are more challenging and require more control than the louder ones.

When a sudden boost in loudness is required to shout, warn, or express extreme emotion, the balance between breath control and phonation becomes even more critical. However, if one can decrease the transglottal pressure drop by varying vocal tract configuration, one can increase it again. Indeed, one of the most impressive aspects of the voice production mechanism is the extreme flexibility of the components of the system, and their appropriate response to the almost constant changes that take place in each of the subsystems during an utterance. The **Ladder Exercise** described in **Box 6-15** illustrates one way to address loudness flexibility.

Ending Therapy

Planning for the end of treatment is a joint decision that requires sophisticated clinical skill (Hersh & Cruice, 2010), especially since there is no direct or single route to the end of the rehabilitation process. Ideally, the patient's expectations of therapy have been acknowledged and incorporated into the development of the goals, anticipated improvement, and the time expected to attain those goals.

"How long will this take?" is often the first question that a patient asks. Your answer depends on many factors, including the patient's adherence to the process, laryngeal pathology and severity of the dysphonia, the current demands on the voice, general health, obstacles to practice, and insurance coverage. Some or all of these considerations will influence your response to this question. While you want to be encouraging regarding the feasibility of the resolution of the voice problem, offering unrealistic expectations will not serve you or your patient's interests well.

As the treatment process unfolds, your understanding of the impact of the voice disorder on your patient's life, hopes, and aspirations deepens. For the patient who achieves a durable, flexible voice that meets all of his communication needs, including shouting and singing, the discharge process may be a straightforward one. As the

Box 6-15

Loudness Inflection Ladder Exercise

The Ladder Exercise begins at a quiet, conversational level (~7–8 cm H_2O), using a phrase that capitalizes on the resonating properties of the vocal tract. We use a turn-taking format that is similar to the one used during the back pressure with a phrase exercises described earlier in this chapter. The exercise incorporates four levels of vocal intensity that are imagined as the rungs on a ladder. As the patient climbs the loudness ladder vocal intensity increases from *quiet → medium loud → very loud, and then returns to the bottom rung, → quiet*. During this exercise it is essential that the patient focus his attention on the sensations of flow and resonance in order to maximize coordination among the subsystems.

The bottom rung (quiet) requires very little air pressure (breath control), and phonation occurs with flow and an awareness of the vibratory buzz described earlier. As vocal intensity increases to the second rung (medium loud), control and resonance are coordinated to produce phonation without laryngeal effort.

The medium loudness level of phonation is one used when we converse in a noisy restaurant, on the street, or subway platform, and requires a strong attention to the connection with the lower abdomen, as well as an increase in the resonant energy experienced by the speaker.

As the third rung (very loud) is reached, the deliberate attention to the balance between resonance and control becomes even more critical in order to avoid extreme laryngeal resistance and stress. This very loud phonation is one used less frequently in daily life, to warn of danger, express extreme anger, or to intimidate, and is not recommended for prolonged periods. The exercise concludes with a release of the control required for the previous trial, and a return to the first rung (quiet) and an easy, flowing manner of phonation. For the purpose of illustration, we will use the phrase, "Many men meet on Monday," but any phrase that includes phonemes with a high back pressure is appropriate during the introductory phase of the exercise. The patient matches each of the clinician's productions at each rung of the loudness ladder.

Nota bene: The Ladder exercise is postponed until the later phases of therapy, when the coordination among the subsystems is optimal.

Clinician: *In a quiet, resonant voice,* "Many men meet on Monday." (quietly)
Patient: "Many men meet on Monday." (quietly)
Clinician: "Many men meet on Monday." (medium loud)
Patient: "Many men meet on Monday." (medium loud)
Clinician: "Many men meet on Monday." (very loud)
Patient: "Many men meet on Monday." (very loud)
Clinician: "Many men meet on Monday." (quietly)
Patient: "Many men meet on Monday." (quietly)

As the patient becomes comfortable incorporating loudness within phrases initiated with phonemes that create a high supraglottal pressure, the complexity of the trials can increase with glides (e.g., /j/) and then vowel-initiated phrases.

Role-play, talking to peers at work, and talking with family and friends will facilitate transfer of loudness inflection. The first scenarios should be basic and straightforward and gradually move toward controversial topics.

During role-play of loud, emphatic utterances and shouts, it is useful to direct the patient's awareness to the sensations in the vocal tract (resonance) as well as to the additional control required from the muscles of expiration. These extreme levels of loudness often trigger unnecessary, extraneous muscle activity in the head, neck, and thorax. To disrupt this reactivated motor pattern, it may be sufficient to draw the patient's attention to it. Alternatively, he may now independently modify the behavior without direction from you.

We have found it useful to engage in conversation with the patient, increasing vocal intensity against a background of loud music played on the radio or a CD. During these interactions the clinician has an opportunity to observe the manner of phonation and intervene to modify effort, if necessary.

new voice patterns stabilize and generalize to more speaking situations, self-efficacy increases, and you move closer to the end of treatment. Therapy may decrease from once or twice weekly to once every two weeks, and then to once per month. If, during that last month, the new motor skills remain stable, discharge from therapy is an appropriate decision. In all likelihood this patient will complete treatment and sustain an effective manner of phonation without additional therapeutic support. Certainly, you will advise the patient that you are available to him if he encounters vocal problems in the future. It is possible that a laryngeal infection with a persistent cough may reactivate old patterns and effort, which may lead to vocal fatigue. If those problems do not resolve within a week, the patient should contact the otolaryngologist before the symptoms worsen and communicate with you for additional treatment, if necessary.

Some patients may not adhere to your treatment recommendations and may discontinue therapy before goals have been attained. It is difficult to know why this happens. As the transtheoretical model (TTM) of behavioral change suggests, there may be a mismatch between the patient's readiness for change and the initiation of treatment. The patient's unrealistic expectations, difficulty attending to sensory information, or lack of experience with any type of therapy may lead him to anticipate a rapid result and loss of interest when his expectations are not met. It may be that he does not adhere to the voice program and becomes impatient with his consequent limited progress. He may lack the tenacity, self-efficacy, and discipline required to participate in a process that requires his very active participation. The cessation of health insurance and relocation for a new job are other possible obstacles to a smooth rehabilitation program.

It can be frustrating when your patient discontinues treatment and does not let you know why. Regardless of the reason, you may feel that his abrupt departure is a reflection on you as a competent clinician. Even after many years of providing treatment for countless patients, self-discharge may be a threat to your self-efficacy. Disappointment and frustration are natural and human responses, however, and are a reflection of your commitment to resolution of the patient's voice problem. As is the case with all patients, if the treatment goals and discharge criteria are planned in collaboration, and you maintain an open, secure atmosphere within the treatment setting, your patient will more likely share his reservations regarding therapy.

It is sometimes the case that a clinically normal outcome is not possible due to an etiology that causes permanent or progressive changes in the larynx (e.g., laryngeal cancer). Spasmodic dysphonia, which is associated with a neurological disorder, can be treated with

botulinum toxin (BoNT) injections and behavioral therapy, but it, too, is chronic and permanent. Discharge criteria under these circumstances are quite different from those related to voice problems associated with muscle tension dysphonia or vocal fold nodules. During your early discussions, you clarify the patient's expectations for improvement and align them with your understanding of the nature of the problem and a realistic outcome that incorporates the patient's goals. The clinician walks a fine line between being a supportive, encouraging partner and maintaining a realistic attitude toward recovery. Irrespective of the anticipated outcome, you will find it helpful to discuss the end of treatment well before the day of discharge to jointly plan your final sessions and discontinue therapy gradually. For those patients who suffer from voice problems that will progressively worsen, adherence to the regimen developed in treatment will increase the likelihood of maintaining their gains. Even more central to these patients is the reassurance that they can contact you, if and when necessary (Hersh & Cruice, 2010).

The discussion in the *Practice as Needed* video emphasizes the importance of interspersing quick practices between the singing teacher's sessions with her students in order to provide periods of "cool down" and set the larynx up for the next hour of demonstration and explanation. In this final session, the patient and clinician discuss carryover and a realistic plan for managing her voice independently.

Summary

Your approach to the patient's voice problem is a function not only of your educational background and familiarity with the specialty of voice itself, but your preferred learning style, your familiarity with a chosen framework, your personal life experiences, and your confidence that the approach you select will effect the changes you seek. Your execution of a procedure will naturally differ from other clinicians, and will vary even with a specific patient depending on your goal within a given session or phase of the treatment process. As you gain clinical experience, you may introduce your own variation of an established procedure or develop a new one that you feel will better address the counterproductive patterns you observe. Furthermore, regardless of how effective you may deem a particular procedure, it will not work for all of your patients. Your patient may not understand the technique, trust it, or possess the necessary motor coordination to execute it easily and efficiently.

References

Abdelli-Beruh, N.B., Wolk, L., and Slavin, D. (2014). Prevalence of vocal fry in young adult male American English speakers. *Journal of Voice*, 28(2), 185–190.

Chapman, J. (2012). *Singing and teaching singing: A holistic approach to classical voice* (2nd ed.). San Diego, CA: Plural.

Ericsson, K.A., Krampe, R.T., and Tesch-Romer, C. (1993). The role of deliberate practice in the acquisition of expert performance. *Psychological Review*, 100(3), 363–406.

Hersh, D., and Cruice, M. (2010). Ending therapy. Beginning to teach the end: The importance of including discharge from aphasia therapy in the curriculum. *International Journal of Language and Communication Disorders*, 45(3), 263–274.

Lessac, A. (1997). *The use and training of the human voice: A practical approach to speech and voice dynamics* (3rd ed.). Santa Monica, CA: McGraw-Hill.

Rogers, C.R. (1951). *Client-centered therapy: Its current practice, implications, and theory.* Boston, MA: Houghton Mifflin.

Titze, I.R. (1983). The importance of vocal tract loading in maintaining vocal fold oscillation. Proceeding of the Stockholm Music Acoustics Conference SMAC 83 (Vol. 1). *Royal Swedish Academy of Music*, 46(2), 61–72.

Titze, I.R. (1988). The physics of small amplitude oscillation of the vocal folds. *Journal of the Acoustical Society of America*, 83(4), 1536–1552.

Titze, I.R. (1994). *Principles of voice production.* Denver, CO: National Center for Voice and Speech.

Titze, I.R. (2001). Acoustic interpretation of resonant voice. *Journal of Voice*, 15(4), 519–528.

Titze, I.R., and Story, B.H. (1997). Acoustic interactions of the voice source with the lower vocal tract. *Journal of the Acoustical Society of America*, 101, 2234–2243.

Titze, I.R., and Verdolini-Abbott, K.V. (2012). *Vocology: The science and practice of voice rehabilitation.* Salt Lake City, UT: The National Center for Voice and Speech.

van Leer, E., and Connor, N.P. (2010). Patient perceptions of voice therapy adherence. *Journal of Voice*, 24(4), 458–469.

Verdolini, K. (1998). *A guide to vocology.* Denver, CO: National Center for Voice and Speech.

Verdolini, K. (2000a). Resonant voice therapy. In J.C. Stemple (Ed.), *Voice therapy: Clinical studies* (2nd ed., pp. 46–61). San Diego, CA: Singular.

Wong, A.W., Whitehill, T.L., Ma, E.P., and Masters, R. (2013). Effects of practice schedules on speech motor learning. *International Journal of Speech Language Pathology*, 15(5), 511–523.

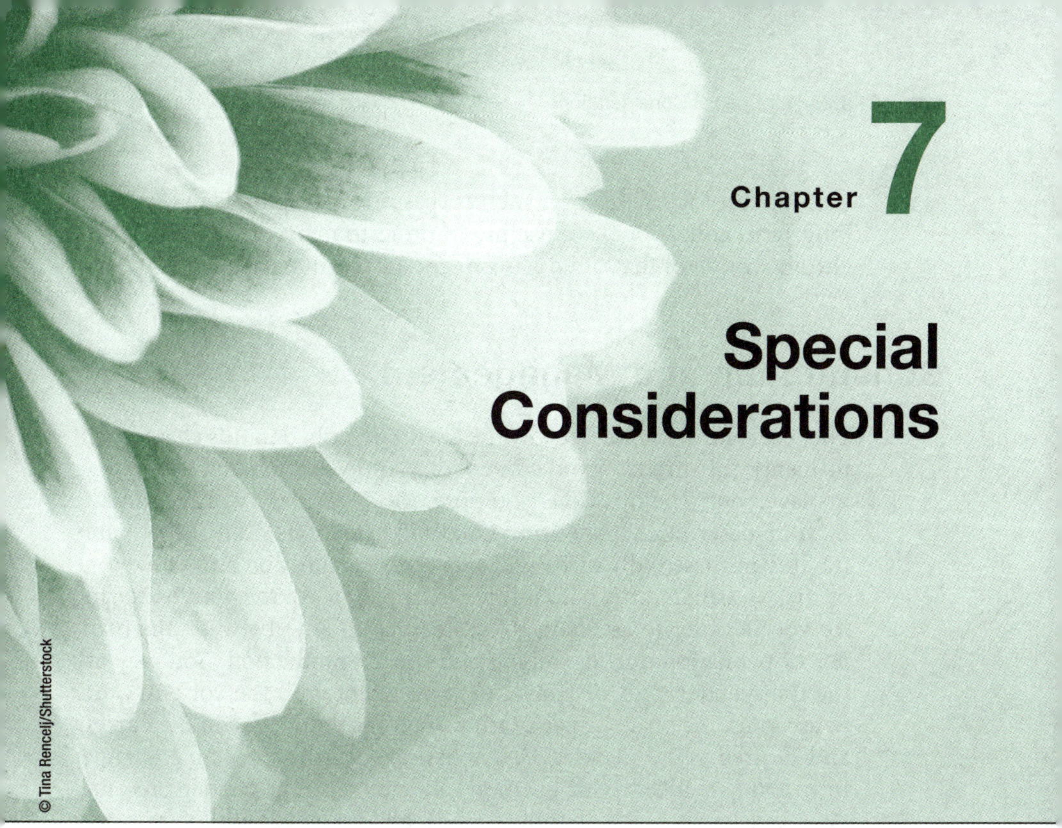

Chapter 7

Special Considerations

"Probably what it is is coordination . . . from the standpoint that you are not pressing in any one place, or forcing in any one area. It's like the really fine bowler . . . it's all in one motion. I had a teacher a long time ago . . . I was kind of tense . . . and he had me pretend to bowl while I was doing my vocalises. I would also pretend to be golfing . . . just something to keep me moving, the golf swing or the tennis swing. I learned to be in motion when I was singing, rather than being very static and rigid."
(McCracken, 1984, p. 157)

Although all of our patients require our clinical and counseling expertise, there are some challenging occupational, cultural, and psychological circumstances that make the work we do especially complex. The intricate interplay between artistic achievement and technical excellence, as well as the career stresses that the singer must manage, and the societal and life-changing stresses that the transsexual client encounters are two such examples. In addition, the patients who face the unpredictable voice disturbances associated with a neurological disorder such as spasmodic dysphonia may require long-term educational counseling in order to manage the stresses of a chronic problem that often has career and social consequences.

Consultation and Management

The disparate obstacles faced by the clients described in this chapter will influence the direction and content of your evaluation and subsequent management. The questions you pose, the vocabulary you incorporate in your descriptions, the individual's expectations, and the possible fragility of these individuals will alter the structure and emotional tone of the assessment. It is relevant, for example, to ask the vocalist to sing for you in order to ascertain the difference (if any) between the manner of phonation during singing and speech production. You may ask the transgender male or female to experiment with the voice in order to ascertain his or her capacity to easily transition between the current and desired vocal persona. A discussion regarding possible changes in mood associated with hormone therapy, current gender presentation, and acceptance by family, friends, and employer will offer insight into the client's relative ease or difficulty with the transition process (Rao, 1997). During diagnostic therapy with a patient who suffers from spasmodic dysphonia, you may provide counseling that addresses the challenges of living with a chronic disorder, provide information regarding the benefits and expected results of botulinum neurotoxin (BoNT) therapy, and explore his attitude toward medical intervention as well as the inclusion of individual therapy sessions to decrease observed compensatory behaviors. Your explanation of the available treatment options assists the patient in making an informed decision.

Counterproductive Behaviors

The singer, the transgender individual, and the patient with a neurological disorder such as spasmodic dysphonia often carry extraneous muscle activity in the head, neck, and upper torso. The clinician's goal is to replace these habituated patterns with a muscular balance that facilitates the freedom to act (Lessac, 1997). The presence of jaw and tongue base stiffness, shoulder rigidity, and misalignment of the neck and torso are especially troublesome when movement plays a crucial role in an effective and credible presentation, as is the case for the performer and transgender client. The professional voice user may fool you initially because he is capable of masking the stiffness he carries with performance values (personality, confidence, authority). When queried, however, the performer often reports problems associated with stiffness and its effect on the voice. The transgender individual may attempt to elevate or lower pitch with laryngeal and supraglottal constriction as well as stiffening of the jaw and tongue base. Given the differences between cisgender males and females with respect to fluidity of movement, the trans woman may require additional work to bring more grace and flexibility to her body if her current movement patterns do not meet the goals she has chosen for herself. In contrast, the trans male may feel that his presentation does not meet the criterion that he has set for a masculine presentation. Finally, patients suffering from **dystonia** often exhibit extraneous stiffness related to the underlying neurological disorder or compensatory stiffness in the head, jaw, neck, and thorax owing to the effort exerted to produce sound. Despite the positive effects of the BoNT injections, these compensatory behaviors may require time and patience to replace, particularly when they have become entrenched. Team collaboration with an otolaryngologist and a neurologist will enhance the effectiveness of the care you provide for this patient.

The Singer

"There is no uniform pattern of abdominal support that is relevant to all speakers and singers."

Many customary voice users identify the voice as a central part of the self; for the vocalist, the voice is the self and the profession. Fear of a chronic or permanent voice disturbance can be overwhelming. The special circumstances that the singer faces—the constant discipline necessary to build and maintain vocal health, learn multiple languages, integrate artistic excellence with technique, interpret musical text, and cope with the stress of auditions—represent ongoing challenges the professional voice user faces during a demanding career. Furthermore, the demands of travel and maintenance of general health require great resilience and tenacity, especially when a voice disorder places financial as well as emotional stress on the patient.

When the vocalist develops a voice problem, it may not be immediately obvious to the performer or voice teacher that the difficulty may be a result of the manner of speaking and unrelated to the singing technique. Even more confusing may be the absence of a laryngeal pathology, swelling, or inflammation when the singer visits the otolaryngologist. At these times it is appropriate to review the manner of phonation used during speech production.

Many of the singers we have treated demonstrate a beautifully integrated vocal technique during voice lessons, coaching, and performance, but do not generalize that technique to the speaking voice, especially in a noisy environment. They complain most frequently of vocal fatigue, laryngeal soreness, deterioration of voice quality with prolonged voice use, and fading at the ends of breath groups. It may be surprising that, given the demands made on the classical singer and the athletic prowess required to meet those demands, the speaking voice may become a source of disturbance, especially because the techniques used to enhance resonance are similar in singing and speech production (Tanner, Roy, Merrill, & Power, 2005). Nonetheless, the resonance techniques used to create the midfacial vibratory sensations during singing are not necessarily or automatically transferred to the production of speech. Although you may not work directly on the singing voice with your patient, your awareness of the similarities (and differences) between the singing and the speaking voice will contribute to the physiological appropriateness of your chosen procedures and your credibility as a voice clinician.

Self-administered questionnaires such as the Singing Voice Handicap Index (SVHI) (Cohen et al., 2007) and the Evaluation of the Ability to Sing Easily (EASE) (Phyland et al., 2013) provide information pertaining to the impact of the voice problem on the singer's occupational and personal daily life. If possible, the client should receive the questionnaire before the assessment to draw his attention to factors that may contribute to his voice problem. Your perusal of the individual's responses on the questionnaire as you begin the consultation brings your attention to specific areas that you might otherwise overlook.

The Singer's Lexicon

The voice clinician collaborates with many experts in order to provide a comprehensive treatment program for the singer. In addition to working with the voice teacher, we share information and gain insight from conductors, stage directors, psychologists, and specialists who work on posture and body alignment (e.g., physical therapy, Alexander, Feldenkrais, Pilates, osteopathy). When you work with a team to provide an integrated approach to voice rehabilitation, you enrich the therapeutic experience by developing special funds of knowledge that inform the decisions you make in partnership with the voice professional. The collaborative relationship is enhanced when you understand the vocabulary of the specialty that complements your work with the singer and coordinates your treatment with the relevant discipline.

If your work as a voice clinician includes rehabilitation of the singing voice it may be useful to expose yourself to the process of vocal training by taking voice lessons or observing your patient's voice lessons. The importance of the relationship between the clinician and the voice teacher cannot be overemphasized. The information and perspectives that you and the voice teacher share will make the rehabilitation process a multidimensional one for the professional singer and facilitate improvement of both the singing and speaking voice. Moreover, when you avail yourself of the opportunity to observe the singer during a voice lesson you become privy to the special communication between student and voice teacher. If you understand and integrate a vocabulary that is meaningful to the singer when you explain a technique, you will not only build a common ground, you will make the information more accessible. The kinesthetic sensibility of the singer is most often quite finely tuned and responsive to a vocabulary that is appreciably different from that of the speech-language pathologist.

It may be necessary at times to recommend a temporary interruption of singing lessons due to the severity of the voice disorder. You and the patient make this determination after discussing the effect of the speaking voice on singing, and keep the voice teacher apprised of progress and an estimation of when voice lessons may resume. It is not unusual for a voice teacher to have concerns, realistic or not, that the voice disturbance may be connected to the singing lessons. When such a situation arises, the collaboration between you and the vocalist's teacher may uncover possible counterproductive motor patterns that contributed to the presenting voice problem. In most instances, we have experienced great generosity and a willingness to cooperate with our efforts from all the professionals who participate concurrently in the care of our professional voice users.

The Role of Listening

Tactile-kinesthetic feedback plays a central role in the direction we believe voice rehabilitation should proceed for the attainment of a voice that easily, efficiently, and effectively communicates the music and message of the speaker. Nonetheless, the singer and stage actor bring a unique set of skills to the process of voice rehabilitation and may represent a special subset of patients who rely on a combination of tactile-kinesthetic feedback and *listening* to produce the optimum sound. Already trained to rely on sensory feedback to manipulate the laryngeal and supralaryngeal structures, these professional voice users benefit from and depend heavily on auditory feedback. The elite voice user needs an astute ear to accurately imitate the pitches prescribed by the composer, attune himself to other singers when performing in a chorus or ensemble (Benninger & Murry, 2009), and reproduce the cadence, intonation, and stress patterns of classical or modern theatre pieces.

The persistence of a voice problem often reinforces counterproductive motor patterns that become chronic and make it difficult for the singer to distinguish between the less preferred voicing patterns and a more efficiently produced sound. When efficient motor patterns are restored and the singer's sensory perception of the sensations in the vocal tract are again active and consistent, that tactile-kinesthetic awareness can then combine with listening to make identification and integration of the preferred manner of phonation possible. Until that sensory integration takes place, however, listening alone remains an *inadequate* strategy for self-monitoring the appropriate manner of phonation (Lessac, 1997). It is never the case that listening replaces the attention to other sensory feedback.

Differences Between Singing and Speaking

A significant difference between singing and speaking resides in the temporal domain. Spoken language consists of rapidly produced phonemes and changes in speech rate that result in alterations in segment duration, articulatory displacement and velocity, and intrasyllabic coarticulation (Gay, 1981). Unlike singing, the stress, rhythms, and temporal patterns of speech are not generally associated with a meter and do not usually contain a periodic beat. It is true that speech may acquire a regular beat in certain contexts, such as counting in regular time, reciting verse, and performing song-speech, but during customary speech production the relative timing of vowels and consonants is subject to changes in stress level and speech rate (Shaffer, 1982). In contrast, the motor events that take place during singing are fixed in time and space by the musical constraints of a score that are external to the (motor events) movements. The timing differences between singing and speaking, as well as the acoustical differences in vowel duration, fundamental frequency, and supralaryngeal adjustments, suggest that the modifications made when shifting from singing to speaking may be more demanding than is often credited, particularly with respect to abdominal breath control. Evidence suggests there is no uniform or standard pattern of breath control that can be assigned to all singers or speakers, especially when we consider anatomical and physiological variability between singers, variation in skill, training, and differences in singing and musical styles (Hixon, 1987; Hoit & Hixon, 1986; Titze, 1994).

Breath Control

Unlike the conflicting opinions pertaining to the importance of breath control during speech production, breath control is always an intrinsic aspect of the development of the singing voice and is integrated in the singing lesson until it becomes efficient and habituated. Although checking action and abdominal control become second nature during *singing*, checking action and the engagement of the expiratory muscles for extended *spoken* utterances or for loudness inflection *may not* be intuitive. When the voice clinician draws the singer's attention to the coordination of placement and controlled exhalation when increasing vocal intensity during speech or producing long and complex utterances, the singer's highly developed kinesthetic sensibility most often facilitates an easy incorporation of control.

When we intervene to develop or modify breath control, we must consider the anatomical and physiological differences between singers, as well as the singer's confidence in a given technique that he developed during voice training prior to your collaboration in voice rehabilitation. The **pear-shape technique** (pear-shape up and pear-shape down) represents an approach to breathing that singers call on to control the voice, and that you will observe as your patient demonstrates varying levels of vocal intensity during speech and singing (Titze & Verdolini-Abbott, 2012). In the case of the pear-shape up technique, the singer maintains a relatively high and stable rib cage to control the voice; the pear-shape down method relies more heavily on a lower abdominal-diaphragmatic breathing pattern. The singer may combine rib cage and lower abdominal control to mitigate against the high elastic recoil pressures generated at the beginning of a long phrase (Titze, 1994) and to maintain the requisite subglottal pressure during a long phrase, a high tessitura, and when dynamic pitch and loudness adjustments occur within a musical score. Inappropriate management of excessive subglottal pressures represents a challenge for the novice singer, and is especially difficult during very quiet singing (marking).

The Ladder Exercise can be used to regulate subglottal pressure as the singer negotiates changes in loudness. Although this procedure is practiced during speech, the rapid and discrete changes in loudness do test flexibility and coordination, and serve as an appropriate introductory challenge before more complex adjustments are presented in singing. The *messa di voce* exercise, for example (in singing), which begins with a soft initiation of phonation, followed by a crescendo and decrescendo, requires control and flexibility in order to coordinate alveolar pressure and laryngeal resistance. When *messa di voce* is produced through a straw, as described in **Box 7-1**, the high back pressure precludes either breathiness or pressed phonation, the duration of phonation increases (owing to semi-occlusion of the vocal tract), and a crescendo is achieved without forceful laryngeal adduction (Titze, 1994). A more advanced version of *messa di voce*, executed without a semi-occluded vocal tract and at varying pitch levels, is usually introduced when the patient has achieved the phonatory control to

Box 7-1

Messa di Voce

- Inhale and sustain a quiet vowel through a straw for two seconds, followed by a smooth crescendo that is sustained for four seconds.
- Proceed effortlessly through the decrescendo portion of the procedure and sustain the quiet vowel through the straw for two seconds.

Nota bene: You will feel both the vibratory feedback and the increase in expiratory drive during the crescendo portion of the exercise. However, the necessary respiratory control is most apparent during the final two seconds of decrescendo.

Data from: Titze & Verdolini-Abbott, 2012.

smoothly and securely move through a wide pitch range with controlled transitions through registers.

Vertical Larynx Height

The relationship between **vertical laryngeal height** and fundamental frequency has received a great deal of attention in the singing literature. When the larynx is low, the tissues between the thyroid and cricoid cartilages are slacker, permitting the singer to achieve high fundamental frequencies with less muscle activity (Sundberg, 1970). Furthermore, a lower laryngeal position appears to facilitate projection of the sound with little effort, whereas a raised larynx is associated with a pressed manner of phonation and excessive medial compression of the vocal folds. Although the intonation patterns of the speaking voice do not require the extreme pitch ranges frequently obtained in singing, a high laryngeal position during speech often co-occurs with muscle tension dysphonia. A quick contraction of the diaphragm during a rapid inspiration may lower the larynx given that there is close mechanical coupling of the subglottal and laryngeal subsystems. When the larynx lowers, the width of the pharynx increases, and the musculature above the hyoid bone releases. The pre-yawn (avoid the full yawn) is recommended as an easy and straightforward technique to facilitate lowering of the larynx (Chapman, 2012).

Tongue Height and Tongue Base Stiffness

Your perceptual voice assessment will be more complete if you monitor tongue and laryngeal position during the motor-sensory examination as you observe the movement of the articulators, manner of phonation, and the respiratory mechanism during speech and singing. The higher fundamental frequencies often required in singing are associated with a more anterior tongue carriage than during speaking. As the tongue tip moves to a forward position during production of the /u/ vowel, for example, the tongue root is drawn downward by a lowered larynx, and the width of the pharynx increases. It is not uncommon to observe inappropriate retroflexion of the tongue base into the pharynx, associated with a singer or speaker's complaint of constriction in the tongue base. In an effort to widen the pharyngeal space the singer may, during inspiration, inadvertently press the tongue base down, which may set off a counterproductive pattern that leads to pressed phonation. The voice clinician must remain observant of possible tightening and stiffening of the tongue root in those singers trained to maintain a lowered larynx and tongue root (Chapman, 2012). You can monitor this pattern by placing your thumb in the soft spot under the chin to detect stiffness in the base of the tongue. Release of this **tongue base stiffness** may be accomplished during the /mhm/, /mhm/, /hu/ series and is enhanced when the tongue is slightly protruded and rests on the lower teeth. In this version the tongue is permitted to fall forward and hang loosely outside of the mouth. With the tongue base released, the laryngeal ventricle and pyriform sinuses widen, and the larynx assumes a lower position in the neck (Sundberg, 1970).

Jaw Opening

The singer modifies the shape and configuration of the vocal tract to project the voice without effort, as well as to navigate the extremes of the pitch range. The high fundamental frequencies often required during singing may be achieved with various articulatory strategies, but a released jaw is essential to sustain and make rapid changes in pitch with **mandibular freedom** and flexibility. The transition through the upper passaggio is a particularly difficult one that is sometimes ineffectively achieved by stiffening or opening the jaw disproportionately. Jaw stiffness and restricted jaw movement often co-occur with voice problems in speaking and singing. Inappropriate tightening of the jaw may be a result of tongue base stiffness, **temporomandibular joint dysfunction** tightness in the floor of the mouth, poor breath control, head–neck misalignment, articulatory variations, and general life stress (Chapman, 2012). Insufficient abdominal control is frequently the source of this counterproductive strategy, causing the singer to depend on the jaw to attain high fundamental frequencies. Although the role of the jaw in articulation is actually a small one, tongue base stiffness or "interdependence" (Chapman, 2012, p. 111) of the tongue and mandible may implicate the jaw in a counterproductive manner of articulation that is a substitute for appropriate tongue-tip movement.

The Singer's Formant

Source-filter theory (Fant, 1970) proposes that the sound generated by the larynx is filtered (modified) by the shape and configuration of the vocal tract. When the resonant frequencies (formant frequencies) of the vocal tract are aligned with those of the voice source the acoustic energy is amplified (Sundberg, 1987; Titze, 1994). This vocal tract transfer function depends on how close the formants are to one another, such that if the distance between them is halved, the transfer of energy increases by 6 dB at the formant frequencies and by 12 dB halfway between them.

The projection of sound without effort is an essential part of vocal longevity for the singer, and can be accomplished with the singer's **formant**, which represents a clustering of the third, fourth, and fifth formants and the amplitude of the partials (the fundamental frequency plus its overtones) between 2000 and 3000 Hz (Sundberg, 1977). The singer's formant, which permits the singer to be heard over a large orchestra without effort, is achieved by lowering the larynx and widening the pharynx in the epilaryngeal region. Nevertheless, although less effort is required to produce sound when the singing formant exists, abdominal control and appropriate alignment of the resonating chamber remain intrinsic aspects of a voice that is produced efficiently.

The Speaker's Formant

The "ring" associated with the singer's formant can be attained in the speaking voice as well, especially for the stage actor, who must project the voice without effort and for extended periods. The energy of the **speaker's formant** is located in the region of 3000 to 4000 Hz, approximately 1 kHz higher than the singer's formant, and represents a cluster of energy in the area of the fourth and fifth harmonic (Bele, 2006). The lowered larynx increases the length of the vocal tract and widens the **hypopharyngeal space** and contributes to the creation of this peak in the spectrum. Although the amplitude of the speaker's formant is somewhat weaker than the singer's formant, it provides the additional acoustic energy that is often associated with trained stage voices, and is commonly referred to as the **actor's formant** (Leino, 1993). The effectiveness of the **Y-Buzz** (Lessac, 1997) and a semi-occluded vocal tract are relevant here because they facilitate not only strong spectral peaks, but appropriate placement and flow phonation. If the stage actor and singer do not capitalize on the semi-occluded vocal tract, the voice may resemble shouting or pressed phonation, and negatively affect timbre and vibrato.

Formant Tuning

The stage actor and the singer use **formant tuning** to increase acoustic energy and intelligibility without the use of an amplification system. Several studies investigating the relationship between formant tuning and the Y-Buzz suggest that when Lessac's (1997) **call technique** is implemented by the actor (the kinesthetic sensations of the half-yawn and vibration along the hard palate and alveolar ridge), F_1 tuning to F_0 is sharper than during customary speech production (Munro, 2002; Raphael & Sherer, 1987). Amplitude of vibration increases as much as 4 to 7 dB in the second harmonic in male voices and the F_0 of female voices.

When the fundamental frequency is high and the harmonics are widely spaced (as in soprano singing), vocal intensity may be augmented by lowering the jaw, which adjusts F_1 to match the F_0 or a harmonic of the source with the frequency of a formant. This formant tuning is specific to high-pitched singing and is not pertinent to singing in the lower pitch range or during everyday speech, when the harmonics are sufficiently close to strengthen the formants (Titze, 1994). For the voice clinician, an understanding of formant tuning and the singer's formant provides a framework for integrating procedures that maximize kinesthetic feedback associated with resonance in "the mask," the hard palate, and the cheek bones. The singer depends on this sensory feedback, not only for an effortless boost in acoustic power, but to achieve an intended tone quality.

Vocal Tract Length and Jaw Opening

The freedom and degree of jaw opening influences not only phonation but the formant frequencies as well. The jaw functions as "one of the anchor points of the larynx" (Sundberg & Skoog, 1997, p. 304), given that the hyoid bone is also attached to the lower mandibular eminence. An increase in jaw opening and some diminishing of vowel intelligibility are typically observed on the /u/ and /i/ vowels in the upper part of the pitch range as the soprano singer ascends a two-octave scale. Great variability has been observed in jaw opening—from 5 mm to 25 mm—especially during the /u/ vowel (Sundberg & Skoog, 1997), which may be a function of vocal training and technique.

The relevance of these anatomic attachments comes into play if the tongue tip and jaw do not move freely and independently during rapid and intricate changes in pitch, loudness, and timbre (tone color). The relationship among vocal tract length, articulation of the lips and tongue, and jaw opening affects the timbre of the voice. Although vocal tract length does not increase to a great extent (~10%) (Titze & Verdolini-Abbott, 2012), the impact on the voice can be quite dramatic. When we lengthen the vocal tract and round the lips the formant frequencies decrease equivalently, and conversely, when we shorten the vocal tract and widen the lips the formant frequencies increase. You will note that the timbre of the singing and speaking voice can be significantly modified with these articulatory modifications. A longer vocal tract tends to darken the voice; a shorter tract produces a brighter sound.

Voice Modification for the Transgender Client

"How do we measure progress for the transgender client?"

Passive Knowledge

Barriers to health care, ostracism by family and friends, employment and social discrimination, misrepresentation, and society's ignorance or transphobia—these obstacles represent only some of the indignities that transgender individuals may endure as they embark on a transition that continues for months or even years. Although you will not directly address these matters, "reading around" the transgender literature will deepen your understanding of the stresses inherent in transition. Accurate empathy contributes to the development of a person-centered, collaborative relationship. A productive partnership is possible only when the clinician acknowledges and respects the other's perspective and the factors that influence adherence and progress. Moreover, the challenges that arise during your work with a transgender client will be more confidently met as the breadth of your knowledge and "cultural competence and humility" deepen (Tervalon & Murray-Garcia, 1998).

Anxiety and stress have been implicated in one's general health as well as the health of the laryngeal mechanism and are factors that the attentive voice clinician considers when these issues potentially hinder the client's participation in the voice modification process. Transgender individuals frequently participate in psychotherapy that is concurrent with the transition and voice modification to cope with these stresses. If your client reports or appears to be highly anxious, and you jointly agree that the anxiety and stress of transition currently have a negative impact on the voice modification process, it is appropriate to contact the consulting psychologist or psychotherapist (with permission from the client). You and the psychologist may discuss the wisdom of pursuing voice modification at this time or strategies that may facilitate the client's continued participation in the process.

Self-administered scales offer a quick and straightforward way to gain information about the individual's perspective on his or her expectations for voice modification. The Transgender Self-Evaluation Questionnaire (TSEQ) (Hancock, Krissinger, & Owen, 2011) and the Transsexual Voice Questionnaire for Male-to-Female Transsexuals TVQ(MtF) (Dacakis, Davies, Oates, Douglas, & Johnston, 2013) are invaluable tools for identifying your clients' attitudes at one moment in time. Of course, these attitudes are in flux. During the transition process, hormone therapy may create changes in the mood similar to those experienced during puberty.

During transition, the transgender client makes many decisions: to select a new name, obtain legal status as the preferred gender, work and live as the preferred gender, begin hormone therapy, and/or undergo sexual reassignment surgery (Currah, Juang, & Minter, 2006). Male-to-female (MtF) individuals may undergo facial surgery to feminize the facial features, electrolysis, hair transplants, tracheal shave to reduce the thyroid notch, surgery to shorten and stiffen the vocal folds, and breast augmentation. Some undergo a penile inversion to construct a vagina. Female-to-male patients may have a double mastectomy, hysterectomy, oophorectomy (ovaries), salpingectomy (fallopian tubes), and vaginectomy (vagina). Many trans men reject a surgically constructed penis owing to the expense and often unsatisfactory result (Solomon, 2012).

The *Standards of Care* published by the World Professional Association for Transgender Health (WPATH) is followed by professionals who work with transgender people. WPATH requires that patients live in the preferred gender for at least a year and participate in psychotherapy before making a commitment to sexual reassignment surgery. The *Standards of Care* provides safeguards to minimize post-operative regret by including two clinicians in the decision process, one of whom is a physician who advises on the medical protocol (Solomon, 2012).

The speech-language pathologist does not work alone during the voice modification process: mental health professionals, endocrinologists, and surgical specialty physicians cooperate to provide comprehensive services. In addition, the university clinic has become a common setting for transgender clients to participate in individual and group voice habilitation, and for student clinicians to apply a theoretical knowledge base that encompasses neuroanatomy, physiology, language, voice, articulation, and counseling.

The Trans Lexicon

Your willingness to immerse yourself in the transgender culture through the literature, panel discussions, and conferences as well as the transgender lexicon will not only deepen your passive knowledge but will reinforce your role as an expert in the area of transgender communication. The following sections provide several of the relevant terms that are currently used to explain the transition process. The terminology in **Box 7-2** and **Box 7-3** was compiled from a variety of sources including Beemyn (2006); Adler, Hirsch, and Mordaunt (2012); and discussions with our clients.

Box 7-2

Terminology of Transition

Bottom surgery: Refers to surgery to modify either the male or female genitalia to the preferred gender.

Cisgender: One who identifies with the gender assigned at birth.

Cross-dresser: An individual who dresses, applies make-up, etc. appropriate for another gender.

FtM: A female-to-male transgender individual, who was assigned the female gender at birth but identifies as a male.

Gender: Refers to the assignment of masculinity and femininity; a specific culture's expectations of masculine and feminine roles; the perception of masculinity and femininity by one's self and others.

Gender dysphoria: One who experiences extreme discomfort with his or her own socially, biologically, or culturally assigned gender role.

Gender expression/presentation: One's choices regarding clothing, hairstyle, voice, etc. to reflect the preferred gender identity.

Gender identity: One's internal appreciation of one's own gender.

Gender identity disorder (GID): The classification for transsexuality in the American Psychiatric Association's *Diagnostic and Statistical Manual of Mental Disorders* (2013).

Genderqueer: An individual who rejects the binary classification of male or female.

Gender reassignment surgery (GRS) or gender confirming surgery: Surgery to alter one's anatomy to conform to the person's gender identity.

Gender variant or gender nonconforming: An individual who does not conform to the binary classification of male or female.

Metoidioplasty: Surgical restructuring of the clitoris.

MtF: A male-to-female transsexual, who identifies as female despite male gender assignment at birth.

Panhysterectomy: Surgical removal of the ovaries and uterus.

Phalloplasty: Surgical construction of a penis.

Scrotoplasty: Surgical creation of a scrotum.

Sexual dysphoria: A disassociation from one's biological sex.

Top surgery: The removal (mastectomy) or augmentation of the breasts.

Tracheal shave: Surgical reduction in the size of the thyroid notch.

Trans / Transgender (TG) / Transsexual: General term used to describe an individual whose identity diverges from the gender assigned at birth.

Transition: The series of changes an individual experiences as he or she achieves congruence with the internal gender identity.

Transphobia: Fear and hatred of transgender individuals.

Vaginoplasty: Surgical construction of a vagina.

Beemyn, 2006; Adler, Hirsch, & Mordaunt, 2012

Box 7-3 provides several of the terms associated with the transgender individual's success blending into society with credible gestures, attire, and voice. These terms are often used among trans men and trans women in their personal and private communication with one another.

Box 7-3

Terminology of "Passing"

Being read (clocked) / Outed: An individual who is recognized as a trans person.

Closeted: A lesbian, gay, bisexual, transgender (LGBT) individual who chooses to keep the gender/sexual identity private.

Hir (pronounced as "here"): A pronoun used to indicate a nonspecific gender individual. The word combines "her" and "him."

Sie or Ze: A nonspecific pronoun that combines "she" and "he."

Beemyn, 2006; Adler, Hirsch, & Mordaunt, 2012

Ambivalence

Over the past 30 years the research in gender identity, access to the internet, film, television, and the expansion of services to the lesbian, gay, bisexual, and transgender (LGBT) community have had a profound influence on the decisions that transgender individuals make with respect to acceptance of a binary system that imposes an exclusive male or female identity. As the paradigm shifts with the emergence of a new generation, gender identity has become far too fluid to fit neatly into this binary scheme. Trans individuals may choose to present themselves along a continuum of masculinity or femininity, and change their persona at various times and in different situations. Furthermore, the individual may choose to incorporate a corresponding gender physical presentation but reject a corresponding voice.

During transition, which can take place over months or years, it is common for the transgender individual to experience **ambivalence**. The decision to transition is neither straightforward nor final. Ambivalence, however, is normal and healthy. It is an inherent part of the transition process that the voice clinician must recognize in order to facilitate the client's willingness to explore the many facets of the vocal personality. This ambivalence may be a reflection of the embarrassment, shame, guilt, and fear of reprisals and rejection that the client feels during the process of transition, and may lead to depression and even suicidal thinking. The burden of presenting as male at work, for example, and female in social situations is a heavy one to bear. Regardless of the persona chosen in these situations, the individual continues to hide or make invisible the other persona, which reinforces guilt and shame. It is for these reasons that the process of transition and its ramifications require our sensitivity and respect for privacy. We acknowledge and support all clients' efforts to make the changes that they decide are relevant to them.

The group participant in the *Ambivalence—Applying for a Job* video describes the "push-pull thing" she continues to feel regarding her transition as well as the difficulty she finds integrating her female voice when she applies for a job.

Congruence of Communication and Persona

Throughout this text, we have emphasized the importance of an easy, efficient, and effective manner of phonation. Nowhere is the coordination of the vocal subsystems more necessary than in your work with the transgender client. The process of modifying the voice to correspond with a male or female persona is a complex one, given anatomical limitations, the individual's kinesthetic awareness, physiological empathy and a good ear. The voice clinician must remain observant of the possible emergence of counterproductive strategies, and be cautious when increasing the complexity of procedures while working with the transgender client to find a voice that not only conveys the chosen persona and meets the communicative requirements but is acknowledged and accepted as true to the self.

The principles of motor learning are equally applicable in your work with the trans speaker, given the necessity for acquiring, shaping, stabilizing, reinforcing, and eventually assimilating new vocal and behavioral motor patterns. The course of motor learning takes time, patience, and repetition in a variety of social and emotional contexts. As is the case with the customary or elite voice user, blocked and random practice are recommended in order to maximize the acquisition and stabilization of the motor skills. The transgender individual may have special difficulty, however, finding an appropriate arena that is not only supportive, but is a safe one to rehearse and reinforce these behaviors. A transgender voice group provides an excellent intermediate and secure environment in which not only to "try on" the behavioral and vocal characteristics of the chosen gender but to receive positive and relevant feedback from peers, and learn from their attempts to integrate these newly acquired motor skills. The group setting is an appropriate one to integrate the vocal and physical presentation with clothing, hairstyle, make-up, and accessories. When the client is capable of incorporating authentic movement and voice within the context of a social gathering, the individual has made great strides in the motor learning process.

In the *Psychological Aspects of Voice* video the transgender voice group discusses the effect of stereotypes and physical appearance on voice, the limitations one imposes on oneself, and the process of building confidence during transition.

Fluidity of Gender Expression

The shift away from a binary sexual classification system has been accompanied by a shift in the area of voice modification. Our profession recognizes that there is no one ideal persona for gender, and that norms differ across ethnic groups and nationalities. When we facilitate the exploration of a comfortable gender expression that aligns with the individual's vision of self, a credible communication style emerges. The importance of pitch to vocal authenticity now appears less central than an inclusion of resonance, timbre, prosody, articulatory precision, speech rate, and loudness inflection when we work with male-to-female or female-to-male transgender clients. The congruence of semantics, syntax, and **pragmatics** further contributes to the effectiveness of communication. As the speech and language characteristics become more integrated, the compatible nonverbal communication factors pertaining to gesture, stance, and facial expression are incorporated to communicate the more subtle aspects of personality.

Pragmatics and Language

So much of the transgender individual's attention is devoted to pitch that the obvious and powerful contribution of language, movement, and gesture to a successful transition may be obscured. Although we may recognize differences that can be identified as more or less typical of the male or female use of language, the most salient linguistic differences might be found in the purpose or intent of the interaction between men and women. Common references are widely made in the general literature to statements that inappropriately simplify and stereotype gender roles such as *men talk to find solutions to problems, while women talk to connect and form alliances*, but the magnitude of the linguistic ingredient in the expression of gender in language may be overstated. One's profession, education, age, socioeconomic status, race, geographical location, and, of course, one's personality, sense of humor, and appreciation of irony contribute to the vocabulary, grammar, syntax, individuality, and even idiosyncrasy of the communication style. The linguistic style of a computer programmer may be precise and concrete, and much of the everyday vocabulary may derive from professional jargon. The actor or writer may use a more florid, descriptive style that includes metaphor and allusions to and quotations from text. The language of the scientist, on the other hand, might be centered about questioning the underlying premises of the communication partner's assumptions or conclusions. The differences we have noted between the individuals we have worked with and the members of our transgender voice groups appear to be a function of their professions, education, and age rather than their gender, and these differences enhance the individual's uniqueness, enrich the linguistic character, and are to be preserved.

Nonverbal Communication

Although your client may recognize the relevance of movement and gesture to a credible presentation, he or she may be unaware that the process of voice modification may include these elements. When the voice, speech, language, and nonverbal aspects of communication are compatible, consistent, and assimilated with the physical presentation, the client has achieved authenticity. Despite the seemingly clear differences ascribed to male and female nonverbal behavior, the goal of habilitation is to achieve an overall impression of femaleness or maleness that matches the individual's self-perception. Nevertheless, the trust between the client and clinician should be well established before broaching the subject of the congruence between the reality of the individual's body size and age, and the chosen attire, hairstyle, and make-up when a disparity exists between them by recognizing culture and individual self-expression.

Nonverbal Communication: Female

Traditionally, women are depicted as soft, gentle, sociable, and nurturing. These conventional characteristics are reflected in the shape of the female body, and make gender recognition often possible from a distance. A woman's silhouette is usually similar to an "S" shape that moves with a shorter, narrower gait and fluid, flowing movements. Gestures tend to be rather small and are made close to the body; hands may gracefully bend at the wrist, with soft, open fingers. When seated, females tend to sit close together, face each other, make eye contact, and attend to social cues (Tannen, 1994). Women may lean in toward the speaking partner, nod the head, smile more often, and are more attracted to those who smile back (Hess, Beaupre, & Cheung, 2002). As a general rule, women express comfort and support by hugging and touching (Nelson & Golant, 2004). When a mixed gender situation calls for a handshake, the woman usually initiates the gesture and executes the handshake with a gentle grasp (Axtell, 1998).

Nonverbal Communication: Male

The stereotypical male figure is portrayed as strong, aggressive, and less demonstrative in his expression of nurturing emotion. The shape of the male body while seated is often somewhat triangular and similar to an "A," occupying more space than its female counterpart (Glass, 1992). Men usually walk with a linear gait and take longer strides that suggest strength and confidence. The trunk and head are often held rather still while listening, and the body tends to lean away from the speaker. While seated, males may cross their legs in a figure four, lean back, and tap their feet, surveying their environment (Tannen, 1994). Generally, male gestures are broader and more angular, and lead from the shoulder with arms moving horizontally or vertically away from the body while keeping the fingers closed and flat. Men may be somewhat more guarded and establish dominance through eye contact (Nelson & Golant, 2004). They more often use a firm grasp when shaking hands with one another, as opposed to a softer and gentler touch when shaking hands with a woman.

Voice Modification: The Transgender Woman

The male-to-female transgender client who expresses an interest in voice modification as part of her transition, may focus on elevating her pitch as the primary and most essential aspect of her new vocal persona. As we suggested earlier, while pitch is certainly an aspect of feminine or masculine identification, it does not, in and of itself, create a voice that possesses the appropriate timbre for the gender. Timbre or voice quality, intonation, and a forward placement are critical ingredients in the perception of vocal femininity, suggesting that head resonance is associated with the female voice and chest resonance is more palpable in the male voice (Adler et al., 2012).

Before she begins voice habilitation, and in an effort to pass, the trans woman may unknowingly produce a fundamental frequency that is inappropriately high and artificial. What is more, clients often use **up-speech** at the ends of declarative utterances. The often-constant use of this prosodic pattern has a negative impact on the listener and detracts from the legitimacy of the message (Adler et al., 2012). When this strategy fails, and she is recognized ("clocked") and addressed as "Sir," frustration, embarrassment, and even despair may provide the impetus to seek professional voice services (Hancock, Krissinger, & Owen, 2011).

The trans speaker in the *Movement—Inflection* video describes the benefits of her modeling experience with respect to movement. Although she acknowledges that her inflection patterns have become more natural, she reports that anxiety sometimes negatively affects her intonation patterns.

The typical adult male has a speaking fundamental frequency range from 85 to 155 Hz, and the typical adult female range is from 165 to 255 Hz (Fitch & Holbrook, 1970). These ranges alter, however, with age, time of day, the presence of allergies, and medication. Although the gap between the male and female fundamental frequency ranges is small, and most males have the vocal capacity to produce a fundamental frequency within the normal range of the female voice, they may do so at the expense of ease, efficiency, and credibility.

The range between 150 and 185 Hz represents a speaking fundamental frequency that is considered a **gender-acceptable pitch range** for the female voice (Adler et al., 2012). As with all voice modification processes, the expansion of the conversational pitch range must be a careful and well-organized one. **Dialogue 7-1** occurs during an early session and focuses on producing a credible pitch with appropriate balance among the vocal subsystems. The back pressure exercise /mhm/

Dialogue 7-1
Fourth Session with a Male-to-Female Transgender Client

The client is a 25-year-old trans woman who has been on hormone therapy for 4 months. This is Ms. J's first experience with voice modification and she is exploring the possibility of using a more feminine manner of phonation. She continues to identify herself with her male name, and has not yet worn female attire, but does often wear earrings and has allowed her hair to grow to shoulder length.

During this session, Ms. J described frustration duplicating the acceptable feminine voice she achieved during the previous one-to-one session when she practiced independently. I suspected that her heavy reliance on auditory feedback was the source of difficulty. During the session, I refocused her on the tactile-kinesthetic, sensory feedback that had previously facilitated a softer, easier, gentler phonation and facilitated a more natural, feminine voice.

"Let's start with the conversation pattern that we have been using. Just follow me. Remember, we talked about physiological empathy, so you want to feel what I am feeling as I produce the /mhm/ and the phrases. Remember to attend to the sensations in your vocal tract and think the glide /j/ onto the vowel /mhm/." *We began a turn-taking exchange using /mhm/ to prepare the larynx for easy phonation, and added phrases that began with the nasal phonemes, then added glides, and, finally, vowel-initiated phrases. During the nasal and vowel-initiated phrases her manner of phonation was appropriate. She reported that she could feel vibration in her face and behind her cheeks, and that she experienced the flowing, gliding feeling of the voice resting easily on the breath.*

Nota bene: The clinician assesses the individual's manner of phonation on each trial, but does not provide feedback on each one.

Ms. J: "/mhm/," *produced with appropriate ease, resonance, and gentle onset of phonation.*

Clinician: "/mhm/."

Ms. J: "/mhm/," *with similar ease.*

Clinician: "/mhm/."

Ms. J: "/mhm/," *maintaining ease.*

Clinician: "Over and over."

Ms. J: "Over and over," *with an easy vowel onset.*

Clinician: "/mhm/."

Ms. J: "/mhm/."

Clinician: "/mhm/."

Ms. J: "/mhm/," *without effort.*

Thus far, Ms. J produced the back pressure and phrase combination easily and effortlessly and she appeared tuned into my model of resonance, flow, and glide. I continued with additional phrases to reinforce and consolidate the attention to the sensory feedback she was now clearly using: "/mhm/, over the Atlantic ocean."

Ms. J repeated the phrase with a gentle onset of phonation, "/mhm/, over the Atlantic ocean/."

To verify that she was, in fact, using kinesthetic feedback, I asked her, "How did those feel so far?"

Thoughtfully, Ms. J replied, "Those felt easy, but I don't know how it sounded."

It was clear that she was still clinging to the auditory mode of evaluating her success. "Today I would like for you to deliberately focus on the sensations in your vocal tract and ignore the sound of your voice. Let's see if we can integrate the tactile-kinesthetic sensations that will facilitate the easy, feminine voice. Would that be okay?"

Ms. J giggled, "I forgot that I was supposed to think about that."

In an attempt to more firmly solidify the sensory component we continued the turn-taking format with further vowel-initiated phrases. I continued, "Deliberately attend to the sensations in your nose and lips, /mhm/."

Ms. J: "/mhm/," *with resonance.*

Clinician: "/mhm/."

Ms. J: "/mhm/," *with continuing resonance.*

Clinician: "/mhm/."

Ms. J: "/mhm/," *with ease.*

Clinician: "Oranges and apples."

Ms. J: "Oranges and apples," *with an easy onset of phonation.*

I noted that she continued to incorporate the goals related to resonance, flow, and ease, and I asked, "How did those feel?"

In an easy, resonant voice Ms. J said, "I felt some vibration here." *She pointed to the midfacial area.*

I was convinced that she was attending to the sensations and proceeded. "Good. Let's see if we can make that feeling more consistent." *We continued with an additional set.* "/mhm/."

Ms. J: "/mhm/," *with resonance.*

Clinician: "/mhm/."

Ms. J: "/mhm/," *with easy onset of the vowel.*

Clinician: "I enjoy oranges."

Ms. J: "I enjoy oranges." *Client's voice breaks into falsetto on the phrase. Looking startled and embarrassed, she said,* "Oh, I guess I overshot that."

I saw an opportunity to help her understand the process by which we develop new motor patterns, and how the components of range and force influence that integration. "You have just demonstrated how it is that it takes time to shape, reinforce, and consolidate a new motor pattern. You have been using your male voice for many years and are now asking the system to do something very different. It is expected that there will be variability as you develop the new motor behavior, but if you continue to focus on feeling, you will develop those patterns without unnecessary and undesirable effort and strain. Let's do some more."

followed by /mʌm, mʌm, mʌm, mʌm/ sets the system up for the forward placement (head resonance) you want the client to experience. This technique creates a semi-occlusion in the vocal tract in order to initiate voicing in an easy and efficient manner. Effective techniques to explore the individual's comfortable pitch range and then begin to expand it implement a variation on the Puffy Cheeks Exercise and voiced lip and tongue trills. The client creates a tight constriction at the lips and inflates the cheeks while producing an upward and downward inflection (Puffy Cheeks), and performs the lip and tongue trills in a similar fashion. With this very high back pressure in place, one can facilitate efficient self-oscillation of the vocal folds through the pitch range.

Just as the *thought* of a yawn may precipitate dilation of the pharyngeal musculature and lift the soft palate to widen the pharynx, thinking *smile* can have a similar effect on the timbre of the voice, creating the impression of a lighter, warmer, and even brighter, more feminine sound. The formant frequencies respond to changes in the shape and configuration of the vocal tract, such that lengthening the tract (by protruding the lips) lowers all formants and shortening the tract (by thinking *smile*) raises them. These resonant frequencies make a significant contribution to the perception of a male or female voice. As you may recall, the first formant (F_1) is associated with **tongue height**, the second formant (F_2) to anterior/posterior placement of the tongue, and the third formant (F_3) to lip spreading (Carew, Dacakis, & Oates, 2007). When one implements a more anterior carriage of the tongue, the second formant is raised, which facilitates the perception of a more feminine voice, and when the vocal tract shortens to produce a slight smile, the third formant raises.

As the vocal transition continues, loudness inflection will become another component of the voice modification process, especially because of the tendency for the trans woman to revert to a male voice when projecting, shouting, or engaging in argument. The principles of back pressure and breath control are extremely relevant here in order to avoid vocal fatigue, vocal tract and laryngeal stiffness, and potential injury to the laryngeal mucosa. Conscious attention to the sensations in the vocal tract builds memory traces and facilitates the consistency and automaticity of the feminized voice. Breath control and loudness exercises such as the Ladder Exercise, *messa di voce*, and Extending the Breath are effective for developing the control and coordination necessary to increase projection and loudness range without effort.

Voice Modification: The Transgender Male

There are several factors to be considered with respect to the use of androgen hormone therapy to lower the speaking fundamental frequency of the voice. If, for instance, the client's typical pitch is lower than the average female before administration of the hormone, an expectation of a significant drop in speaking fundamental frequency is an unrealistic one (Adler et al., 2012). The lowering of pitch occurs over time with continued use of the androgens, and even with a change that is less than one octave the client may achieve a significant "perceptual" (p. 157) result.

The transgender male may benefit from voice habilitation to eliminate any extraneous effort he has implemented to exaggerate the male voice. In addition, changes that occur following hormone therapy take time and are often less dramatic than expected. In an attempt to produce an authoritative, commanding voice, the transgender male may force the mechanism to lower the pitch by using a pressed manner of phonation, which reduces air flow and squeezes the arytenoid cartilages together, leading to laryngeal fatigue, difficulty projecting the voice, and over time, deterioration of voice quality. In all likelihood, the extreme pressure on the laryngeal mechanism will deprive the voice of its resonance characteristics. Under these counterproductive circumstances, projection and loudness inflection may actually diminish and lead to voice or upward pitch breaks. Again, your work will involve establishing appropriate coordination among the subsystems, and to that end you may incorporate the concepts of back pressure and breath support. To reinforce a more masculine voice quality in an efficient manner the individual may lower the larynx, which will lengthen the vocal tract, lower all formants, widen the hypopharyngeal space, and shift the resonance from the more feminine head voice to chest resonance. Although one does experience chest resonance on the nasal phonemes, the awareness of the resonance in the chest intensifies with the voiced fricatives /v/, /ð/, /z/, and /ʒ/.

Progress

How do we measure progress for the transgender client? Is it the number of trials during which the client maintained a F_0 of 187 Hz? Or is it that the client experiments with the voice to find the most efficient, effective manner of phonation and physical presentation that correlates with and enhances the perception of the chosen persona, and is sustainable across varying social and emotional contexts? Our bias is always in favor of the most natural and credible expression of the individual's self. To accomplish this goal, the client and clinician explore the vocal repertoire, integrate the nonverbal elements of the persona into the chosen procedures, and provide a supportive environment in which the client comes to appreciate the realistic parameters of change that are within reach.

With ambivalence so often in the background of transition, it is one's resilience, tenacity, self-efficacy, and positive self-regard that represent the inner resources that are central to one's readiness for change.

It is often the case that the transgender client does not recognize these traits within himself or herself. Your collaborative, person-centered attitude plays a significant part in facilitating the client's access to and appreciation of these attributes. As the client incorporates the facets of the male or female persona, receives positive feedback from peers, and enjoys the success of passing at work and in the social milieu, these individual qualities will be reinforced and trusted.

Spasmodic Dysphonia (Focal Laryngeal Dystonia)

"The efficacy of behavioral voice therapy is influenced by the patient's response to BoNT injections."

History and Recognition of Spasmodic Dysphonia

The patient with spasmodic dysphonia comes to you with concerns regarding the voice symptoms associated with his neurological diagnosis. Together, you explore the available treatment options. Diagnosis and treatment of individuals with spasmodic dysphonia is more effective when the voice clinician has a working knowledge of the underlying neurological disease and can discuss its causes, possible accompanying medical signs, the patterns of onset and progression, medical treatments, and possible side effects of these treatments. The clinician then observes the patient to identify possible counterproductive patterns in order to offer treatment choices within an objective framework that allows the patient to make an informed treatment decision.

Passive knowledge of the medical vocabulary associated with spasmodic dysphonia helps to build professional credibility with the physician. To translate this medical information into the patient's vocabulary requires a familiarity and ease with the medical jargon, the subtle meanings of the terminology, and the confidence to restate the information in lay terms. A patient may have an incorrect or incomplete understanding of the diagnosis and not recognize that the perceptual changes in his voice reflect the underlying changes in the neurological system. Due to the inconsistency of the voice symptoms (e.g., worsening under stress, improvement with consumption of alcohol), it is not unusual for a patient to deny the neurological diagnosis and respond negatively to the fear and stigma associated with neurological disorders. Your knowledge and counseling skills will facilitate the patient's understanding, acceptance, and successful compensation for the associated voice symptoms.

Spasmodic dysphonia has been recognized for many years as a distinctive voice disorder (Schnitzler, 1875; Traube, 1871). In 1968 Aronson et al. described the spasmodic nature of the symptoms and coined the term *spasmodic dysphonia*. Numerous researchers have described neurological symptoms that frequently accompany spasmodic dysphonia, including involuntary blinking of the eyes or neurological writer's cramp. In 1991 Blitzer and Brin recognized the underlying neurological condition as a dystonia and classified spasmodic dysphonia as a focal laryngeal dystonia. Other types of **focal dystonia**, including blepharospasm (involuntary closing of the eyelids), cervical dystonia (involuntary movement and postures in the neck and shoulders), oromandibular dystonia (involuntary opening or closing of the jaw), graphomotor dystonia (involuntary movements in the hand during skilled movement), and Meige (a combination of blepharospasm and oromandibular dystonia) may accompany and exacerbate the symptoms and treatment of spasmodic dysphonia (Blitzer & Brin, 1991; Fahn, 1988).

Focal dystonia is slightly more common in females, usually develops in adulthood, can have a sudden or gradual onset, and worsens over a period of several months or up to three years before the symptoms stabilize. Spasmodic dysphonia may co-occur with generalized dystonia (affecting the entire body), which begins in childhood and progresses over many years. Additional dystonic symptoms are not uncommon in patients with spasmodic dysphonia. It is necessary, therefore, to screen for co-occurring focal dystonias, and to make a referral to a neurologist when these symptoms are observed.

Patients often ask about the cause of their dystonia in an attempt to understand why and how it happened to them. Dystonia is either the primary problem or a secondary symptom of another problem. If it is the sole problem, it is usually idiopathic (unknown cause) or genetic and the involuntary movements are usually "action-induced" (activated by learned movement such as speech). If it is a secondary symptom of another neurological disorder such as Wilson's disease, Leigh's disease, or Huntington's disease, or in reaction to environmental causes such as head trauma, brain lesions, infection, medication (phenothiazines, dopamine), or chemical toxins there will likely be other symptoms in addition to the dystonia (Marsden, 1988).

The patient in the *Description of Voice Problem* video, was diagnosed with adductor spasmodic dysphonia following this session. He describes the progression of his voice problem and "muscling through" in order to make sound. He now reports that he connects words without the struggle previously experienced.

A diagnosis of spasmodic dysphonia may be a devastating one because it represents a permanent neurological disorder. If the patient fears that the dysphonia is due to a deep-seated neurosis, however, the confirmation of a diagnosis other than a psychological one can sometimes be a relief. In contrast, a patient who believes his voice disorder to be a result of an inappropriate manner of phonation may be shocked to discover that he has a neurological disorder; the full impact of its etiology, progression, remission, as well as the potential for its genetic consequences can be overwhelming. Regardless of the patient's response to the diagnosis, you begin your therapeutic relationship by acknowledging his concerns and providing information about the dystonia and its associated symptomology. An in-depth understanding of spasmodic dysphonia, its causes, progression, and treatments provides the passive knowledge you need to address the demands of this complex disorder.

Special Considerations

Spasmodic dysphonia is a chronic neurological voice disorder that does not resolve with behavioral or medical treatment. All available treatments address the symptoms but do not treat the underlying etiology or neurological changes that are a consequence of the dystonia. As a result, the patient's decision to accept or reject treatment of the symptoms is a personal one that is a function of the impact of the disorder on the individual's life, his coping strategies, his communicative needs, and his understanding of the medical treatments available to him.

The Voice Handicap Index—Spasmodic Dysphonia (VHI SD) (Wingate et al., 2005) and the Disease-Specific Self-Efficacy in Spasmodic Dysphonia (SE-SD) (Hu et al., 2012) are self-administered scales designed specifically for individuals who suffer from spasmodic dysphonia. They provide information pertaining to the patient's response to the disorder.

The differences between spasmodic dysphonia and other voice disorders pertain to the involuntary nature of the motor component of the dystonic symptoms. During the laryngeal examination the structures usually appear to be normal and without lesions. The movement of the vocal folds is typically unremarkable when the patient is breathing, sustaining a single note, or singing. The involuntary hyperadduction and abduction of the vocal folds is observed when connected speech is produced in the customary fashion (Arnold, 1959; Blitzer, Brin, Fahn, & Lovelace, 1988).

When conscious attention is applied to the sensations of the muscles in the larynx to override and possibly disrupt the normal sequence of motor patterns, the patient may gain control of the symptoms. It is relatively rare that the patient will implement this deliberate behavioral control as the primary therapeutic tool due to the high level of sustained concentration required, but we have treated patients who have chosen the behavioral route in lieu of the BoNT therapy. Most individuals rely on the BoNT injections to ameliorate their spasmodic symptoms. The patient may incorporate gentle onsets, a breathy voice, semi-occlusion of the vocal tract, or speak during inhalation as supplementary techniques to the injections.

Given that spasmodic dysphonia is a neurological disorder, the vocal symptoms usually worsen under physiological or emotional stress. A patient may report that his speech is acceptable in all situations except when he is speaking on the telephone or when giving a lecture. In treatment, he may want to focus on specific speaking situations to improve his effectiveness at work or within social interactions.

Perceptual Voice Symptoms

The symptoms of spasmodic dysphonia are usually action induced. The movements that trigger these symptoms are associated with customary speech production. Vegetative sounds and less frequent modes of speaking (whisper, speaking in a high pitch, using a foreign accent, or singing) are relatively preserved, and vocalizations such as laughter, cough, throat clearing, yawn, and sigh are usually less affected or possibly unaffected by the dystonia. The contrast between improved phonation during laughter and disturbed phonation during conversation can be unnerving, eliciting concern that the disorder is a psychological one. Unfortunately, this pattern is simply part of the phenomenon of spasmodic dysphonia. These phonatory tasks can be used to differentially distinguish dystonia from voice problems in which a laryngeal pathology is absent.

The patient in the *Awareness of Effort* video describes feeling "locked-up" in the throat when he pushes to make sound. Your physiological empathy will heighten your awareness of his high levels of effort.

The voice symptoms associated with spasmodic dysphonia are usually classified and described by the involuntary action of the vocal folds during connected speech as opposed to the description of a laryngeal pathology, which is identified by changes in the cover, transition, or body of the vocal fold (Aronson, 1990). Regardless of the type of spasmodic dysphonia, patients often report that the most troubling symptom is the high level of effort required to produce voice. **Adductor spasmodic dysphonia** is more common and results in intermittent, involuntary hyperadduction and stiffening of the vocal folds with a choked, rough, strained-strangled voice quality and effortful, and abrupt phonation breaks. The less common **abductor spasmodic dysphonia** is characterized by intermittent, involuntary abduction of the vocal folds associated with an effortful, breathy, or whispered voice; breathy voice breaks; and possible hyperventilation often associated with the production of voiceless consonants. Occasionally, individuals present a *mixed* spasmodic dysphonia, exhibiting symptoms of both the adductor and abductor type or a respiratory dystonia that occurs during inhalation. The **Unified Spasmodic Dysphonia Rating Scale (USDRS)** (Stewart et al., 1997) is a perceptual voice measure that is used to assess the overall severity and specific characteristics of voice production, including responses to those vocal tasks that are associated with enhancement and exacerbation of an individual's vocal symptoms.

The place, manner, and voicing of initial sounds in syllables influence the severity of the symptoms (Izdebski, Dedo, & Boles, 1984). For those with adductor spasmodic dysphonia, the preset hyperadduction of the vocal folds sets the larynx up for greater medial force, which is further exacerbated by voiced sounds (vowels and voiced consonants, such as "Rainey Island Avenue"). The hyperadduction is partially ameliorated on phrases that contain voiceless sounds that partially abduct the vocal folds (e.g., Harry's hat). Conversely, those with abductor spasmodic dysphonia exhibit a preset, abducted vocal fold posture. Symptoms are exacerbated when phrases contain voiceless sounds during which the vocal folds are abducted. The type of phonatory breakdown (on voiced or voiceless sounds) is fairly consistent in a given speaker's voice, but the emergence of the symptoms on any specific syllable is highly variable such that speech fluency is difficult to predict. Problems may be present at the onset of one syllable and not during the next. This variability in symptom severity makes it difficult for the patient to predict his fluency.

The patient with spasmodic dysphonia may exhibit a co-occurring vocal **tremor** that originates in the diaphragm, intrinsic or extrinsic laryngeal muscles, head, or mandible. The tremor may be rhythmical or arrhythmical. A co-occurring tremor may not be noticeable during the initial assessment due to the masking effects of the other voice symptoms. It may reveal itself following an injection or voice therapy when the symptoms have diminished.

Injections of Botulinum Neurotoxin (BoNT)

Treatment of spasmodic dysphonia changed abruptly in 1991, when Drs. Blitzer and Brin identified injections of botulinum neurotoxin (BoNT) as a treatment that would reduce the involuntary contractions in the laryngeal muscles. They reported that individuals who receive BoNT notice improved phonation that lasts typically from one to six months. When the benefit from the injections weakens, the treatment is readministered. The role of the speech-language pathologist typically includes diagnosis, assessment of the patient's response to BoNT injections, counseling related to expected outcomes, and therapy to reduce the counterproductive behaviors that may have developed in response to the chronic voice problem. Most individuals with spasmodic dysphonia elect to participate in a treatment regimen of BoNT injections and have a satisfactory response to the treatment.

For adductor spasmodic dysphonia, BoNT is injected under electromyographic guidance (EMG) into the **thyroarytenoid muscle**, and the neurotoxin chemically blocks the release of acetylcholine to reduce the strength of the closure of the glottis and the stiffness of the vocal folds. The most common transitory side effects are breathiness, reduced loudness, and the potential for aspirating thin liquids. With abductor spasmodic dysphonia, BoNT is injected into the posterior cricoarytenoid muscle to reduce the involuntary abduction of the vocal folds. The most common transitory side effects are vocal stridor and shortness of breath. When the side effects have subsided, the benefits of the injection begin and the patient may achieve near-normal phonation. At times, the injection into the posterior cricoarytenoid muscle is supplemented with surgery to medialize one of the vocal folds and strengthen glottal closure.

It is possible that following the first injection (for adductor SD), the strained-strangled voice quality and compensatory effort the patient used prior to the injection will persist. The patient may need a supplemental injection to further weaken the vocal folds. In contrast, when the patient's vocal folds become excessively weak following the injection, although this breathiness is temporary, he may compensate for it with extreme effort that leads to a similar (the previous) strained-strangled voice quality. The patient's response to the sound of his voice (the strained-strangled quality) sometimes prompts a request for an additional injection because he does not understand the difference between the compensatory strategy and the original symptom. In this case, after the clinician has determined that there has been a response to the BoNT, the clinician explains that the vocal folds are sufficiently weak and that an additional injection is unnecessary. With time and voice therapy, the counterproductive compensations abate. During the postinjection phase of temporary breathiness, voice loss, and mild dysphagia, the patient is advised to use confidential voice, diminish expiratory drive, and to exercise caution when swallowing thin liquids (i.e., take small sips, and possibly use a chin tuck procedure) to protect the airway.

Behavioral Voice Procedures

The counseling skills you bring to the assessment and treatment of the individual suffering from spasmodic dysphonia are central to a comprehensive management plan. The patient may not have accepted or integrated the reality of a chronic, neurological disease into his self-image. Coping strategies such as seeking information about dystonia, denial, anger, frustration, blame, or questions of "why me," may permeate the treatment session. These strong responses are not only normal human reactions to a difficult situation, but are expected given the significant change this will mean in the patient's life. It may be within your skill set to talk with the patient and offer general support to help him face these concerns. Conversely, if the individual is overwhelmed by his feelings or if you feel uncomfortable, it is appropriate to ask the patient if he would like a referral to a psychologist, social worker, or religious counselor. Reassure the patient that everyone needs support at some time, and that this is one of those times.

A few patients decide that they prefer to follow a behavioral treatment approach and seek voice therapy rather than the BoNT injection. The efficacy of **behavioral voice therapy** for spasmodic dysphonia is influenced by the patient's response to BoNT injection, the severity and habituation of the counterproductive patterns the patient has developed, the severity of the spasmodic dysphonia, and the patient's self-efficacy.

Voice therapy for both adductor and abductor spasmodic dysphonia does not treat the underlying involuntary motor pattern associated with the disorder, but focuses on minimizing the resulting counterproductive, compensatory vocal behaviors to maximize the efficiency of voice production. Many patients with adductor or abductor spasmodic dysphonia use excessive expiratory drive during phonation. Those with the adductor type use high subglottal pressure to counteract the hyperadduction and stiffening of the vocal folds, while those with the abductor type compensate for the glottal opening by using higher than expected glottal airflow. Regardless of the glottal configuration, the high expiratory drive places an additional strain on the larynx. Therapy to reduce these counterproductive compensations can enhance voice production in conjunction with and independently of BoNT injections. The expiratory drive can be reduced with the introduction of confidential voice, which improves voice production in many patients. In addition, back pressure exercises such as the airway reflex, Puffy Cheeks, and straw phonation decrease extraneous muscle activity and shift the sensory attention to the facial mask, tricking the larynx to release and disrupting the spasmodic pattern. This shift grants the speaker some control over voice production. It is necessary to vary these procedures in order to avoid their loss of effectiveness as novelty diminishes.

Techniques that rely on vegetative functions or nonhabitual manners of phonation can act as **sensory tricks** and are valuable for reducing the stiffness in the laryngeal area and facilitating continuous phonation for individuals who have either adductor or abductor spasmodic dysphonia. Procedures such as sniffing, yawning, gargling, speaking on inhalation during laughter or sighing, using a higher or lower pitch, speaking with an unfamiliar accent (Sapir & Aronson, 1985), and Froeschel's chewing technique reduce stiffness in the larynx and automatically facilitate a decrease in effort for most individuals. Given that the symptoms of dystonia are often action induced during the usual and customary production of a movement, and sensory tricks reduce or eliminate these dystonic symptoms, speaking in an unexpected manner often improves phonation. The use of resonance, which shifts the sensory attention to the facial mask, actually tricks the larynx to release and disrupts the spasmodic pattern, granting the speaker some control over voice production. It is necessary to vary these sensory tricks in order to avoid their loss of effectiveness as novelty diminishes.

When a patient is diagnosed with spasmodic dysphonia, it can be easy to overlook risk factors (e.g., laryngopharyngeal reflux, smoking, allergies, and talking in noisy environments) that have a negative effect on the patient's voice. Since the symptoms of dystonia fluctuate (e.g., with stress, situations, fatigue), the risk factors may masquerade as part of the neurological disorder. Unfortunately, if risk factors remain undiagnosed, they may exacerbate the voice problem and minimize the effects of the BoNT or behavioral voice therapy.

The clinician in the *Sip and Yawn* video demonstrates the stretch in the pharyngeal area that triggers the pre-yawn, which releases the muscles in the hypopharynx.

Summary

Voice habilitation and rehabilitation are unified by motor learning considerations, underlying physiological patterns, hypothesis testing, a patient-centered environment, and goals that foster generalization of new motor behaviors. Although we have chosen only three specific client groups to describe some of the special demands placed on the voice clinician by disparate patient/client needs and expectations, the similarities among voice patients and procedures are more notable than the differences between them.

References

Adler, R.K., Hirsch, S., and Mordaunt, M. (2012). *Voice and communication therapy for the transgender/transsexual client: A comprehensive guide* (2nd ed.). San Diego, CA: Plural.

American Psychiatric Association. (2013). *Diagnostic and statistical manual of mental disorders* (5th ed.). Arlington, VA: Author.

Arnold, G.E. (1959). Spasmodic dysphonia. *Logos*, 2, 3–14.

Aronson, A.E., Brown, J.R., Litin, E.M., and Pearson, I.S. (1968). Spastic dysphonia. II. Comparison with essential (voice) tremor and other neurologic and psychogenic dysphonias. *Journal of Speech & Hearing Disorders*, 33, 219–231.

Aronson, A. (1990). *Clinical voice disorders: An interdisciplinary approach*. New York, NY: Decker.

Axtell, R.E. (1998). *The do's and taboos of body language around the world*. New York, NY: John Wiley and Sons.

Beemyn, B.G. (Ed.). (2006). *Transgender resource guide*. National Association of Student Personnel Administrators. Ohio State. New York: GLBT Student Services, The Multicultural Center.

Bele, I. (2006). The speaker's formant. *Journal of Voice*, *20*(4), 555–578.

Benninger, M.S., and Murry, T. (2009). *The singer's voice*. San Diego, CA: Plural.

Blitzer, A., and Brin, M.F. (1991). Laryngeal dystonia: A series with botulinum toxin therapy. *Annals of Otology Rhinology & Laryngology*, *100*(2), 85–89.

Blitzer, A., Brin, M.F., Fahn, S., and Lovelace, R.E. (1988). Localized injections of botulinum toxin for the treatment of focal laryngeal dystonia (spasmodic dysphonia). *Laryngoscope*, *98*, 193–197.

Carew, L., Dacakis, G., and Oates, J. (2007). The effectiveness of oral resonance therapy on the perception of femininity of voice in male-to-female transsexuals. *Journal of Voice*, *21*(5), 591–603.

Chapman, J. (2012). *Singing and teaching singing: A holistic approach to classical voice* (2nd ed.). San Diego, CA: Plural.

Cohen, S.M., Jacobson, B.H., Garrett, C.G., Noordzij, J.P., Stewart, M.G., Attia, A., . . . Cleveland, T.F. (2007). Creation and validation of the singing voice handicap index. *Annals of Otology Rhinology & Laryngology*, *116*(6), 402–406.

Currah, P., Juang, R.M., and Minter, S.P. (2006). *Transgender rights*. Minneapolis, MN: University of Minnesota Press.

Dacakis, G., Davies, S., Oates, J.M., Douglas, J.M., and Johnston, J.R. (2013). Development and preliminary evaluation of the transsexual voice questionnaire for male-to-female transsexuals. *Journal of Voice*, *27*(3), 312–320.

Fahn, S. (1988). Concept and classification of dysphonia. *Advances in Neurology*, *50*, 1–8.

Fant, G. (1970). *Acoustic theory of speech production*. The Hague, Netherlands: Monton.

Fitch, J.L., and Holbrook, A. (1970). Modal vocal fundamental frequency of young adults. *Archives of Otolaryngology*, *92*, 379–382.

Gay, T. (1981). Mechanism in the control of speaking rate. *Phonetica*, *38*, 148–158.

Glass, L. (1992). *He says, she says: Closing the communication gap between the sexes*. New York, NY: G.P. Putnam and Sons.

Hancock, A.B., Krissinger, J., and Owen, K. (2011). Voice perceptions and quality of life of transgender people. *Journal of Voice*, *25*(5), 553–558.

Hess, U., Beaupre, M., and Cheung, N. (2002). To whom and why—cultural differences and similarities in the function of smiles. In M.H. Abel (Ed.), *The smile: Forms, functions, and consequences*. New York, NY: The Edwin Mellen Press.

Hixon, T.J. (1987). Respiratory function in speech. In T.J. Hixon (Ed.), *Respiratory function in speech and song*. Boston, MA: Little Brown.

Hoit, J.D., and Hixon, T.J. (1986). Age and speech breathing. *Journal of Speech and Hearing Research*, 30(3), 351–366.

Hu, A., Isetti, D., Hillel, A.D., Waugh, P., Comstock, B., and Meyer, T.K. (2012). Disease-specific self-efficacy in spasmodic dysphonia patients. *Otolaryngology—Head and Neck Surgery*, 148(3), 450–455.

Izdebski, K., Dedo, H.H., and Boles, L. (1984). Spastic dysphonia: A patient profile of 200 cases. *American Journal of Otolaryngology*, 5, 7–14.

Leino, T. (1994). Long-term average spectrum study on speaking voice quality in male actors. In A. Friberg, J. Iwarsson, E. Jansson, & J. Sundberg (Eds.). *SMAC 93 (Proceedings of the Stockholm Music Acoustics Conference 1993)* (pp. 206–210). Stockholm, Sweden: Royal Swedish Academy of Music Sweden, No. 79..

Lessac, A. (1997). *The use and training of the human voice: A practical approach to speech and voice dynamics* (3rd ed.). Santa Monica, CA: McGraw-Hill.

Marsden, C.D. (1988). Investigation of dystonia. *Advances in Neurology*, 50, 35–44.

McCracken, J. (1984). James McCracken. In J. Hines (Ed.), *Great singers on great singing*. (pp. 156–163) Pompton Plains, NJ: Limelight Editions.

Munro, M. (2002). *Lessac's tonal action in women's voices and the "actor's formant": A comparative study* (Unpublished doctoral thesis). Potchefstroom, South Africa: Potchefstroom University.

Nelson, A., and Golant, S.K. (2004). *You don't say: Navigating nonverbal communication between the sexes*. New York, NY: Prentice Hall.

Phyland, D.J., Pallant, J.F., Benninger, M.S., Thibeault, S.L., Greenwood, K.M., Smith, J.A., and Vallance, N. (2013). Development and preliminary validation of the EASE: A tool to measure perceived singing voice function. *Journal of Voice*, 27(4), 454–462.

Rao, P. (1997). Adult neurogenic communication disorders. In T.A. Crowe (Ed.), *Applications of counseling in speech-language pathology and audiology* (pp. 238–261). Baltimore, MD: Lippincott Williams & Wilkins.

Raphael, B.N., and Sherer, R.C. (1987). Voice modification of stage actors: Acoustic analysis. *Journal of Voice*, 1, 83–87.

Sapir, S., and Aronson, A.E. (1985). Clinical reliability in rating voice improvement after laryngeal nerve section for spastic dysphonia. *Laryngoscope*, 95, 200–202.

Shaffer, L.H. (1982). Rhythm and timing in skill. *Psychological Review*, 89(2), 109–122.

Solomon, A. (2012). *Far from the tree: Parents, children and the search for identity*. New York, NY: Scribner.

Stewart, C.F., Allen, E.L., Tureen, P., Diamond, B.E., Blitzer, A., and Brin, M.F. (1997). Adductor spasmodic dysphonia: Standard evaluation of symptoms and severity. *Journal of Voice*, *11*(1), 95–103.

Sundberg, J. (1970). Formant structure and articulation of spoken and sung vowels. *Folia Phoniatrica*, 22, 28–48.

Sundberg, J. (1977). Studies of the soprano voice. *Journal of Research in Singing*, 1(1), 25–35.

Sundberg, J. (1987). *The science of the singing voice*. De Kalb, IL: Northern Illinois Press.

Sundberg, J., and Skoog, J. (1997). Dependence of jaw opening on pitch and vowel in singers. *Journal of Voice, 11*(3), 301–306.

Tannen, D. (1994). *Gender and discourse*. New York, NY: Oxford University Press.

Tanner, K., Roy, N., Merrill, R.M., and Power, D. (2005). Velopharyngeal port status during classical singing. *Journal of Speech, Language and Hearing Research, 48*, 1311–1324.

Tervalon, M., and Murray-Garcia, J. (1998). Cultural humility versus cultural competence: A critical distinction in defining physician training outcomes in multicultural education. *Journal of Health Care for the Poor and Underserved, 9*(2), 117–125.

Titze, I.R. (1994). *Principles of voice production*. Denver, CO: National Center for Voice and Speech.

Titze, I.R., and Verdolini-Abbott, K.V. (2012). *Vocology: The science and practice of voice rehabilitation*. Salt Lake City, UT: The National Center for Voice and Speech.

Wingate, J.M., Ruddy, B.H., Lundy, D.S., Lehman, J., Casiano, R., Collins, S.P., . . . Sapienza, C. (2005). Voice handicap index results for older patients with adductor spasmodic dysphonia. *Journal of Voice, 19*(1), 124–131.

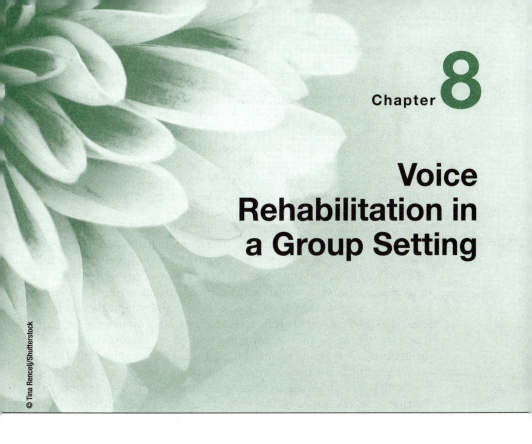

Chapter 8

Voice Rehabilitation in a Group Setting

"As you're introducing yourselves, see if you can use some of the techniques you've been working on in your own sessions, okay?"

Group therapy for adults has been a widely recognized approach to treatment for at least a century. Initially, **group therapy** was created to provide support for people suffering from tuberculosis, and it was later used extensively in psychotherapy and counseling for individuals suffering from alcoholism or drug abuse, cancer, visual impairment, mental disability, or chronic illness. According to Gordon (1965), a group consists of "two or more persons who have a psychological relationship to each other" (p. 323). This proposition "re-emphasizes the notion that the behavior of members of a group affects the behavior of other members" (p. 324).

In the realm of speech pathology, the group setting was originally used to serve the needs of soldiers who had sustained brain injuries during World War II. With limited staff available to cope with the growing number of veterans, the group format provided an efficient and practical environment to conduct aphasia therapy (Kearns & Elman, 2001). During the last half-century, the use of group therapy to supplement and enhance individual voice, speech, and language intervention has gained increased favor not only for aphasia, but for stuttering, traumatic brain injury, deafness, laryngectomy, spasmodic dysphonia, and transgender voice modification.

Traditionally, voice therapy takes place in a one-to-one setting over a period of time determined by factors that include laryngeal diagnosis, chronicity, ongoing occupational demands, general medical considerations, and psychological/emotional/social circumstances. Individuals who suffer from a voice problem, however, often talk about feeling isolated because people do not understand their problem. They feel excluded from conversations, and often avoid social functions owing to the limitations imposed on them by the voice disturbance. Despite the counseling that takes place in the individual sessions, patients may not have the opportunity to discuss their feelings with peers who share a common complaint, or to use the voice in the many diverse situations that have played a role in the development of the voice problem. The interaction between participants in a group allows not only for peer modeling, feedback, and the opportunity to learn from members of the group, but for emotional support, empathy, and mutual concern. Although group voice therapy continues to be relatively uncommon, we have found this setting to be extremely useful as a stand-alone treatment or as an addition to the individual therapy sessions we provide.

Philosophical Underpinnings of Group Voice Therapy

The principles of **cooperative learning**, which was designed as a team-oriented approach (Avent, 1997, 2004), provide the framework for the voice rehabilitation groups we have organized for our patients. The participants in the group share information, work together on procedures within a small group context (four to six individuals), discuss problems associated with practice and adherence, and benefit from one another's strategies to persevere and maintain motivation during the rehabilitation process. Given the opportunities for generalization, peer support and feedback, and peer modeling, the group context offers a relevant working environment to integrate the skills developed in the individual milieu, to acknowledge the long-term changes necessary to maintain a healthy voice, and to better understand therapy as a process that occurs over time.

Historically, cooperative group treatment was organized by similar levels of severity or similar deficits within a particular aspect of language impairment (Avent, 1997). The homogeneity of the group, therefore, was most often based on a diagnostic label. Yet groups that share a diagnosis cope with differences among members pertaining to education, values, occupation, etc. Although we have integrated the cooperative learning model with respect to size and group objectives, the organization of our voice groups includes patients with different etiologies and severity levels because the diagnostic differences between members of the voice group appear to us to be less significant than the similarities between participants. These similarities pertain to the profound negative effects a voice disorder may have on the individual (i.e., isolation, anxiety, and embarrassment), as well as the difficulty that all participants describe in implementing appropriate and efficient techniques during activities of daily living and professional voice use. It appears that what binds group members is the similar impact a voice disorder has on their performance in social interactions and the workplace, rather than the specific diagnosis they have received from the otolaryngologist. Teachers, for instance, face exceptional and specific challenges, which could potentially be addressed in a group context where the participants have a strong and uniting bond.

Patient-Centered Group Therapy

The most effective voice groups are conducted in tandem with individual therapy, which identifies and addresses the patient's individual goals that will then be addressed within the group setting to facilitate carryover. The group format offers a unique challenge for the voice clinician, especially when a client-centered approach is applied to its organization. The principles of accurate empathy, positive regard, and recognition of the patient's capacity to find solutions to his voice problem are especially relevant within a group where the problem-solving process is played out among its participants (Rogers, 1946). If your experience in a group setting is limited, it may be tempting to apply a more directive education model in order to cope with the disparate personalities and attitudes of the group participants. In an effort to maintain control of the group you may call on familiar strategies that encourage patients to seek answers from you rather than through interaction with other group participants. Although you may recognize the importance of cooperative problem solving, the patient's perspective, and self-efficacy, the confidence to allow patients to find their own solutions within the group context takes time to build. The inclination to persuade or convince patients can be a strong one that should be resisted, because when change does not originate from the patient it is likely to be ephemeral, at best.

The specific organization of a voice group derives from its primary goal: to provide a safe and supportive environment in which patients cooperate to integrate and generalize the techniques developed in individual therapy within a variety of social and professional circumstances. These sessions may consist of discussion interwoven with procedures already familiar to the participants, and those that capitalize on the group format. Role-play and presentations, as well as self-monitoring manner of phonation during discussion, provide a variety of opportunities to facilitate generalization. A specific session might begin with a group warm-up to release the jaw, connect with the breath (basic breathing exercises), and reinforce semi-occlusion of the vocal tract (tongue and lip trills). Participants have the opportunity to offer constructive feedback to their peers based on their growing kinesthetic awareness and knowledge of the characteristics of an effective voice, as well as to benefit from the opportunity to implement newly acquired motor patterns into a less structured format than the individual therapy sessions. Some of the categories of procedures that can be used effectively in group voice therapy are presented in **Figure 8-1**.

It may be useful for the clinician to categorize the types of communication that take place in the group setting in order to facilitate the interaction among its participants. The leadership of the group is imperceptible when the clinician holds in mind the specific areas that represent the goals of the group members, and observes their verbal and behavioral interplay in order to evaluate (i.e., engage in **meta-discussion**) whether the interaction represents the goals mutually identified by the clinician and participants. The questions and responses provided by the clinician influence the discussions and interchanges that take place. If, for example, your goal is to encourage peer and independent *problem solving*, you might query the group regarding the strategies they have successfully implemented to address perseverance and adherence (*accountability*). When you actively listen and wait for **peer feedback** and **peer support**, you have indirectly facilitated an interactive formant within which the members find solutions to common problems. Given that the group offers an opportunity for participants to share their concerns and strategies, they benefit from the knowledge that they are not alone in the struggle to modify long-term, counterproductive motor behaviors, and to *generalize* these newly acquired skills to unfamiliar circumstances. When you organize the discourse utterances into specific categories, the structure and direction of the group emerges more tangibly, providing easier access to your role as a facilitator (patient-centered *counseling*), instead of a director or sole source of information. The categories in **Figure 8-2** will facilitate classification of the discourse utterances of group members according to the nature of interaction (Avent, 2004).

Figure 8-1

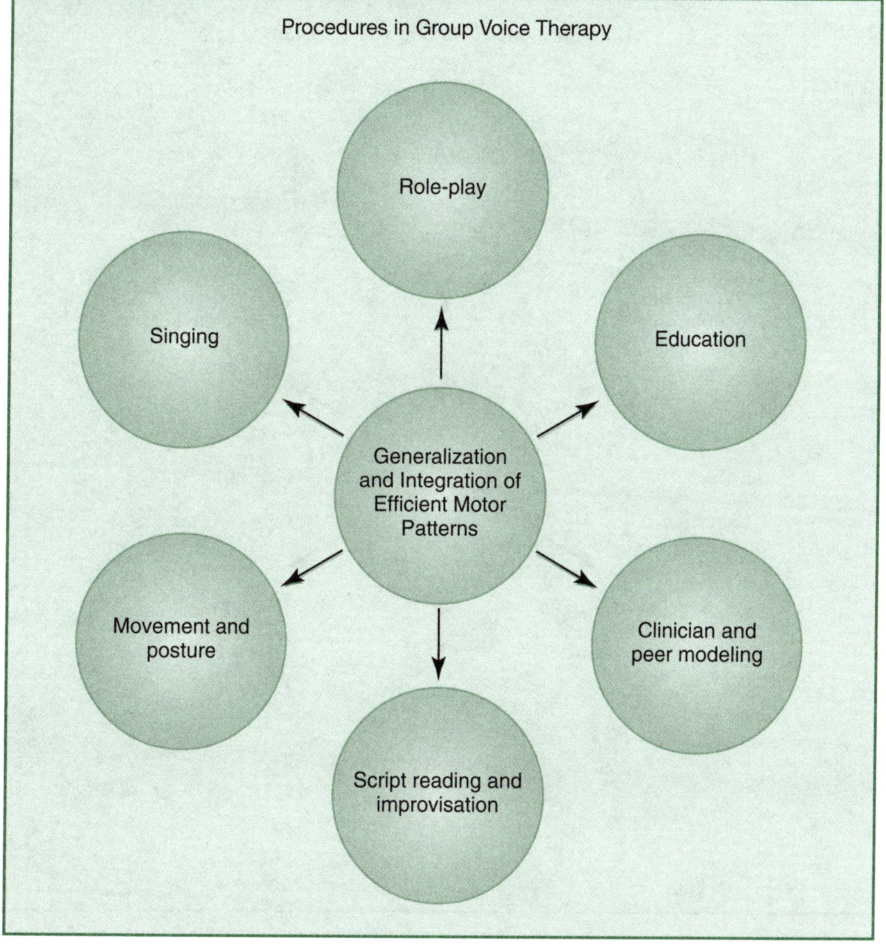

Given that group therapy is a dynamic interaction, the excerpt in **Dialogue 8-1**, taken from an initial group meeting, may be illustrative of the clinician's role and the communication among the group participants. This group consisted of three patients (all of whom happen to be female) and a speech-language pathologist who served as the group leader. During this first session, the clinician set the tone for an open environment by encouraging the participants to describe the difficulties they encountered during the therapeutic process and the strategies that allowed them to persevere despite the obstacles they faced. The speech-language pathologist implemented a patient-centered approach to facilitate the individual narratives and interaction among participants, rather than a **clinician-directed format**. The clinician

Figure 8-2

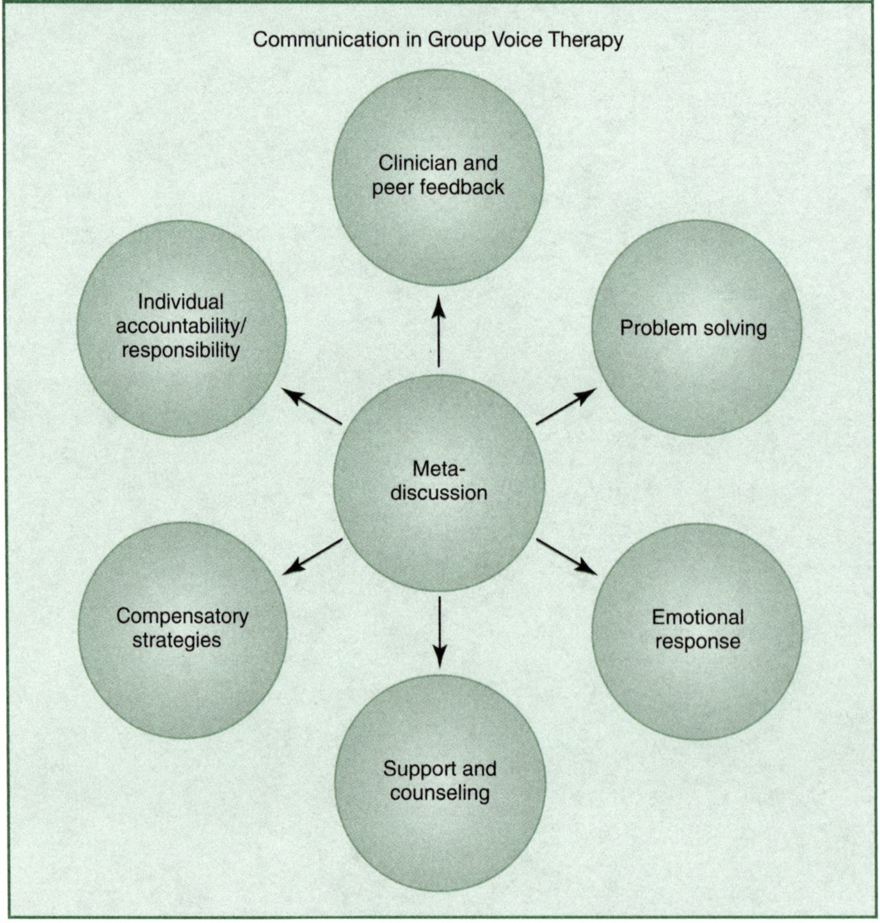

monitored the participants' verbal descriptions of their manner of phonation in order to avoid language that implied self-criticism. When one participant used the word "incorrectly" to describe a difficult transfer experience, the leader suggested that a better focus might be "to note the presence of effort." This subtle shift from "judging" to "noticing" may increase the patients' insight and willingness to carry over the techniques developed in the individual sessions.

The group described in Dialogue 8-1 developed a warm and supportive camaraderie. Those who had progressed further in therapy supported the newer member. This group context allowed the three participants to practice their skills and receive the feedback necessary to generalize the techniques to more cognitively loaded situations.

Dialogue 8-1
Excerpt from Voice Group Session #1 (Three Participants)

I began with an open question, "Have you met each other?"

All three patients responded as one, "No."

Encouraging the patients to talk with one another, I said, "Why don't you introduce yourselves?"

Ms. S began with little use of flow phonation, " I'm S. I'm a graduate student, and I've been in voice therapy for three months. I had vocal cord nodules and now they are gone. I'm scared to start talking louder."

I recognized that the patient was not integrating the technique addressed in the individual sessions, and I wanted to focus the group on the process of transferring their skills, "As you're introducing yourselves, see if you can use some of the techniques you've been working on in your own sessions, okay?"

Ms. W spoke next and applied resonant phonation to her speech, "I'm W, and I lost my voice because of vocal nodules as well. I'm a professor, and I had to give up teaching for the semester. When other remedies didn't work, I started voice therapy."

Noting the easy, effortless flow of her voice, "And where are you in your therapy? What's changed since you've started?"

She continued with an effective manner of phonation, "A lot. My nodules have gone away, and I'm working on soft starts to my vowels and sustaining my breath. I haven't yet started to work on loudness."

All three patients laughed.

Laughing, I restated, "The big 'L.'"

With quiet, controlled phonation throughout, Ms. N introduced herself, "I'm N, and my voice has gotten very hoarse. Today is a good example. I'm learning how to use my voice differently. My vocal cords are very thin. It's the only part of me that's very thin [Laughter]. So, I'm learning how to treat them kindly and produce a better sound quality."

Pleased with Ms. N's personalization of the goals of therapy, "So what's one of the things that you've been doing to 'treat them kindly?' What's changed for you?"

Using confidential voice, Ms. N continued thoughtfully, "Well, speaking in a confidential voice, which isn't natural for me. I didn't realize it, but I had a very hard-edged voice. So I'm speaking confidentially, and concentrating on soft vowels at the beginning of what I'm saying."

I was impressed with her deliberate focus on the sensations in her vocal tract. "Well, you have some other challenges in your life that were making you use your voice . . .

Ms. N blurted out, "Incorrectly."

I feared that the conversation could slip into self-criticism, and I quickly changed its direction, "Well, maybe not incorrectly, but with a lot of effort. What are some of those challenges?"

Thoughtfully, and continuing to use deliberate self-monitoring, Ms. N continued, "Oh, well, my husband is hard of hearing, and he didn't want to accept that. He kept on saying, 'Speak louder.' I fell into that trap [laughing]. But I'm not doing it now. I feel very good about that. I just repeat what I said at the same level, and he seems to get it. I think maybe he gives up sometimes. But, it's not affecting me. It's not aggravating my voice. So that's it."

Ms. W jumped into the conversation, and focused on her manner of phonation, Ms. W added, "Oh, I had a family problem, too. I just had some cousins in from out of town with some little kids. It's very distracting with kids around, so it's hard to pay attention to this stuff."

I recognized an opportunity to facilitate group problem solving, "I was wondering if sometimes your voice problem is isolating in a way. The number of people who have voice problems is far fewer than people who have other kinds of speech problems. They don't often get to talk to one another and find out how it is that you solve a problem and what strategies work best. This is something that might be useful to talk about here. You've been through a fair amount of voice therapy, and you're pretty much almost finished. I mean, we're just putting the icing on the cake here, right? You've worked very hard and have been disciplined and very consistent, which I think is part of what it takes. And that's another aspect of therapy that's difficult. To be consistent and do the exercises. What sorts of things were hard for you in the beginning?"

After a moment of thought and now incorporating ease and flow, Ms. S slowly offered, "Okay, it's all about breaking habits. Confidential voice was impossible for me. I was teaching preschool. So you can imagine. I had 17 2-year-olds, so you can imagine the—"

Instantaneously, and with appropriate inflection and ease Ms. N said, "Oh, absolutely."

Continuing to maintain her easy manner of production, Ms. S affirmed, "The contrast. And that was the first challenge. That was so hard. The phone was probably the hardest. My parents always put me on speakerphone. And I just had to say, 'I can't, I can't do it.' When you're on speakerphone, it's so much harder to hear the other person. Your reaction is to talk louder. I work in a library. I asked my boss to 'Remind me to talk quietly' and she did. It was a very supportive environment. That was my first big challenge. Then easy onsets were the second one, because that's another habit to break. It's so unnatural to have to add a silent /h/ before your words. It's really hard. So just learning to break your habits is really hard. And then remembering to practice. I put notes everywhere. In fact, I have a note on my cell phone here."

In an easy and effective voice, Ms. N questioned, "What does that say?"

Ms. S giggled and displayed her phone, "'Easy onsets.' So, I have reminders everywhere. Because I would realize when I wasn't using them, but it was too late. So all I do is feel guilty about it."

Ms. W joined in producing a resonate voice, "That's really a good idea."

Her attention slipped and Ms. S's voice became slightly pressed, "So yeah, that worked well."

Wanting to verify if they had the same instructions, Ms. N queried, "Did you have an hourly practice regimen? Were you supposed to do something every hour?"

Ms. S focused carefully on the resonance of her voice and said, "Yeah. It changed throughout, but I started with—I forget the names of all the exercises. What are they?"

Pleased about the client interaction and support, I recognized an opening to provide specific information about treatment, "The first ones you practiced, which you're all doing, the /mhm/ one is called a back pressure exercise."

Ms. S took advantage of the group setting to explore her experience and integrate an appropriate manner of phonation. She said a bit more. "Okay, so I started with that, and I was doing it every hour."

Seeking affirmation about the difficulty with practice, Ms. N asked, "And did you have trouble doing it every hour?"

Ms. S shook her head, chuckled, and produced an easy, resonant voice, "Yeah, I was supposed to do it every hour, and it was hard. There were times when I just couldn't do it. You said that you can do it on the train and stuff. But I found I really couldn't practice on the train, because, the /hu/ part is . . . [laughter]. I worked it into my morning and evening routines. I did it when I'd wake up, I'd do it in the shower, I'd do it frequently. I don't know if there was harm in doing it too much, but I did it as much as possible when I was home. I couldn't do it while I was at work, or when teaching my classes. I wasn't going to leave class to do back pressure exercises, you know, so yeah, I wasn't *that* consistent. But I was very consistent while I was home by myself, or on the weekends."

This safe environment is also necessary for transgender individuals who are in the process of transferring the vocal persona and experimenting with different speaking styles.

The Transgender Voice Group

Although it is more common for voice patients to receive individual and group voice therapy concurrently, transgender voice clients often choose to participate exclusively in one or the other process. Clients who participate in both individual and group sessions appear to have a richer experience because they can share their ambivalence with one another and discuss the commonality that exists among them with respect to the transition process. These discussions often lead to the realization that one's goals are as fluid as the continuum of gender. The group experience allows the individuals to explore these ongoing concerns in a safe environment that encourages mutual problem solving as well as an exploration of communicative styles that are compatible with the persona they wish to project.

In contrast, during the individual sessions clients access a gender-acceptable and effective pitch range, develop easy and efficient patterns of breath control, and learn to capitalize on the resonating characteristics of the vocal tract. Those clients who participate concurrently in the group and individual sessions find that the peer feedback and camaraderie of the group sessions enhance the work of one-to-one sessions as well as the process of generalizing.

An effective transgender voice group offers a multidimensional setting that integrates all aspects of voice and communication, with special attention to physical presentation, posture (Franco et al., 2014), gestures, and movement. Only when the process includes the whole person does the voice become an authentic, credible part of the individual's identity. A believable physical presentation may be difficult for the individual to determine on his or her own. The group offers a protected environment where the client can integrate the physical presentation with the voice modification work. Some may bring their clothing and change into the gender-appropriate apparel immediately prior to a group session so they can practice wearing the gender-appropriate clothing as they practice and have a more integrated experience. When all of these elements combine, the prosodic patterns, the gestures, and the movement of the chosen gender are more naturally and easily sustained.

A background in theatre and singing can be extremely useful to the clinician who works with trans speakers in a voice group. In a group of male-to-female participants, the inclusion of film and television clips of women whose voices are feminine but not necessarily high-pitched dramatizes the various qualities and range of the female voice. Films with actresses from previous generations—among them Marlene Dietrich, Lauren Bacall, Joan Crawford, Barbara Stanwyck, and Rosalind Russell—and from this generation—including Cate Blanchett, Kathleen Turner, Scarlett Johansson, Kirstie Alley, and Angelina Jolie—demonstrate that pitch is not the sole arbiter of femininity. The analysis of the characteristics and use of the female actor's communicative style reveal the significance of these feminine attributes to the desired persona.

A participant in the transgender voice group in the *Self-Evaluation of Comedy Performance* video is pleased that she now integrates breath control and "a feminine energy" during her comedy performances.

The client in the *Practice Regimen: Projecting the Voice* video describes her practice routine with an emphasis on attention to rhythm and intonation rather than imitation.

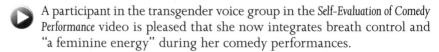

Attention to the actor's facial expression, eye movements, and gestures in combination with intonation patterns, speech rhythm, and rate provide useful visual and **auditory feedback** that can be applied to the reenactment of scenes that are then played by the group participants. Group procedures that incorporate script, role-play, and improvisation allow the group members to explore gender roles, vocal emotion, accents, and the dynamic range of their voices. Sometimes an accent or role provides access to a more feminine voice, posture, and use of gestures. A southern accent, for example, with its slow, vowel-to-vowel lilting, and even slightly breathy quality often facilitates the prosodic elements that enhance the female persona. This is not to say that a southern accent is the goal of the trans speaker, but that imagery can be incorporated to achieve the softer, more fluid, flowing voice of a woman. Variations on these procedures might include taking turns with the delivery of a line from a film to illustrate the many possible prosodic features available to the speaker. It is always a surprise to our group members that the same line enacted by several speakers can be delivered in so many different ways. This practice again reinforces the idea that pitch is only a part of the female voice, and that the perception of femininity is multifaceted. Each individual explores his or her own distinctive and authentic way to communicate.

The client in the *Discussion of Projection and Speech Rate* video recognizes the connection between giving the body time to breathe, the preparation required to project the voice, and the effectiveness of communication.

The clinician in the *Integration of Techniques: Script Reading* video prepares the group to perform a commercial with suggestions regarding each participant's objective and action during the reading. The participants in the film clip integrate intonation, singing, and accent to bring the commercial to life.

In the same way that prosody varies between female speakers, posture, gesture, and facial expression are quite individual. Emulating the movements of a film or television actor contributes to the repertoire available to the client as she integrates these features to make them congruent with the characteristics she wishes to embody. With repetition and reinforcement, these aspects of femininity become valuable assets to the physical presentation.

The poem, written and performed by the group member in the *Poem: "Imagine"* video, describes her difficult transition, feeling "different," and her recognition that she must accept herself in order to continue the process.

Imagery provides access to the sensibility and sensations that are associated with the envisioned persona. The imagination allows one to integrate voice, prosody (intonation, rhythm, rate), body language, posture, and gesture with clothing, jewelry, hairstyle, and make-up. The internal picture created by the individual then becomes active during role-play, script reading, and improvisations that incorporate the appropriate emotions and responses of the character with the chosen gender. The ultimate goal is to integrate all aspects of communication into a unified whole, to reinforce the newly acquired motor patterns, and to encourage exploration of a credible self.

The participants in the *Group Impressions of Breathing Exercises* video discuss the importance of breath control to facilitate the feminine intonation patterns and loudness ranges that are a part of everyday communication. They emphasize the significance of repetition to integrate these sophisticated motor patterns and acquire automaticity and flexibility of breath management.

We encourage our transgender clients to discuss their outside experiences using the techniques developed in the group setting. When a trans woman client is frustrated and distressed because she was addressed as "Sir," the group members offer support as well as concrete examples of the techniques they use to circumvent these occasions. When the group includes clients of varying ages and cultural backgrounds, the discussion includes divergent perspectives on what transition means (Freeman, 1993). More and more frequently, the younger clients in our voice groups express their indifference to passing in the traditional, binary classification system. They value the freedom to merely "be" rather than "pass." Their attitudes are often antithetic to those older clients who more often want acceptance in the chosen gender 100% of the time. Despite the diversity of these viewpoints, the influence of each on the other appears to be beneficial. Younger clients appreciate the tenacity and courage that older participants have shown, and the more seasoned participants welcome and recognize the value of taking risks to be oneself and live in a more fluid continuum of gender expression.

A group member in the *Being "Sirred"* video, emphasizes how important one's attitude is with respect to "being sirred." She notes the tendency to regress without practice of the characteristics that feminize her voice and describes special difficulty on the telephone. She uses humor to dissipate some of the embarrassment and hurt she has experienced.

The group participant in the *Self-Evaluation* video, has achieved a sense of comfort with herself that the video she produced demonstrates to her. She has struggled with negative feelings about her physical appearance and the credibility of her voice, but has begun to recognize her many assets.

The psychosocial aspects of transition and their relevance to voice modification and its effective long-term integration into one's daily life represent a primary focus of these group discussions. In the end the recognition that ". . . there are many ways of life and many truths . . ." and that "true 'advance' is the development of the human being as an integrated whole" (Berlin, 1998, p. 409) is what we hope to bring to our clients.

Summary

A group format is a recent phenomenon that has proven to be a very effective one for voice habilitation and rehabilitation because it provides a transition between a structured context and the more demanding, spontaneous speaking situations that patients will eventually face. The group setting is not recommended as a substitute for the individual work, but as an opportunity to transfer the techniques developed during the one-to-one sessions to a less structured context. Certainly, the group format does not suit all personalities or requirements. Individuals may be reluctant to join a group because of shyness and a reticence to incorporate newly acquired motor patterns into an environment that is foreign to them. Nevertheless, for those patients who choose the group as an interim stage, this setting can represent a powerful impetus to the process of generalization.

References

Avent, J. (1997). *Manual of cooperative group treatment for aphasia*. Boston, MA: Butterworth and Heinemann.

Avent, J. (2004). Group treatment for aphasia using cooperative learning principles. *Topics in Language Disorders*, 24(2), 118–124.

Berlin, I. (1998). *The proper study of mankind: An anthology of essays*. New York, NY: Farrar, Straus, and Giroux.

Franco, D., Martins, F., Andrea, M., Fragoso, I., Carrao, L., and Teles, J. (2014). Is the sagittal postural alignment different in normal and dysphonic adult speakers? *Journal of Voice*, 28(4), 523.e1–523.e8.

Freeman, S.C. (1993). Client-centered therapy with diverse populations: The universal within the specific. *Journal of Multicultural Counseling and Development*, 21(4), 248–254.

Gordon, J.E. (1965). Project cause, the federal anti-poverty program, and some implications of subprofessional training. *American Psychology*, 20, 334–343.

Kearns, K., and Elman, R. (2001). Language intervention strategies in aphasia and related neurogenic communication disorders. In R. Chapey (Ed.), *Group therapy for aphasia: Theoretical and practical considerations* (4th ed., pp. 316–337). Baltimore, MD: Lippincott Williams & Wilkins.

Rogers, C.R. (1946). Significant aspects of client-centered therapy. *American Psychologist, 1*, 415–422.

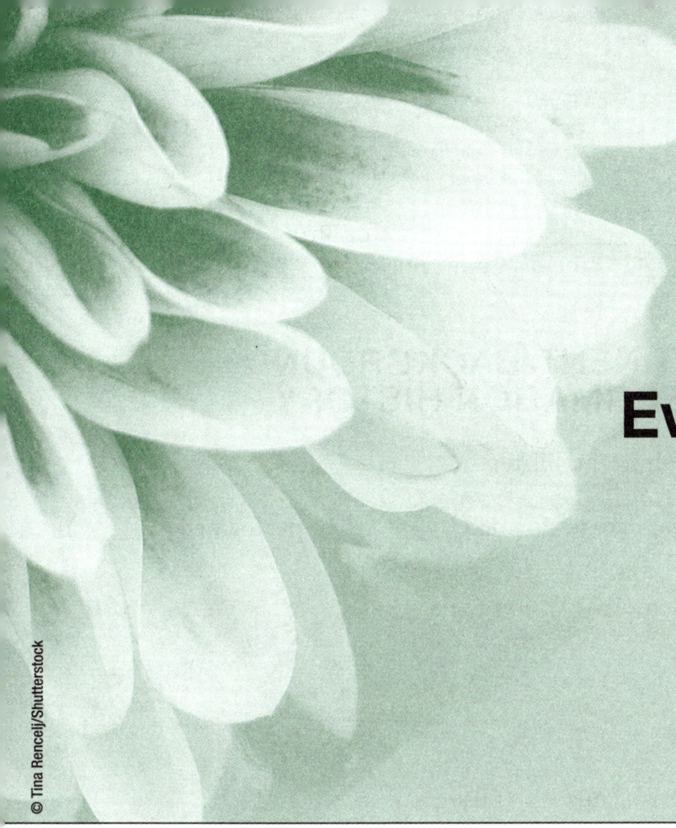

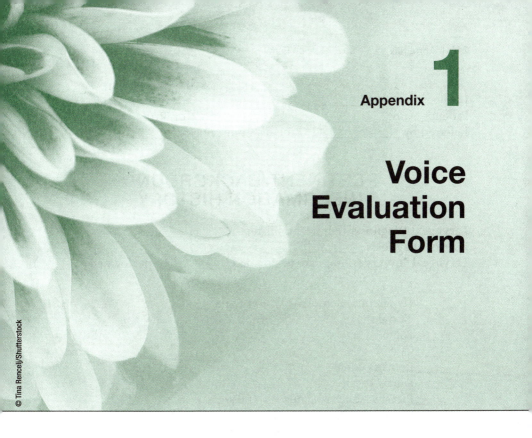

Appendix 1

Voice Evaluation Form

I started with an open-ended question: "How did your voice problem begin?"

A voice assessment offers an opportunity for us to appreciate the voice problem from the patient's point of view, and to evaluate his current manner of phonation. Diagnostic therapy during this initial meeting yields information regarding the ease with which the individual modifies effort with clinician cues and models. We begin the treatment process by integrating these observations with our fund of knowledge of the anatomy and physiology of the voice production subsystems, motor learning theory, patient-centered care, and evidence-based practice.

Date of Evaluation _______________
Patient's Name ___________________________ Date of Birth ____________
Referred by ______________ Patient's Complaint(s) ______________________

PERTINENT/BACKGROUND INFORMATION HISTORY

Laryngeal Diagnosis (left, right, bilateral)
Date of Diagnosis _______________
Laryngeal Surgery (none, date performed ______, to be performed _______)

_____ Edema
_____ Hyperemia, hemorrhage, erythema
_____ Nodule
_____ Polyp
_____ Cyst
_____ Reinke's edema
_____ Sulcus vocalis
_____ Paresis/paralysis (unilateral/bilateral)
_____ Spasmodic dysphonia
_____ Paradoxical vocal fold motion (PVFM)
_____ Tremor
_____ Glottic insufficiency (bowing)
_____ Presbylarynx (atrophy/bowing)
_____ Muscle tension dysphonia
_____ Other (specify)____________________________

Pertinent Medical History/Risk Factors
How long has the problem persisted? ______________________________
Onset (gradual, sudden) ______________________________
Course of symptoms (stable, worsening, improving) ______________________________
Pain or discomfort ______________________________
General surgery ______________________________
Medications ______________________________
Alcohol, tobacco, recreational drug(s) ______________________________
Asthma/ COPD/emphysema ______________________________
Allergies/sinusitis ______________________________
Dyspnea ______________________________
Chronic cough ______________________________

Throat clearing ______________________________
Laryngopharyngeal reflux (LPR)/Gastroesophageal reflux disease (GERD) ______________________________
Neurological diagnosis ______________________________
Hearing loss (self, significant other) ______________________________
Excessive stiffness in the head, neck, shoulders, thorax ______________________________
Grinds teeth ______________________________
Exercise regimen ______________________________
Family history of voice disorders ______________________________
Psychological/emotional factors ______________________________
Other medical history ______________________________

Daily Voice Use

Occupation________________
Is dysphonia/aphonia a handicap in occupation? Yes/No
How is it a limitation? ______________________________

_____ Extensive social talking
_____ Extensive phone use
_____ Lectures/meetings
_____ Classroom teaching
_____ Singing performances/concerts
_____ Inappropriate loudness
_____ Noisy environment
_____ Effortful laughing or crying
_____ Vocal fatigue
_____ Extensive travel
_____ Air pollution (type)
_____ Airborne irritants
_____ Exacerbating behaviors
_____ Behaviors that improve voice
_____ Other (specify)____________

Self-Assessment Questionnaires

Voice Handicap Index (VHI) ______________________________
Voice-Related Quality of Life (V-RQOL) ______________________________
General Self-Efficacy Scale (GSES) ______________________________
Reflux Symptom Index (RSI) ______________________________
The Evaluation of the Ability to Sing Easily (EASE) ______________________________
Singing Voice Handicap Index (SVHI) ______________________________
Transgender Self-Evaluation Questionnaire (TSEQ) ______________________________
Transsexual Voice Questionnaire for Male to-Female Transsexuals TVQ (MtF) ______________________________
Effects of Sex Hormones on Attitudes and Behaviors ______________________________
Voice Handicap Index—Spasmodic Dysphonia (VHI SD) ______________________________
Disease-Specific Self-Efficacy in Spasmodic Dysphonia (SE-SD) ______________________________

DIRECT OBSERVATION

Severity of Dysphonia (none, mild, mild-to-moderate, moderate, moderate-to-severe, severe)

Severity of Perceptual Voice Symptoms
(none, mild, mild-to-moderate, moderate, moderate-to-severe, severe)

___ Rough
___ Breathy
___ Strident
___ Strained-strangled
___ Hypernasality
___ Hyponasality
___ Back quality
___ Persistent falsetto
___ Virilization

___ Abrupt initiations
___ Fading at end of breath groups
___ Vocal fry
___ Creaky voice
___ Pressed phonation
___ Inappropriate loudness
___ Inappropriate loudness variability
___ Limited loudness range

___ Inappropriate pitch variability
___ Limited pitch range
___ Pitch breaks
___ Voice breaks
___ Aphonia, continuous
___ Aphonia, intermittent
___ Tremor
___ Other (specify)

Prosody (normal, mild, mild-to-moderate, moderate, moderate-to-severe, severe)

___ monotone ___ inappropriate inflection patterns ___ inappropriate stress

Other Perceptual Symptoms **Behavioral Symptoms**
(none, mild, mild-to-moderate, moderate, moderate-to-severe, severe)

___ Effortful phonation
___ Excessive expiratory drive
___ Limited expiratory drive
___ Stridor (inhalation/exhalation)

___ Extraneous muscle activity (head, neck, thorax)
___ Extensive clavicular motion during inhalation
___ Behavioral TMJ
___ Tongue posteriorization
___ Posture (lordosis, kyphosis)
___ Other (specify) _______________

Respiratory Function

Mean vital capacity ___________ cc

Mean maximum phonation time /a/ ____ sec

Phonation quotient ___________ (Vital capacity ÷ maximum phonation time for /a/)

Mean duration /s/___________ sec

Mean duration /z/___________ sec

s/z ratio __________

Mean flow _________ cc/sec

Breaths per minute _____________

Acoustic Analysis

Mean F_0 vowel ______Hz

Mean F_0 continuous speech _____ Hz

Frequency perturbation (vowel) _______ Hz

Amplitude perturbation (vowel) _______

Harmonics-to-noise ratio (vowel) ___

Spectrum of a vowel (vowel) _______

Broadband analysis (vowel) ________

Intensity vowel ____ dB

Intensity continuous speech _____ dB

Diagnostic Voice Tokens	**Appropriate (✓)**	**Inappropriate (✓)**
/mhm/	___________	___________
/hu/ downward inflection	___________	___________
Voiced sigh	___________	___________
Yawn/sigh	___________	___________
Glissando /a/ (low to high, high to low)	___________	___________
Falsetto (male) / whistle register (female)	___________	___________
Vocal fry	___________	___________
Shout ("taxi")	___________	___________
Quiet voice ("shh, the baby is sleeping")	___________	___________
Whisper ("shh, the baby is sleeping")	___________	___________
Cough	___________	___________
Laugh (unelicited)	___________	___________

Discrimination/Identification of Effortful Versus Easy Manner of Phonation

(Y/N) ___ in evaluator ___ in self

Modification of Effort (Model one or more of the Diagnostic Therapy Tokens)

Token 1 _____ (Patient modified production [Y/N]) _________________

Token 2 _____ (Patient modified production [Y/N]) _________________

Structure and Function of the Speech Mechanism
(Within normal limits or remarkable)

___ Lips ______________________________

___ Jaw ______________________________

___ Tongue ______________________________

___ Hard palate ______________________________

___ Soft palate ______________________________

SCREENINGS

Hearing	___ Within normal limits	___ Remarkable
Cognition and Language	___ Within normal limits	___ Remarkable
Articulation and Fluency	___ Within normal limits	___ Remarkable
Swallowing	___ Within normal limits	___ Remarkable

IMPRESSIONS AND RECOMMENDATIONS

Diagnostic Impressions (Diagnostic Hypotheses) ______________________________

____

Prognosis ______________________________

____

Recommendations ______________________________

____

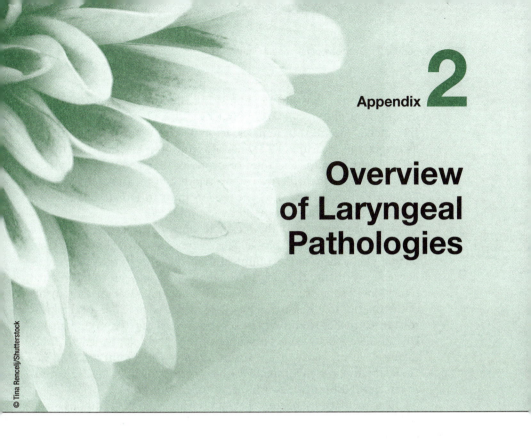

Appendix 2

Overview of Laryngeal Pathologies

When a patient comes to you for a voice evaluation he may have questions about the laryngeal diagnosis, etiology, progression, and possible negative outcomes if the condition is left untreated. It is often our responsibility to provide information that addresses his concerns (appropriate or inappropriate) that often pertain to whether the lesion is life-threatening or will permanently affect his voice. In the following tables we provide an overview of the laryngeal anatomy and physiology and the most common laryngeal pathologies typically treated in the voice clinician's practice.

The Larynx: Structure and Function

The larynx is much smaller and more delicate than you may realize. It varies across individuals much like the size of a nose, ears, and feet and is larger in males than in females. The laryngeal structure grows in length and diameter during normal development, with significant changes taking place during puberty. According to Sappey (1872), the mean height of the adult larynx is 1.73 inches (44 mm) in males and 1.42 inches (36 mm) in females. Its transverse diameter is similar to its height and measures 1.7 inches (43 mm) in males and 1.61 inches (41 mm) in females. The anterior-posterior diameter of the larynx is slightly smaller than the transverse width and measures 1.42 inches (36 mm) in males and 1.02 inches (26 mm) in females. This small structure houses the even smaller vocal folds.

The vibrating edge of the vocal fold (anterior 2/3), composed of the vocal ligament, is soft and pliable. This membranous structure is bordered on one end by the anterior commissure and the other by the vocal prominence. It is difficult to measure the length of the fold due to the gradual transitions of soft tissue into cartilage (Titze, 2006). Mean measurements of the anterior to posterior length of the medial edge of the vocal folds at rest are .63 inches (16 mm) in males and .39 inches (10 mm) in females. Due to the elasticity and compliance of the vocal fold, its length easily increases during pitch changes from .22 inches (5.6 mm) to .59 inches (15.0 cm) in males and from .02 inches (.6 mm) to .50 inches (12.6 mm) in females (Nishizawa, Sawashima, & Yonemoto, 1988).

The medial edge of the vocal fold is comprised of gelatinous material and does not contain muscle fibers. The cover of the fold has an overall thickness of .037 inches (.93 mm) in males and .038 inches (.96 mm) in females (Titze, 2006). During vibration, the glottis opens and closes in an upward rocking motion and the glottal opening at the maximum striking zone varies from a fraction of a millimeter at low subglottal pressures to nearly .196 inches (5 mm) at high subglottal pressures (Titze, 2006).

The larynx is a complex valve constructed of fast moving and delicate structures—its position above the trachea and below the pharynx allows air to pass through to the articulators above. The primary function of the larynx is to protect the airway from foreign matter by mechanically blocking and forcefully expelling items that have been aspirated. The secondary function of the larynx, producing voice, is the focus of this text. As you can imagine, all laryngeal pathologies that affect the closure of the glottis can result not only in a voice problem but the potential threat of aspiration.

The thyroid cartilage and the cricoid cartilage are composed of hyaline cartilage and form the scaffolding for the larynx. The cricothyroid joint dwells between these cartilages and is manipulated to control pitch. Two arytenoid cartilages made of both hyaline and elastic cartilage are located on top of the cricoid cartilage and articulate along the cricoarytenoid joint to adduct and abduct the vocal folds. Two corniculate cartilages and two tiny cuneiform cartilages made of elastic cartilage rest on top of the arytenoid cartilages and do not appear to have an impact on voicing or swallowing but are visible as small bumps in the aryepiglottic fold. The fifth and final cartilage, the epiglottis, is a large, leaf-shaped structure made of elastic cartilage that supplements the protection of the airway during swallow. The larynx is suspended from the hyoid bone, which attaches to several strap muscles and provides support for the tongue root. The suprahyoid and infrahyoid muscles are responsible for elevating and lowering the larynx (Zemlin, 1998). We pay attention to this muscle activity because we often note extraneous involvement in these extrinsic laryngeal muscles when our patients use an effortful manner of phonation.

The intrinsic laryngeal musculature is responsible for forming the membranous portion of the vocal folds, for adducting and abducting the folds, and for tilting the thyroid cartilage to facilitate changes in pitch. All of these actions are necessary for both the production of the voice and protection of the airway. The paired vocal folds are made up of two bundles of striated fibers—the thyromuscularis muscle and the more medial thyrovocalis muscle. The vocal folds move quickly to close the glottis (to protect the airway), but they are delicate and should not be pressed tightly together for prolonged periods. The posterior cricoarytenoid is the primary abductor of the vocal folds and the lateral cricoarytenoid (the antagonist to the posterior cricoarytenoid muscle) facilitates increases in vocal intensity. The interarytenoid muscles adduct the vocal folds. The cricothyroid muscle is the intrinsic muscle responsible for increasing the fundamental frequency and the thyroarytenoid muscle contributes to active lowering of pitch.

The interior of the larynx, with the exception of the vibrating portion of the true and false vocal folds, is lined with ciliated columnar epithelium, and the medial edge of the vocal fold is covered with the more durable squamous cell epithelium. The vocal folds are a multilayered structure that is clinically divided into the *cover*, *transition*, and *body* (Hirano, 1981). The *cover* of the vocal folds includes the squamous cell epithelium and the gelatinous superficial layer of the lamina propria. This represents the flexible, medial edge of the larynx that generates the mucosal wave and is responsible for the complex and beautiful tone of a normal voice. Damage to this area may result in disruption of the mucosal wave and changes in the pitch, loudness, and quality of the voice. Laryngeal pathologies in the cover are usually observed easily when viewing the larynx with instrumentation such as videostroboscopy or ultra-high-speed photography. The vocal fold *transition* is made up of the elastic fibers of the intermediate layer of the lamina propria and the collagenous fibers of the deep layer of the lamina propria. The *body* of the vocal fold is stiffer than the cover or transition and is composed of the thyroarytenoid muscle, which has two sections—the more medial thyrovocalis and the lateral thyromuscularis. The arytenoid cartilages are adducted to phonation neutral position and remain in this position during production of all voice sounds. The vocal folds abduct during voiceless sounds and quiet inhalation and exhalation.

Pathologies of the Larynx

Given the small dimensions of the vocal folds, it is easy to understand that a vocal nodule the size of a grain of sand or a period at the end of a sentence can change the compliance, weight, and stiffness of the vocal fold and alter the vibratory pattern. When a lesion develops in the vocal fold cover it often results from an inappropriate manner of phonation and occurs in the midmembranous portion of the vocal folds (i.e., the primary striking zone) (Hochman, Sataloff, Hillman, & Zeitels, 1999) because the greatest kinetic forces take place here. The diagram in **Box A2-1** identifies this zone. The anterior (anterior commissure) and posterior (arytenoid cartilages) portions of the membranous vocal fold provide anchors during phonation, permitting the midmembranous portion of the vocal fold to make lateral and medial excursions. The middle of this zone makes the greatest excursions (like a jump rope); thus the term **primary striking zone**.

Absence of Medical Pathology

When an individual encounters a vocal problem associated with a temporary upper respiratory infection, a severe episode of reflux, excessive and forceful coughing, laughing, or sobbing, he may compensate ineffectively by pushing the voice, using the ventricular vocal folds to make sound, or adducting the vocal folds during inhalation. These counterproductive behaviors probably began as a short-term strategy to maintain vocal intensity and clarity during a period of vocal, anatomic, or physiologic stress and then developed into a chronic, habitual problem (See **Table A2-1**).

It is not always the case that your patient brings a report with a specific laryngeal diagnosis from the otolaryngologist (Table A2-1). Dysphonia is often a symptom of an incipient, developing problem that shows no visible lesion except perhaps minor inflammation of the vocal fold. Nonetheless, voice production may be sufficiently compromised to require intervention. During assessment and treatment, you will consider the possible sources of the presenting problem and work with your patient to reverse and eliminate these counterproductive or phonotraumatic events. Nonetheless, our goal is not to eliminate esion—although this often occurs as an added benefit. *The goal of therapy is to improve the ease, efficiency, and effectiveness of the voice and strive for ptimal coordination among the respiratory, phonatory, resonation, and articulation ystems of voice production for a given task.*

Box A2-1

Adduction/Abduction and Vibration of the Vocal Folds

Abduction of Vocal Folds During Inhalation

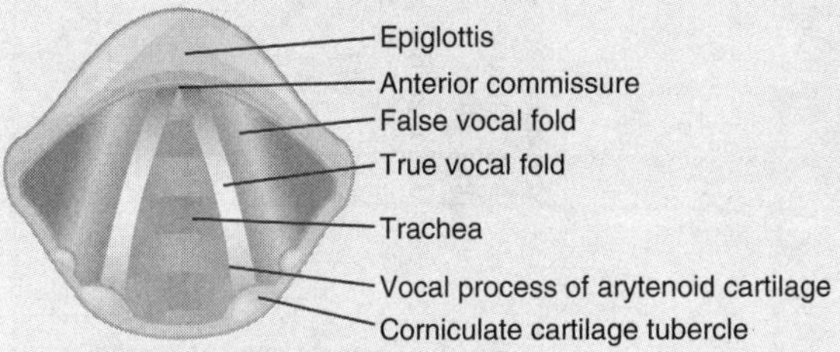

During inspiration, which almost always precedes phonation, the vocal folds are abducted to allow air to pass through unimpeded. The arytenoid cartilage cannot be seen, but the corniculate seen as a small mound rests atop it.

Adduction of Vocal Folds to Phonation Neutral Position

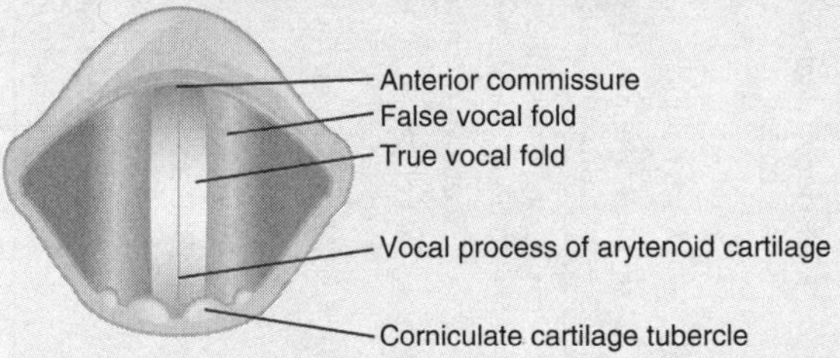

At the onset of phonation, the arytenoid cartilages adduct the vocal folds to phonation neutral position (~3 mm separates the cartilages) (Zemlin, 1998).

Excursions of the Vocal Folds During Phonation

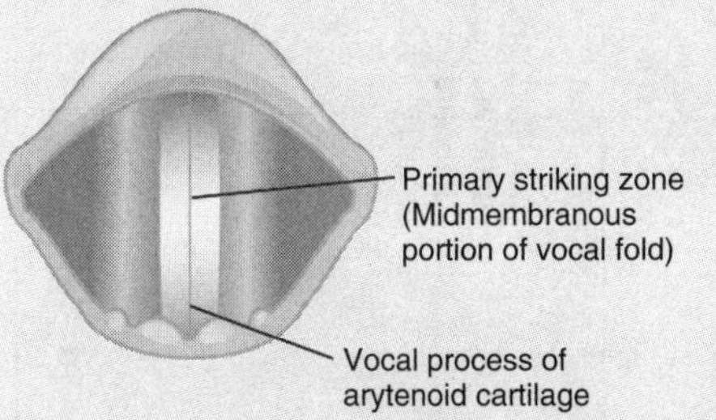

At the initiation of phonation, the membraneous portion of the vocal folds is sucked toward the midline due to the Bernoulli effect. The arytenoid cartilages remain in phonation neutral position while the membranous portion vibrates.

When the air pressure below the glottis exceeds ~3 to 4 cm H_2O (for quiet phonation), the membranous portions of the vocal folds are blown apart. The arytenoid cartilages remain in phonation neutral position.

Development of Lesion at the Primary Striking Zone

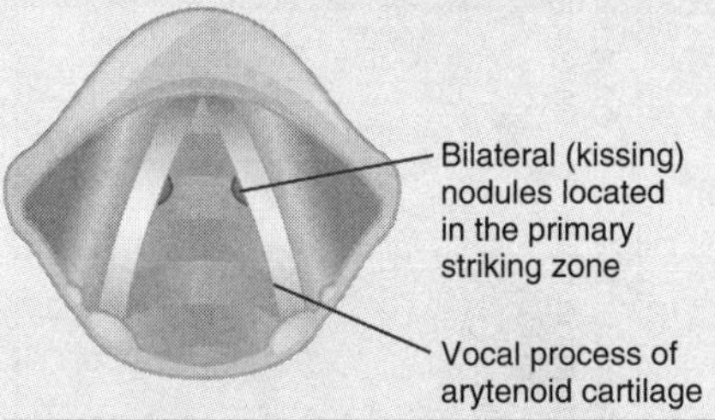

Lesions in the cover of the vocal fold usually develop in the primary striking zone due to the increased friction at this point of maximum lateral excursion and medial contact.

Data from Zemlin, 1998.

Table A2-1 Vocal Symptoms in the Absence of Laryngeal Pathology

Laryngeal Diagnosis	Anatomical/ Physiological Changes	Etiology	Typical Symptoms	Potential Treatments
Idiopathic/unknown	• None visible	• Manner of phonation • Idiopathic • Voice problem usually begins gradually and worsens over time	• Roughness • Breathiness • Stridency • Intermittent aphonia • Reduced pitch and loudness range(s) • Strain • Vocal fatigue • Deterioration of voice quality with prolonged use	• Voice therapy to reduce effort to facilitate easy manner of phonation • Minimize risk factors
Counterproductive Compensation and muscle tension dysphonia	• Absence of laryngeal pathology	• Idiopathic • May be response to sudden or gradual deterioration of voice quality	• Extraneous muscles activity in head, neck, and thorax • Excessive or limited expira-tory drive • Pressed phonation • Abrupt initiati on of phonation • Roughness • Breathiness • Stridency • Intermittent aphonia • Reduced pitch range • Inappropriate loudness	• Voice therapy to reduce effort to facilitate easy manner of phonation • Minimize risk factors

Plicae ventricularis	• Phonation produced by adducting and vibrating the ventricular folds	• Idiopathic • May be learned behavior • Possible compensation for damage to true vocal fold (paralyzed or paretic vocal fold)	• Low pitch • Roughness • Diplophonia • Breathiness • Reduced loudness • Reduced pitch and loudness range(s) • Strain	• Voice therapy to reduce effort to facilitate easy manner of phonation • Ventricular phonation may be an appropriate compensation when normal vocal fold vibration is not possible • Minimize risk factors
Paradoxical vocal fold motion	• Vocal folds adduct involuntarily during inspiration and block airflow through the glottis • Adduction of the anterior two-thirds of vocal folds with diamond-shaped chink in the posterior glottis	• Idiopathic • May be learned behavior • Reflux can exacerbate the symptoms • Induced by exercise • Induced by irritants • Often misdiagnosed as asthma	• Symptoms are usually frightening to the patient and those around them • Often occurs during sports or exertion • Dyspnea • Wheezing on inhalation • Inhalatory stridor • Tightness in the throat • Cough	• Anti-anxiety medication • Anti-reflux medication • Respiratory procedures to normalize breathing • Movement-stretching, relaxation techniques • Increase awareness of warning signs • Reduction of throat clearing and coughing • Intubation or tracheotomy in rare cases • Minimize risk factors

Data from: Angsuwarangsee & Morrison, 2002; Aronson & Bless, 2009; Boone, McFarlane, Von Berg, & Zraick, 2010; Colton, Casper, & Leonard, 2011; Ferrand, 2012; Hicks, Brugman, & Katial, 2008; Morris, Perkins & Allan, 2006; van Houtte, van Lierde, & Clayes, 2011; Vertigan, Gibson, Theodoro, & Winkworth, 2007.

Lesions Restricted to Vocal Fold Cover

Many laryngeal pathologies that develop within the cover of the vocal folds are associated with excessive expiratory drive and hyperadduction of the vocal folds. The high resistance offered by the vocal folds against an elevated subglottal pressure represents an effortful and counterproductive manner of phonation. The high expiratory drive results in excessive lateral excursions and medial compression of the vocal folds during each glottal pulse and over time contributes to irritation, inflammation, and even the development of a lesion. The laryngeal pathologies described in **Table A2-2** typically occur in the cover (i.e., epithelium and superficial layer of the lamina propria).

Lesions Affecting Cover, Transition, and Body

The presence of a laryngeal pathology that crosses all layers of the larynx may threaten not only voice quality but the general health of the patient (see **Table A2-3**). A laryngeal web, stenosis, or cancer of the larynx may compromise the airway, causing shortness of breath and extreme anxiety or even panic in association with air hunger. In order to sustain life, the treatment of choice may be surgical, but given the natural tendency for the patient to introduce counterproductive strategies during the development of these problems, voice therapy to stabilize manner of phonation and minimize these behaviors is appropriate when the life-threatening situation is resolved.

Lesions Affecting the Body of the Vocal Fold

Atrophy, or deconditioning, of the body of the vocal fold (vocalis muscle) may be a result of aging (presbyphonia) or a neurological problem (e.g., vocal fold paralysis, Parkinson's disease). These conditions may be progressive (e.g., dysarthria, glottal insufficiency) and require a joint approach that includes surgery, laryngeal injections, or medications in conjunction with voice therapy to minimize the development of counterproductive strategies to cope with the condition (see **Table A2-4**). Under these circumstances the goal of voice rehabilitation is the facilitation of the most efficient manner of phonation considering the limitations imposed by these anatomical and physiological changes. These conditions are often accompanied by dysphagia and changes in respiration, articulation, and resonance. As is the case with all voice problems, the changes associated with aging and neurological challenges may have a profound impact on your patient's capacity to function in his vocation and social milieu.

Table A2-2 Lesions Restricted to the Vocal Fold Cover

Laryngeal Diagnosis	Anatomical/Physiological Changes	Etiology	Typical Symptoms	Potential Treatments
Edema/ swelling	• Swelling and stiffening located on the medial edge of the midmembranous portion of vocal folds • Swelling may extend along the length of the membranous portion of the fold	• Manner of phonation • Effort during speaking or singing for prolonged periods may produce inflammation and swelling of vocal fold cover • Usually begins as a localized swelling in the primary striking zone • Swelling may abate and the vocal folds may well return to normal • If effortful phonation continues and the folds remain swollen, anatomic changes may develop	• Roughness • Breathiness • Voice and pitch breaks • Reduced pitch and loudness range(s)	• Voice therapy to reduce effort to facilitate easy manner of phonation • Modified voice rest • Increase hydration • Minimize risk factors
Ectasia	• Proliferation of tortuous blood vessels	• Phonotrauma • Vocal fatigue • Anticoagulants • Hormone therapy • Reflux	• Loss of pitch range • Roughness • Minimize risk factors	• Voice rest • Voice therapy to reduce effort to facilitate easy manner of phonation • Increase hydration • Avoidance of anticoagulants • Cessation of hormone therapy and/or contraceptive medications • Anti-reflux medication • Surgery • Minimize risk factors

(*continues*)

Table A2-2 Lesions Restricted to the Vocal Fold Cover (*continued*)

Laryngeal Diagnosis	Anatomical/Physiological Changes	Etiology	Typical Symptoms	Potential Treatments
Varix	• Prominent dilated vein or blood vessels • Rupture of vein	• Phonotrauma • Vocal fatigue • Anticoagulant • Hormone therapy • Reflux	• Loss of pitch range • Roughness	• Voice rest • Voice therapy to reduce effort to facilitate easy manner of phonation • Increase hydration • Avoid anticoagulants • Cessation of hormone therapy and/or contraceptive medications • Anti-reflux medication • Surgery • Minimize risk factors
Hyperemia or hemorrhage	• Collection of blood may stiffen the vocal fold cover at the location of a hemorrhage • May spread (bleed into) to a larger area	• Manner of phonation • Effortful phonation may rupture the delicate blood vessels in the vocal fold and it may bleed into the cover of the vocal fold • A bruise may develop when the vocal folds strike each other with excessive force during shouting, loud singing, or effortful coughing • Permanent scarring is possible with continued effort and abrupt contact	• Roughness • Breathiness • Pain (at time of pre-cipitating event) • Intermittent aphonia • Reduced pitch and loudness range(s)	• Voice rest • Voice therapy to reduce effort to facilitate easy manner of phonation • With reduction in effort vocal fold heals and the blood is carried away as debris • Minimize risk factors

Vocal fold nodule(s)	• Located on medial edge of midmembranous portion of vocal folds • Benign unilateral or bilateral callous-like, fibrous mass that stiffens the cover of the fold • Typically starts as a soft, unilateral swollen area in the primary striking zone and develops into well-defined, firm, callous-like growth	• Manner of phonation • Effort during speaking or singing for prolonged periods may produce inflammation and swelling of the cover that transforms into a nodule • Friction between the folds may contribute to development of a contact lesion on the opposite fold	• Roughness • Breathiness • Stridency • Abrupt initiation of phonation • Pressed phonation • Intermittent aphonia • Reduced pitch and loudness range(s) • Vocal fatigue • Deterioration of voice quality with prolonged speaking • Lump in the throat	• Voice therapy to reduce effort to facilitate easy manner of phonation • Surgical removal • Minimize risk factors
Sessile or pedunculated vocal fold polyp	• Fluid-filled sac located on medial edge of midmembranous portion of vocal fold, which stiffens the cover of the fold • With bleeding, stiffness may develop in vocal fold cover • Sessile (broad based, fluid-filled sac) • Pedunculated (fluid-filled sac hanging by a thin stem)	• Manner of phonation • Prolonged effortful phonation may thicken the cover of the folds • Left untreated the irritation may develop into polypoid degeneration of the larynx (Reinke's edema)	• Roughness • Breathiness • Intermittent aphonia • Reduced pitch and loudness range(s) (sessile polyp) • Voice breaks (pedunculated polyp) • Lump in the throat	• Surgical removal • Voice therapy to reduce effort to facilitate easy manner of phonation • Minimize risk factors

(*continues*)

Table A2-2 Lesions Restricted to the Vocal Fold Cover (*continued*)

Laryngeal Diagnosis	Anatomical/ Physiological Changes	Etiology	Typical Symptoms	Potential Treatments
Reinke's edema	• Swelling in the superficial layer of lamina propria • Translucent, gelatinous lesion that may extend along the length of the membranous portion of the vocal fold, bilaterally	• Manner of phonation (prolonged, effortful phonation) may thicken the cover of the folds • Chronic smoking • Gastroesophageal reflux • Hormonal changes (hypothyroidism) • With prolonged and continuous effort the cover may thicken and change permanently	• Lowered pitch • Roughness • Breathiness • Stridency • Intermittent aphonia • Reduced pitch range • Shortness of breath (with narrowing of the airway)	• Surgical removal • Voice therapy to reduce effort to facilitate easy manner of phonation • Minimize risk factors
Epidermoid cyst	• Fluid contained within a closed membranous sac • May occur deeper near the vocal ligament • Usually sessile (broad base) • May protrude into vibratory margin of vocal folds and increase vocal fold stiffness • When the membrane forms it becomes difficult for the fluid to reabsorb	• Phonotrauma • LPR • Upper respiratory tract infection • May be congenital or acquired	• Roughness • Breathiness • Vocal fatigue • Intermittent aphonia • Reduced pitch range	• Surgery • Voice therapy to reduce possible contribution of effort to development of cyst • Minimize risk factors

Papilloma	• Wart-like thickening and growth may occur at any point on the vocal fold and can spread throughout the airway • Stiffens the cover of the fold(s)	• Exposure to the human papilloma virus (HPV) • Often recur following surgical removal	• Roughness • Pressed phonation • Lower than customary pitch • Reduced pitch range • Reduced loudness • Strain	• Microlaryngeal surgical or carbon dioxide laser removal of the growth • Anti-viral medications • Voice therapy to reduce possible contribution of effortful use of voice • Cessation of smoking • Anti-reflux diet • Minimize risk factors
Nonspecific granuloma or contact ulcer	• Ulceration of the tissue covering the vocal processes of the arytenoid cartilages • The body protects the area by forming granuloma tissue to cover the lesion (ulcer)	• Intubation • Reflux • Excessive rocking and grinding together of arytenoid cartilages associated with low-pitched phonation and extreme vocal intensity • Persistent abrupt initiation of phonation • Chronic throat clearing, forceful coughing, uncontrolled reflux, or effortful manner of phonation	• Roughness • Breathiness • Pressed phonation • Abrupt initiation of phonation • Excessively low pitch • Vocal fatigue • Pain reflected to ear	• Microsurgery or carbon dioxide laser removal of the ulcer • Voice therapy to facilitate easy manner of phonation • Confidential voice • Anti-reflux diet • Minimize risk factors

(*continues*)

Table A2-2 Lesions Restricted to the Vocal Fold Cover (*continued*)

Laryngeal Diagnosis	Anatomical/ Physiological Changes	Etiology	Typical Symptoms	Potential Treatments
Sulcus vocalis	• Groove, furrow, depression with stiffening along the medial margin of the vocal fold(s) • Furrow may extend from part to full length of vocal fold • May be unilateral or bilateral	• Etiology and history of development of the sulcus is unclear • May be congenital • May develop when a cyst ruptures • May develop as a result of poor healing following a hemorrhage • May be associated with counter-productive manner of phonation	• Roughness • Breathiness • Intermittent aphonia • Higher than normal pitch	• Surgical transplantation of autologous fat or injection of other bulking substance (e.g., collagen) • Voice therapy to reduce effort to facilitate easy manner of phonation • Minimize risk factors
Leukoplakia	• Thickened, white, plaque-like lesions on mucosal surface of the vocal folds • May vary in extent and location on the vocal fold • Can spread throughout the airway • At risk for development of carcinoma	• Cause is unknown • May be associated with tobacco and alcohol use • Reflux • Genetic predisposition	• Roughness • Breathiness • Stridency • Intermittent aphonia • Reduced pitch and loudness range(s)	• Voice therapy to reduce effort to facilitate easy manner of phonation • Cessation of smoking and alcohol consumption • Anti-reflux diet • Minimize risk factors

Data from Aronson & Bless, 2009; Boone, McFarlane, Von Berg, & Zraick, 2010; Colton, Casper, & Leonard, 2011; Ferrand, 2012; Fried & Ferlito, 2009; Hirano, 1981; Nemecek, 2009.

Table A2-3 Lesions Affecting the Cover, Transition, and Body of the Vocal Fold

Laryngeal Diagnosis	Anatomical/Physiological Changes	Etiology	Typical Symptoms	Potential Treatments
Vocal fold scar	• Scar may occur at any point on the vocal fold • Stiff, disorganized tissue, decreased visco-elasticity around the scar, and decreased mucosal wave	• Sequelae to vocal fold surgery • A ruptured cyst or surgical removal of a growth may lead to scarring	• Roughness • Breathiness • Stridency • Intermittent aphonia • Reduced pitch and loudness ranges • Diplophonia	• Surgical removal of scar • Voice therapy to reduce effort and facilitate easy manner of phonation • Minimize risk factors
Laryngeal or subglottic stenosis	• Injury to epithelial lining of airway • Constriction or narrowing of the airway between the glottis and first tracheal ring • Abnormal growth of tissue	• Can be congenital or acquired • Irritation from laryngeal trauma (intubation) • Radiotherapy • Inhalation of foreign body	• Inhalatory or exhalatory stridor • Shortness of breath • Roughness • Breathiness • Stridency • Cough	• Surgical removal of foreign body • Anti-inflammatory medications • May require tracheotomy • Voice therapy to reduce effort and facilitate easy manner of phonation • Minimize risk factors
Laryngeal web	• Excessive, pliant or stiff tissue located on the medial edge of the vocal folds extending across the glottis	• Congenital laryngeal stenosis/atresia • Congenital webs develop during the seventh and eighth weeks of gestation and may be the result of genetic mutations or incomplete maturation of the developing larynx • Laryngeal trauma (intubation)	• Inhalatory or exhalatory stridor • Roughness • Shortness of breath • Higher than typical pitch	• Surgical removal of thin webs with endoscopic laser or serial dilations • Thicker webs may require more aggressive surgery • Voice therapy to reduce effort and facilitate easy manner of phonation • Minimize risk factors

(*continues*)

Table A2-3 Lesions Affecting the Cover, Transition, and Body of the Vocal Fold (*continued*)

Laryngeal Diagnosis	Anatomical/Physiological Changes	Etiology	Typical Symptoms	Potential Treatments
Epithelial hyperplasia and dysplasia (precancerous conditions)	• Precancerous lesions of the mucosa or lesions that penetrate into the intermediate and deep layers of the lamina propria • Irregular thickening and darkening of the vocal fold mucosa • Can spread throughout the airway	• Chronic laryngeal irritation • Alcohol consumption • Smoking • Exposure to irritants and fumes • Chronic reflux • Manner of phonation • Minimize risk factors	• Inhalatory stridor • Chronic roughness • Cough • Sore throat • Pain radiating to the ear	• Surgical removal of the lesions • Radiotherapy • Cessation of smoking and consumption of alcohol • Avoidance of irritants • Treatment to reduce reflux • Voice therapy to reduce effort and facilitate easy manner of phonation
Carcinoma	• Irregular thickening and cancerous overgrowth of vocal fold tissue • Most laryngeal cancers are squamous cell carcinomas • Develops at the anterior or posterior commissures • Can be glottal, subglottal, or supraglottal • Tumors may invade deep structures	• Smoking • Alcohol consumption • Combined effect of smoking and drinking alcohol • Minimize risk factors	• Inhalatory and/or exhalatory stridor • Shortness of breath • Roughness • Breathiness • Stridency • Intermittent aphonia • Reduced vocal pitch and loudness range(s) • Dysphagia	• Surgical removal of cancerous tissue • Chemotherapy • Radiotherapy • Voice therapy following treatment to develop compensatory strategies • Dysphagia treatment • Minimize risk factors

Carcinoma with subsequent partial laryngectomy	• A tracheostomy is constructed to maintain the airway • Tracheostomy tube is removed, stoma closes, phonation is reestablished	• Cancer of the larynx	• Possible aphonia • Intermittent aphonia • Roughness • Breathiness • Reduced pitch and loudness range(s) • Breathing may be temporarily compromised • Dysphagia may occur and require treatment	• Goal of surgery is to preserve essential functions of larynx • Conservation surgery limited to the epiglottis or part of one vocal fold • Primary limiting factors for surgery are the size and location of the lesion and the need to protect the airway • Voice therapy following treatment to develop compensatory strategies • Dysphagia treatment • Minimize risk factors
Carcinoma with subsequent total laryngectomy	• Results in separation of the digestive tract from the airway and complete blockage of airflow from the lungs to the mouth and nose • Creation of a permanent tracheostomy allows the patient to breathe through an opening in the neck (stoma) • Breathe, sneeze, yawn, sigh, and laugh through the stoma		• Aphonia	• The larynx is removed due to advanced cancer to preserve life • May be performed when patients have severe, unmanageable dysphagia • Surgical construction of a tracheoesophageal puncture with placement of a prosthetic, one-way air valve that directs air from the lungs through the vocal tract • Electrolarynx produces an electronic sound source • Esophageal voice therapy: esophageal speech is produced by volitionally injecting air into the esophagus and then releasing it • Minimize risk factors

(*continues*)

Table A2-3 Lesions Affecting the Cover, Transition, and Body of the Vocal Fold (*continued*)

Laryngeal Diagnosis	Anatomical/Physiological Changes	Etiology	Typical Symptoms	Potential Treatments
Carcinoma with post radiotherapy damage or fibrosis	• Tissues in larynx, neck, lower face, and upper thorax become firm, fibrotic, and stiff in response to radiotherapy	• Radiotherapy to prevent metastasis • Radiotherapy may be used as a stand-alone treatment prior to surgery to shrink a tumor, or as a postoperative treatment to destroy any remaining cancer cells	• Roughness • Breathiness • Stridency • Intermittent aphonia • Reduced pitch and loudness range(s) • Dysphagia	• Voice therapy to reduce effort and facilitate easy manner of phonation • Dysphagia therapy • Minimize risk factors

Data from Aronson & Bless, 2009; Boone, McFarlane, Von Berg, & Zraick, 2010; Colton, Casper, & Leonard, 2011; Ferrand, 2012; Fried & Ferlito, 2009; Nemecek, 2009.

Table A2-4 Lesions Affecting the Body of Vocal Fold

Laryngeal Diagnosis	Anatomical/Physiological Changes	Etiology	Typical Symptoms	Potential Treatments
Glottal insufficiency (bowed vocal folds)	• Low tone in the vocal fold(s) results in weakness in the membranous portion of the fold • Muscular atrophy	• Aging • Parkinson's disease • Atrophy of the vocalis muscle	• Roughness • Breathiness • Stridency • Intermittent aphonia • Monopitch • Monoloudness • Strain • Variable speech rate (Parkinson's disease) • Aspiration (dysphagia)	• Surgical medialization of vocal fold • Vocal fold implants • Voice therapy to reduce effort and facilitate easy manner of phonation • Dysphagia therapy • Minimize risk factors
Vocal fold(s) paresis or paralysis	• Reduced adduction and abduction of one or both vocal folds • Vocal fold(s) flaccidity	• Damage or trauma to the recurrent laryngeal nerve (possible side effect of cardiac and thyroid surgery, tumor, etc.) • Often nerve will regenerate and re-establish movement of the fold • Viral infection • Neurological conditions (stroke, ALS, etc.)	• Roughness • Breathiness • Intermittent aphonia • Reduced pitch and loudness range(s) • Shortness of breath • Hyperventilation • Dizziness • Weak, ineffective cough increases risk of aspiration and pooling of saliva in pyriform sinuses • Insufficient glottal closure resulting in difficulty protecting the airway during swallow	• Spontaneous recovery is possible • Surgical reconstruction of nerve • Surgical medialization of vocal fold • Voice therapy to reduce effort and improve closure of glottis • Dysphagia therapy • In rare cases, permanent, complete, bilateral paralysis may require drastic measures such as a total laryngectomy to protect the airway • Minimize risk factors

(*continues*)

Table A2-4 Lesions Affecting the Body of Vocal Fold (*continued*)

Laryngeal Diagnosis	Anatomical/Physiological Changes	Etiology	Typical Symptoms	Potential Treatments
Laryngeal dystonia AKA Adductor spasmodic dysphonia and Abductor spasmodic dysphonia	• Involuntary adduction or abduction of both vocal folds during customary speech	• Neurological disorder	• Short-term variations in severity of the symptoms but overall severity stabilizes • Action induced (symptoms noticeable when the individual talks in his customary manner) • Symptoms diminish with sensory tricks **Adductor SD** • Strained-strangled voice • Roughness • Intermittent aphonia **Abductor SD** • Breathy voice breaks • Intermittent aphonia • Reduced loudness • Roughness • Breathiness	• Injections of BoNT • Voice therapy to reduce effort and facilitate easy manner of phonation **Sensory Tricks** • Speak on inhalation • Speak at higher or lower pitch • Speak with unfamiliar accent • Speak while laughing or yawning

Tremor	• Involuntary oscillatory movements of the larynx, head, jaw, lips, tongue, pharynx, or diaphragm	• Hereditary factors • Parkinson's disease • Essential tremor • Ataxia • Dystonia • Alcoholism • Neuropathy	• Oscillations in the pitch and loudness of the voice due to tremor in head, jaw, larynx, or diaphragm • Symptoms worsen under stress or fatigue **Resting Tremor** • Parkinson's disease • Occurs during quiet breathing and often disappears during phonation **Postural Tremor** (e.g., Essential tremor) • Occurs during sustained vowels (singing, maximum phonation time maneuver, glissando) **Kinetic Tremor** • Occurs during customary speech **Idiopathic Dystonic Tremor** • Irregular tremor • Usually action induced	• Voice therapy to reduce effort and facilitate easy manner of phonation • Increase speed of articulation to camouflage symptoms • Increase pitch to mask the oscillations • Medication • Minimize risk factors

(*continues*)

Table A2-4 Lesions Affecting the Body of Vocal Fold (*continued*)

Laryngeal Diagnosis	Anatomical/Physiological Changes	Etiology	Typical Symptoms	Potential Treatments
Dysarthria	• Impairment in motor control of laryngeal structures • Muscle weakness • Changes in muscle tone • Involuntary movements	• Flaccid dysarthria • Spastic dysarthria • Ataxic dysarthria • Hypokinetic dysarthria • Hyperkinetic dysarthria • Mixed dysarthria	• Symptoms depend on underlying neurological disorder, but can be remarkably similar at the onset of the disorder • Roughness • Breathiness • Imprecise articulation • Slowed speech rate • Decreased intelligibility • Dysphagia is common	• Medications or surgery to minimize symptoms • Voice therapy to reduce effort and facilitate easy manner of phonation • Minimize risk factors

Data from Aronson & Bless, 2009; Boone, McFarlane, Von Berg, & Zraick, 2010; Colton, Casper, & Leonard, 2011; Ferrand, 2012; Fried & Ferlito, 2009; Nemecek, 2009.

Problems Affecting the Laryngeal Joints

The larynx contains two major joints that have widely different functions: the cricoarytenoid joint and the cricothyroid joint. The bilateral cricoarytenoid joints are adjusted by two sets of muscles that allow the arytenoid cartilage to pivot and move laterally to abduct and medially to adduct the vocal folds. Damage to one or both cricoarytenoid joints results in decreased adduction or abduction of the vocal folds. The interarytenoid muscles regulate the strength of the vocal fold adduction and the lateral cricoarytenoids support adduction. Decrease in the adductory forces may result in breathiness, reduced loudness, or even aphonia (see **Table A2-5**).

Damage to the cricothyroid joint results primarily in difficulty changing pitch but can also limit loudness inflection. When the cricothyroid muscle contracts it moves the cricothyroid joint and passively stiffens and lengthens the vocal folds, thus raising the pitch. If the range of motion of the joint is restricted, difficulty lengthening and stiffening the vocal fold results in restricted pitch ranges, especially notable during singing.

The underlying problem, whether it is inflammatory (autoimmune disease), reflux, infection, or blunt trauma, may require collaboration with a team of professionals. Voice therapy is relevant to minimize inappropriate vocal behaviors and maximize voice production.

Presbyphonia

With aging, normal changes occur in the structures of the larynx. The voice may continue to meet the individual's needs, however, if he maintains an easy, efficient, and effective manner of phonation (see **Table A2-6**). Both males and females experience these changes, but males tend to exhibit more significant changes than females. For both genders, the layers of the lamina propria become stiffer, less elastic, and thinner, resulting in a diminished mucosal wave and atrophy of the vocalis muscle, which may contribute to bowing and insufficient closure of the glottis. In addition, cartilage ossifies and becomes stiffer and heavier.

Summary

Our voice rehabilitation plan reflects our understanding of the underlying physiology of voice production. Voice problems may emerge with or without a laryngeal pathology or prolonged, inappropriate manner of phonation, in response to systemic medical conditions (e.g., arthritis, cancer, neurological disease), or aging. These conditions may be associated with

Table A2-5 Problems Affecting the Laryngeal Joints

Laryngeal Diagnosis	Anatomical/Physiological Changes	Etiology	Typical Symptoms	Potential Treatments
Ankylosis of cricoarytenoid joint	• Decreased adduction and/or abduction of vocal folds • Upper airway obstruction with respiratory restrictions	• Rheumatoid arthritis • Crohn's disease • Systemic lupus • Reiter's syndrome • Erythema • Strep infection	• Symptoms develop as underlying disease progresses • Nocturnal stridor, stridor on exertion • Air hunger • Breathy voice breaks • Intermittent aphonia • Roughness • Reduced pitch and loudness range(s) • Aspiration • Aspiration pneumonia • Pain	• Anti-inflammatory and analgesic medications, and antibiotics • Surgery • Injections of fat or other substance to approximate the vocal folds • Voice therapy to reduce effort and facilitate easy manner of phonation • Use abrupt onset to increase adductory force • Speak on inhalation • Minimize risk factors
Intubation-related joint fixation	• Decreased adduction or abduction of vocal folds • Upper airway obstruction with respiratory restrictions	• Arytenoid cartilage is dislocated from the cricoarytenoid joint during intubation • Vocal folds do not adduct or abduct following intubation	• Nocturnal stridor, stridor on exertion • Breathy voice breaks • Intermittent aphonia • Roughness • Breathiness • Reduced pitch and loudness range(s) • Aspiration • Pneumonia	• Surgery to restore the cartilage to appropriate alignment and location • Minimize risk factors

Data from Aronson & Bless, 2009; Boone, McFarlane, Von Berg, & Zraick, 2010; Colton, Casper, & Leonard, 2011; Ferrand, 2012; Fried & Ferlito, 2009; Nemecek, 2009.

Table A2-6 Normal Vocal Changes Associated with Aging

Laryngeal Diagnosis	Anatomical/Physiological Changes	Etiology	Typical Symptoms	Potential Treatments
Presbyphonia (aging)	• The vocal folds thin and atrophy • Lamina propria becomes edematous and thicker • Hyaline cartilage ossifies, becomes heavier and less compliant • Laryngeal joints may stiffen • Decreased elasticity of the respiratory system	• Aging	• Reduced loudness inflection and projection • Limited vocal endurance • Lowering of fundamental frequency in women • Elevation of fundamental frequency in men • Breathy voice breaks • Roughness • Breathiness • Reduced control and range of singing (tremolo, wobble, bleat) • Diminished vital capacity	• Voice therapy to reduce effort and facilitate easy manner of phonation • Minimize risk factors

Data from Aronson & Bless, 2009; Boone, McFarlane, Von Berg, & Zraick, 2010; Colton, Casper, & Leonard, 2011; Ferrand, 2012; Fried & Ferlito, 2009; Nemecek, 2009.

changes in the underlying anatomy and physiology of the vocal fold or may reflect general changes in the body. Planning for treatment requires an understanding of the relationship among voice, anatomy and physiology of the vocal folds, and the overall health of the individual.

References

Angsuwarangsee, T., and Morrison, M. (2002). Extrinsic laryngeal muscular tension in patients with voice disorders. *Journal of Voice*, 16, 333–343.

Aronson, A.E., and Bless, D. (2009). *Clinical voice disorders: An interdisciplinary approach*. New York, NY: Thieme.

Boone, D.R., McFarlane, S.C., Von Berg, S.L., and Zraick, R.I. (2010). *The voice and voice therapy* (8th ed.). Upper Saddle River, NJ: Pearson.

Colton, R., Casper, J.K., and Leonard, R. (2011). *Understanding voice problems: A physiological perspective for diagnosis and treatment* (4th ed.). Baltimore, MD: Lippincott Williams and Wilkins.

Ferrand, C.T. (2012). *Voice disorders: Scope of theory and practice*. Boston, MA: Pearson Higher Education.

Fried, M.P., and Ferlito, A. (2009). *The larynx* (3rd ed., Vol. 2). San Diego, CA: Plural.

Hicks, M., Brugman, S.M., and Katial, R. (2008). Vocal cord dysfunction/paradoxical vocal fold motion. *Primary Care and Clinical Office Practice*, 35, 81–103.

Hirano, M. (1981). *Clinical examination of voice*. New York, NY: Springer-Verlage.

Hochman, I., Sataloff, R.T., Hillman, R.E., and Zeitels, S.M. (1999). Ectasias and varices of the vocal fold: Clearing the striking zone. *Annals of Otology, Rhinology and Laryngology*, 108(1), 10–16.

Morris, M.J., Perkins, P.J., and Allan, P.F. (2006). Vocal cord dysfunction: Etiologies and treatment. *Clinical Pulmonary Medicine*, 13, 73–86.

Nemecek, O. (2009). *Laryngeal diseases: Symptoms, diagnosis and treatments*. Hauppauge, NY: Nova Science.

Nishizawa, N., Sawashima, M., & Yonemoto, K. (1988). Vocal fold length in vocal pitch change. In: O. Fujimura (Ed.), *Vocal fold physiology: Voice production, mechanisms and functions* (pp. 75–82). New York: Raven Press.

Sappey, P.C. (1872). *Traité d'anatomie descriptive*. Paris: Delahaye.

Titze, I.R. (2006). *The myoelastic aerodynamic theory of phonation*. Iowa City, Iowa: National Center for Voice and Speech.

van Houtte, E., van Lierde, K., and Clayes, S. (2011). Pathophysiology and treatment of muscle tension dysphonia: A review of the current knowledge. *Journal of Voice*, 25, 202–207.

Vertigan, A.E., Gibson, P.G., Theodoror, D.G., and Winkworth, A.L. (2007). A review of voice and upper airway function in chronic cough and paradoxical cord movement. *Current Opinions in Allergy and Clinical Immunology*, 7, 37–42.

Zemlin, W.R. (1998). *Speech and hearing science: Anatomy and physiology* (4th ed.). Needham Heights, MA: Allyn and Bacon.

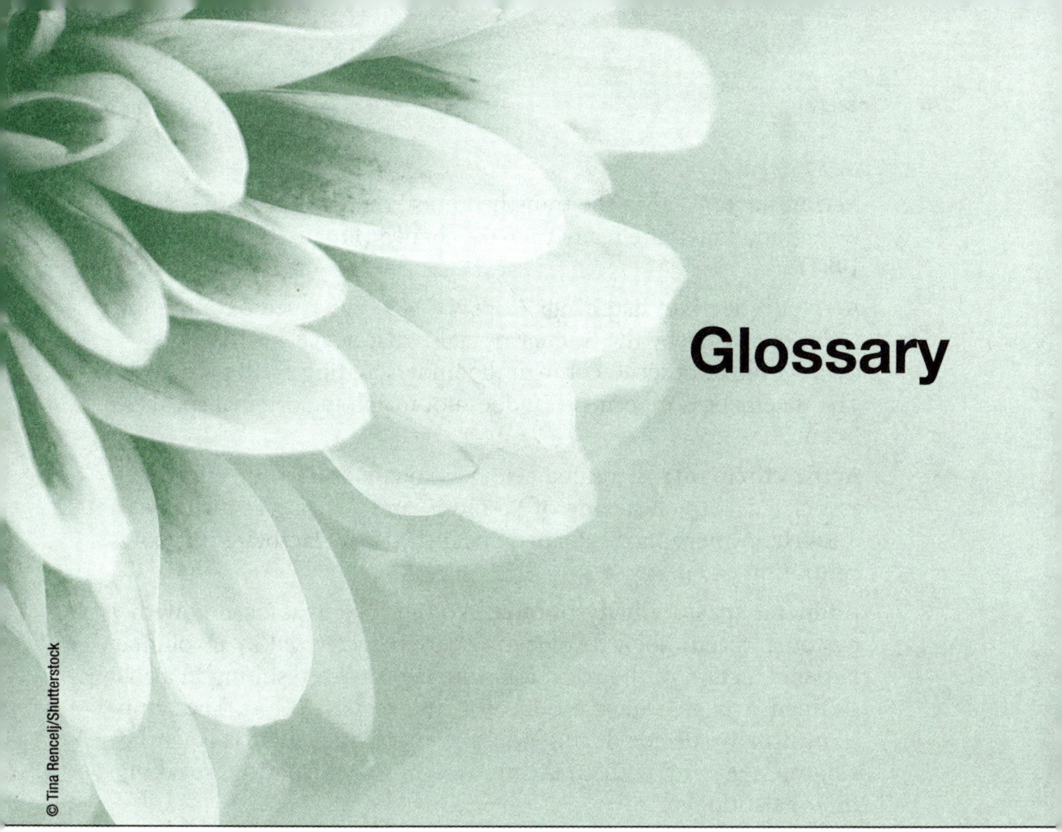

Glossary

Abductor spasmodic dysphonia: Voice problem associated with dystonia, a neurological disorder, characterized by involuntary abduction of the vocal folds during speech resulting in a weak, breathy voice. The symptoms usually diminish during nonspeech activities such as laughing, singing, speaking with an accent, coughing, whispering, speaking on inhalation, etc.

Abrupt onset of phonation: Sudden, forceful initiation of phonation associated with complete closure of the glottis and blockage of airflow prior to the initiation of phonation.

Accurate empathy (evocative empathy): The clinician's appreciation of the patient's perspective and experience of the (voice) problem.

Acoustic analysis: Instrumental measurement of frequency, intensity, and duration of sound.

Acoustic energy: Transmission of energy associated with the compression and rarefaction of air molecules.

Action stage: Within the transtheoretical model (TTM), the phase when individuals are ready to make change (Prochaska & DiClemente, 1984).

Active (reflective) listening: Rogers (1959) described a counseling technique whereby the listener restates what he has heard in his own words in order to confirm the understanding of all participants. The statement is modified if it does not match the original speaker's intent.

Actor's formant: A trained actor's resonant voice projection is associated with clustering of F_4 and F_5 and a strong acoustic peak at 3.5 kHz. A megaphone-shaped vocal tract may facilitate this concentration of energy.

Adductor spasmodic dysphonia: Voice problem associated with dystonia, a neurological voice disorder characterized by involuntary hyperadduction of the vocal folds during speech resulting in a rough, strained-strangled voice produced with excessive effort. The symptoms usually subside during nonspeech activities such as laughing, singing, speaking with an accent, coughing, whispering, speaking on inhalation, etc.

Adherence: In voice therapy, following through with recommendations for treatment (e.g., practice, attending scheduled appointments).

Aerodynamic assessment: The process of measuring air pressure and flow during phonation onset and ongoing vocal productions.

Alexander technique: A technique designed to facilitate alignment of the spine and avoid unnecessary levels of muscular stiffness and mental tension during everyday activities.

Ambivalence: These feelings emerge with all voice patients as they progress through the various stages of voice rehabilitation. The trans speaker often experiences conflicting emotions during voice modification as he or she works to achieve a credible voice.

Aphonia: Involuntary cessation of voice in response to interruption in the vibration of the vocal folds.

ASHA's Principles of Ethics: A charge from the American Speech-Language-Hearing Association that calls for the members of the association to recognize that other cultures are valuable and should be honored and respected.

Assessment: The evaluation and estimation of the etiology, development, symptoms, severity, and prognosis for remediation of a voice disorder.

Attend to: Conscious attention to the sensations of phonation or resonance.

Auditory feedback: Listening to the sound of the voice.

Back pressure: Within a narrow tube (e.g., vocal tract), an obstruction produces resistance in response to the flow of the fluid.

Back pressure exercise: In voice rehabilitation, a technique that creates a semi-occluded vocal tract and increases resistance in the supraglottal space (can be achieved with /mhm/ or straw phonation, etc.).

Behavioral voice therapy: In voice treatment, it is a focus on the learned behaviors that contribute to the voice disorder. These behaviors may be activated by environmental challenges.

Bernoulli effect: In the case of an ideal fluid, as velocity of fluid flow increases, pressure decreases, so long as the total energy remains constant. Pressure is perpendicular to the direction of flow. (Zemlin, 1998).

Biomedical model: A framework used by many physicians and healthcare workers that focuses exclusively on the physical or biological aspects of medical treatment and views the physician as the authority on the presenting problem.

Blocked practice: Drill that emphasizes repetition and consistency before variation is introduced.

Botulinum toxin (BoNT): The bacterium *Clostridium botulinum* manufactures a protein neurotoxin that may cause botulism poisoning, a serious and life-threatening illness in humans and animals. A purified and titrated version of this toxin is injected into specific muscles to chemically block the flow of neural impulses causing a chemically induced weakening of the strength of contraction of the selected muscles.

Breath control: Conscious regulation of the flow of air to slow the exhalation phase during speaking or singing.

Breath group: An utterance produced during one breath.

Call technique: Refers to the train conductor's call, "All aboard," which capitalizes on the resonating properties of the vocal tract to project the voice efficiently and effectively (Lessac, 1997).

Checking action: The continued engagement of the muscles of inhalation to slow the exhalation phase.

Chest voice: Describes the lower notes of the vocal range; it is associated with the sympathetic vibrations resonated in the chest. Chest resonance is encouraged in the male trans speaker.

Chronic obstructive pulmonary disease (COPD): General term for a group of progressive respiratory problems that result in persistent shortness of breath, poor airflow, cough, increased mucus production, and a wet vocal quality.

Client-centered approach (patient-centered approach): Carl Rogers (1946, 1951) described a method used in treatment to improve adherence by recognizing a patient's insight and capacity to take responsibility in the decision-making process of therapy.

Clinician-directed format: A treatment plan that is conceived and directed by the therapist.

Closed-loop theory: A cognitive theory proposed by Adams (1971) that uses feedback to describe the acquisition of motor skills.

Cognition: The use of executive function, reasoning, judging, and remembering.

Cognitive work: The intellectual resources recruited to perform a function.

Congruence: In transitions associated with gender, an abstract term that suggests a state of similarity or concordance of the internal gender and the external manifestations of that gender.

Contemplation stage: In the transtheoretical model (TTM) (Prochaska & DiClemente, 1984), this phase signals the patient's awareness and deliberation about a problem, but not a decision to take action.

Cooperative learning: A group dynamic that encourages participants' joint learning through discussion, development of strategies and possible outcomes. The clinician's role is to facilitate rather than control.

Counterproductive compensation: An ineffective, possibly detrimental behavior, that is used consciously or unconsciously to cope with negative physiological challenges.

Cricothyroid muscle: Intrinsic laryngeal muscle that attaches to the cricoid cartilage and the thyroid cartilage. Contraction of this muscle tilts the thyroid cartilage forward to stretch and stiffen the thyroarytenoid muscle and modify pitch.

Cultural humility: Belief that all societies and communities are valuable and equal (Tervalon & Murray-Garcia, 1998).

Decision-making process: In voice treatment, a process by which the clinician and patient choose a course of action for the rehabilitation program.

Degrees of freedom: The number of independent ways a dynamic system can move without violating the inherent limitations of the system.

Deliberate practice: Ericsson, Krampe, and Tesch-Romer (1993) proposed that simply repeating a motor act in a drill-like fashion does not result in skilled performance. A motor skill improves with thoughtful attention and consideration of individual movements during practice.

Diagnostic hypothesis: Logical statement pertaining to a possible cause.

Diagnostic impression: In voice therapy, a concise description of the voice problem and its etiology, prognosis, and management plan.

Diagnostic therapy: In voice treatment, trial therapy to assess the patient's response to exercises introduced by the clinician.

Disease-oriented approach: A medical model that relies on experts to make decisions.

Dystonia: A neurological disorder manifested by involuntary muscle contractions that are usually action induced. The movements are large enough to move a body part.

Ease/easy: In voice treatment, the production of voice without strain or effort.

Effective voice: A voice that meets one's needs.

Efficiency: The ratio of the output of a system to the input.

Emotional-physiological state: The biological arousal experienced in response to stimuli.

Empathy: To appreciate or identify with another individual's feelings.

Empirical observation: A process whereby information is acquired through observation.

Epilarynx: A space in the vocal tract immediately above the larynx. Also known as the aryepiglottic space, it can be narrowed by the muscles that surround it. When narrowed sufficiently, it becomes a high-frequency resonator.

Evidence-based practice: The interaction of (1) clinical expertise and experience, (2) scientific evidence, (3) client/patient and caregiver perspectives to provide high-quality care. A treatment approach that relies primarily on qualitative research studies to make decisions about the efficacy of treatment.

Excessive laryngeal valving: Effortful adduction of the vocal folds to produce grunts, coughs, and throat clearing that may irritate the laryngeal mucosa.

Exhalation: The flow of breath from the body.

Expiratory reserve volume: Air remaining in the lungs following a normal exhalation. This air can be exhaled by contracting the expiratory muscles.

Extraneous muscle activity: Unnecessary stiffness or movement that occurs in conjunction with voice production. Usually involves structures in the head, neck, and thorax.

Falsetto: The highest of the vocal registers, produced with very thin vocal folds.

Feels: In voice therapy, the awareness of the sensations related to resonance, the difference between ease and effort, postural alignment, etc.

Feldenkrais Method: A somatic educational system designed to reduce pain or limitations in movement, improve physical function, and promote well-being by increasing kinesthetic and proprioceptive self-awareness of functional movement (Nelson & Blades-Zeller, 2002).

Focal dystonia: Dystonia that affects a single body part (e.g., focal laryngeal dystonia/spasmodic dystonia).

Forced vital capacity: The maximum volume of air that can be exhaled following a maximum inhalation.

Formant: A concentration of acoustic energy around a particular frequency in the speech wave.

Formant tuning: Manipulating the shape and configuration of the vocal tract to concentrate the acoustic energy at specific frequencies in order to amplify sound (Sundberg, 1970).

Freedom to act: A physical state of relaxation that exists between the body's most lax position and its stiffest resulting in an efficient use of the musculature (Lessac, 1997).

Freeway space: Small opening between the upper and lower teeth (Fenn, Liddelow, & Gimson, 1961).

Fundamental frequency: The lowest frequency of vibration of the vocal folds and the slowest frequency of a quasi-periodic waveform.

Gastroesophageal reflux disease (GERD): Chronic symptoms or mucosal damage resulting from abnormal backflow of stomach fluids into the esophagus.

Gender-acceptable pitch range: Adler, Hirsch, and Mordaunt (2012) suggest that a speaking fundamental frequency between 150 to 185 Hz is acceptable for the female voice.

Generalized dystonia: A neurological disorder that begins in childhood and affects the entire body.

Generalized motor program: Within Schmidt's schema theory (1975a), the generalized motor program is an abstract representation of the order, relative timing, and force of movements.

Glissando: The vocal ascent and descent of a musical scale.

Group therapy: In voice, a form of treatment where a small group of patients and a group leader meet regularly to integrate and generalize the strategies and techniques developed in the individual sessions.

Head voice: Refers to the upper part of the vocal range and is produced with a light registration, but is supported, unlike pure falsetto. The trans female speaker is encouraged to rely on head resonance to produce voice in an easy, effortless, and effective manner.

Hierarchy: In voice therapy, a system of goals and procedures ranked one above another based upon complexity.

Hypopharyngeal space: An anatomical section of the airway extending from the esophageal inlet (lower margin of the cricoid cartilage) to the oropharynx (hyoid bone).

Hypothesis development: The process of integrating empirical observation with theory and one's fund of knowledge.

Hypothesis-driven therapy: Treatment that relies upon hypothesis development and testing.

Inertance: The impeding effect of the sluggishness of the air molecules on the transmission of sound through a tube.

Inertia: Newton's third law of motion: the tendency of a body at rest to remain at rest, or when in motion to continue that motion, unless acted upon by an external force.

Inhalation: The flow of air into an organism.

Initiation of phonation: The onset of voicing associated with vocal fold vibration.

Inspiratory checking: Deliberate reduction in the alveolar pressure and airflow from the lungs as a result of engagement of the primary muscles of inhalation.

Inspiratory reserve: Additional air that can be inhaled following a tidal inhalation.

Intermittent aphonia: Momentary breaks in phonation.

Internal assessment: One's personal consideration of the appropriateness of manner of phonation.

Intervention process: The plan for remediation that includes one's hypothesis, goals, and procedures.

Kinesthetic awareness: The body's sense of its relative position in space and time.

Ladder Exercise: In voice therapy, a procedure that exploits the resonating properties of the vocal tract to increase loudness and projection.

Laryngopharyngeal reflux (LPR): Known as silent reflux due to absence of heartburn for most people; gastric acid that enters the pharyngeal area and comes into contact with the posterior larynx.

Learning theory: Conceptual frameworks that explain the process of acquiring and retaining motor or cognitive information.

Less effort: In voice treatment, less demand and strain on the subsystems of voice production.

Listen: In voice, listening refers to the perception of the voice solely through the acoustic information received by the ears. Voice patients often emphasize the importance of the auditory signal, ignoring the kinesthetic feedback central to the modification of effort.

Lombard effect: Unconscious tendency to increase vocal intensity when speaking in noisy environments.

Loudness control: In voice therapy, the subjective regulation of vocal intensity is practiced and monitored through sensory feedback.

Loudness inflection: Refers to the modification in vocal intensity necessary to cope with varying communication intent and environment.

Lung capacities: Cubic capacity of the respiratory mechanism.

Lung volume: The quantity of air in the lungs.

Maintenance stage: In the transtheoretical model (TTM) (Prochaska & DiClemente, 1984), a stage during which the changes made by the patient become consolidated.

Mandibular freedom: In voice production, rigidity in the jaw and surrounding areas may negatively affect voice production during speech or singing. Reduction of stiffness in the jaw often facilitates an easier manner of phonation.

Manner of phonation: The skill with which the subsystems of voice production (respiration, phonation, resonation, articulation) are balanced to produce voice. This may be easy, efficient, and effective, or effortful.

Mask: The area of the face surrounding the eyes, nose, and mouth. Singers are often directed to sing in the mask in order to maximize resonance.

Mastery experience: The skilled performance of a behavior or task. Bandura (1986) proposed that the best way to enhance one's sense of self-efficacy is through the achievement of proficiency.

Maximum phonation time: A clinical measurement of the longest phonatory duration of a vowel or consonant.

Medial compression of vocal folds: The strength with which the membranous portion of the vocal folds touch during the closed portion of the vibratory cycle. The contact is determined by several factors, including the adduction of the arytenoid cartilages, the expiratory drive, the manner of voice onset, and the coordination of the vocal subsystems.

Memory trace: In motor learning theory Schmidt (1975a) suggests that following a skilled movement an imprint of the motor act remains. When a motor act is repeated, the imprint becomes stronger.

Mental practice: Gabriele, Hall, and Lee (1989) suggest that a memory trace can be developed or strengthened when an individual visualizes or imagines performing a motor act.

Messa di voce: An increase and decrease of vocal intensity on a single pitch.

Meta-discussion: An analysis of a discussion.

Model: In voice therapy, a vocal stimulus produced by the clinician to be imitated by the patient.

Modification: In voice rehabilitation, a measurable change that occurs during voice production or the management of risk factors.

Motivational interviewing (MI): A directive, client-centered counseling style for eliciting changes in behavior through the exploration and resolution of ambivalence (Rollnick & Miller, 1995).

Motor archetype: Schmidt (1975a, 1975b) proposed that learned movements are formed in memory through the accumulation and refinement of memory traces that identify shared rules for programming the timing, sequence, and strength of performance.

Motor learning theory: Schmidt and Lee (2011) attribute the acquisition of a skilled movement to deliberate repetition of a motor act.

Motor program: A theoretical (conceptual) or actual neural, hard-wired organization that serves to organize and constrain the degrees of freedom of a system.

Muscle tension dysphonia: Voice is produced with excessive laryngeal effort, stiffness, and/or expiratory drive in the absence of a laryngeal pathology.

Myoelastic-aerodynamic theory of voice production: Vocal fold vibration is a result of the interaction of muscular, elastic recoil, and aerodynamic forces (Muller, 1843; van den Berg, 1958).

Open-loop theory: A cognitive theory proposed by Adams in 1971 to describe a motor control system with preprogrammed instruction that does not use feedback.

Pascal's law: Pressure applied within a closed structure is transmitted throughout the structure.

Passaggio: The area of transition between vocal registers.

Patient-centered therapy: Carl Rogers (1951) introduced a philosophy of therapy that emphasizes the patient's capacity to make decisions and solve problems. It recognizes and values the patient's knowledge and experience of the illness, and includes the patient as a partner in the process of change.

Pear-shape technique: Titze and Verdolini-Abbott (2012) describe two breathing styles used by singers to support the breath: pear-shape up (high stable thorax) and pear-shape down (lower abdominal-diaphragmatic control).

Peer feedback: In group therapy, feedback is shared between participants.

Peer support: In group therapy, participants may share experiences, emotional responses, ways to practice, or strategies to cope with challenging (vocal) situations.

Phonation: The production of a quasi-periodic vibration at the level of the vocal folds resulting in the production of sound.

Physiological empathy: In voice therapy, a clinician and patient use careful observation and kinesthetic awareness to create a vicarious experience of a motor act and to modify the patient's effortful manner of phonation.

Physiological framework: In voice therapy, the clinician's reliance on an understanding of the underlying physiology of the voice problem to develop an appropriate management plan.

Physiological model: In voice therapy, a treatment plan based on integrating empirical observation with an understanding of normal anatomy and physiology.

Physiology of respiration: The movement of air that takes place as a result of the underlying functions of the lungs and chest wall.

Pitch break: Sudden, involuntary shift in pitch.

Pleural linkage: The mechanism by which the lungs are "linked" to the thoracic wall, allowing movements of the chest wall to be transmitted to the lungs.

Positive regard: Carl Rogers (1951) introduced the concept of unconditional acceptance and support of the patient.

Pragmatics: In voice therapy, the use of pitch, inflection, vocabulary, gestures, facial expression, and other verbal and nonverbal communication.

Precontemplation stage: In the transtheoretical model (TTM), the phase when the patient is either unaware of an existing problem or, despite awareness, is uninterested in making change (Prochaska & DiClemente, 1984).

Preoperative voice therapy: Voice rehabilitation services that are provided prior to laryngeal surgery.

Preparation stage: In the transtheoretical model (TTM), this phase represents a time when the patient plans to take action within the foreseeable future, but has not yet initiated action (Prochaska & DiClemente, 1984).

Primary striking zone: Refers to the middle of the membranous portion of the vocal fold. The strongest collision forces are believed to take place in this region (Hochman, Sataloff, Hillman, & Zeitels, 1999).

Procedural memory: Verdolini (2000a) suggests that motor patterns are developed without conscious awareness, but require attention, repeated practice, and sensory attention.

Professional voice user: The reliance on the vocal mechanism to fulfill the demands of one's profession (singers, actors, ministers, lawyers, speech-language pathologists, etc.).

Prognosis: In voice treatment, a prediction of the likely outcome of therapy.

Proprioceptive feedback: Refers to one's awareness of posture, movement, and changes in equilibrium.

Prototype: An original representation from which others evolve.

Psychotherapy: A treatment involving verbal interaction with a psychiatrist, psychologist, or other mental health provider to address mental, emotional, and adjustment problems.

Quiet tidal volume (QTV): The amount of air inhaled and exhaled during quiet breathing.

Random practice: In voice therapy, practice might include varying factors such as the phonemic context, cognitive and linguistic complexity, conversation partners, and communication environment while incorporating a specific vocal technique (Sherwood & Lee, 2011).

Recall schema: Schmidt and Lee (2011) proposed that repetition of a motor act builds a representation of the motor program. The recall schema is used to program a motor act.

Recognition schema: Schmidt and Lee (2011) proposed that repetition of a motor act builds a template of the motor program. The recognition schema is used to evaluate and monitor the efficiency and accuracy of a movement.

Reflux (backflow): A flowing back; a process of refluxing. Within the context of swallowing it refers to the flow of food or stomach contents back into the esophagus, pharynx, larynx, and/or mouth, usually associated with relaxation of the lower esophageal sphincter.

Reflux Symptom Index (RSI): Questionnaire probing the types and degree of severity of patient-perceived symptoms of reflux in the aerodigestive tract (Belafsky, Postma, & Koufman, 2002).

Rehabilitation hypothesis: In voice therapy, a rehabilitation hypothesis is used to develop and test theories that propose to facilitate an appropriate manner of phonation.

Relaxation pressure: Intrapulmonic pressure due to tissue elasticity, torque, gravity, and intra-abdominal pressure (Zemlin, 1998).

Reliability: The extent to which a procedure produces the same results on repeated trials. The consistency of the patient's response.

Resistance: Resistance and drag as air passes through a tube; pressure opposing airflow; back pressure.

Resonance: Dynamic changes in the shape and configuration of the vocal tract that create resonant frequencies in the vocal tract and allow for the differentiation of speech sounds.

Resonant voice: Term used to describe a voice produced with the least possible muscular effort and lowest possible collision forces between the vocal folds; the resistance by which the vocal tract assists the sound source in producing acoustic energy (Titze & Verdolini-Abbott, 2012).

Resting expiratory level (REL)/resting lung volume (RLV): A state of equilibrium exists in the respiratory system at approximately 38% of vital capacity due to the coupling of the chest wall–lung unit. The exhalatory pull of the lungs is balanced by the inspiratory pull of the chest wall, and any movement away from REL requires muscular activity.

Retroflection of the tongue base: In an effort to widen the pharyngeal space and lift the soft palate a singer may inadvertently press the tongue base down during inspiration. This behavior may lead to tongue base tension and pressed phonation.

Risk factors: In voice, an activity or predisposition that increases the probability of developing a voice problem.

Schema theory: Schmidt and Lee (2011) proposed that motor learning occurs when a model that predetermines the order, strength, and duration of the contraction of the muscles is built in memory.

Self-efficacy: Belief in one's capacity to affect one's own behavior (Bandura & Adams, 1977).

Self-esteem: One's overall evaluation of his self-worth; contributes to the individual's adherence to voice rehabilitation and to one's self-efficacy.

Self-perception: The beliefs that one holds about oneself. Self-perception contributes to the individual's adherence to a regimen and to one's self-efficacy.

Self-regulation: The control of negative forces that interfere with perseverance.

Self-sustained oscillation: Titze (1994) postulated that a nonlinear, interactive source-filter that incorporates the inertive reactance of the vocal tract with the airflow and pressures at the level of the glottis facilitates self-sustained vibration of the vocal folds.

Semi-occluded maneuvers: Voice exercises that increase supraglottal pressure and decrease the transglottal pressure drop (Titze & Verdolini-Abbott, 2012).

Semi-occluded vocal tract: An increase in air pressure above the vocal folds due to a narrowing of the vocal tract. This increase in back pressure facilitates self-oscillation of the membranous portion of the vocal folds, thus reducing impact stress (Titze & Verdolini-Abbott, 2012).

Sensory awareness/feedback: In voice therapy, attention to and reliance on the resonating characteristics of the vocal tract.

Sensory trick: An idiosyncratic movement (e.g., touching the side of the face, pulling on the corner of the mouth, speaking in a higher pitch, speaking on inhalation) that temporarily interrupts the dystonia symptoms. Some individuals attain fleeting periods of near normal voice production when using a sensory trick, and may use it to briefly cope with the involuntary movements and postures associated with spasmodic dysphonia.

Simultaneous initiation of phonation: Coordinated adduction of the vocal folds to phonation neutral position with airflow to initiate phonation with an easy onset.

Source-filter theory: Speech production system consists of the sound source (vocal folds) and the filter or resonator (the vocal tract) (Fant, 1970).

Speaker's formant: In a trained actor's voice, projection is associated with clustering of acoustic energy at F_4 and F_5 and a strong acoustic peak at 3.5 kHz. May be related to an inverted megaphone-shaped vocal tract (Bele, 2006).

Subglottal pressure: Term used to describe the air pressure beneath the vocal folds.

Supraglottal pressure: Term used to describe the air pressure above the vocal folds.

S/Z ratio: Method to evaluate the relative duration of the maximum phonation of the phonemes /s/ and /z/. It is used to assess the integrity of glottal closure.

Tactile-kinesthetic feedback: In voice therapy, the attention to and reliance upon sensory feedback.

Temporomandibular joint dysfunction (TMJD): A general term describing pain, popping, or clicking in the temporomandibular joint and/or the muscles of mastication.

Tessitura: Refers to the *texture* of a song or role; the range within which the majority of the pitches lie; the tessitura of a song may or may not match the tessitura of a voice.

Theoretical framework: When considering voice problems we use theory to frame the processes of voice assessment and treatment.

Therapeutic hypothesis: Logical statement regarding a possible course of treatment including ways to test the effectiveness of the proposed treatment.

Thyroarytenoid muscle: The paired thyroarytenoid muscle is attached to the thyroid and arytenoid cartilages and forms the body of the vocal fold. It shortens the vocal folds.

Timbre: The color or tone of the voice provided by the harmonic overtones.

Tongue base: The posterior one-third portion of the tongue.

Tongue base stiffness: Excessive rigidity, firmness, and inflexibility in the posterior one-third of the tongue.

Tongue height: Distance that the tongue is elevated toward the roof of the mouth.

Transglottal pressure differential/Transglottal pressure drop: Reduction in air pressure as air flows across the glottis. When a vowel is articulated, the transglottal pressure differential is similar to the subglottal pressure, but when a constriction occurs to produce a consonant the supraglottal pressure is elevated and the transglottal pressure differential diminishes. Zemlin (1998) provides the following formulae to calculate the transglottal pressure differential (subglottal pressure – supraglottal pressure = transglottal pressure differential).

Transtheoretical model (TTM): Prochaska and DiClemente (1984) developed a model to identify and classify an individual's readiness for change and provided strategies to facilitate that change.

Tremor: A rhythmic oscillation around a central point. Voice tremor results in changes in pitch and loudness.

Unified Spasmodic Dysphonia Rating Scale (USDRS): A rating scale developed to identify the severity and symptoms associated with spasmodic dysphonia (Stewart et al., 1997).

Up-speech: A characteristic feature of some regional dialects of American English that use a rising pitch at the end of a declarative statement.

Validity: The extent to which a tool measures the intended variable.

Velopharyngeal competence: Adequate closure of the velopharyngeal port by elevation of the soft palate and constriction of the posterior pharyngeal wall. All consonants in American English except /m/, /n/, and /ŋ/ are produced with a closed velopharyngeal port.

Verbal persuasion: The attempt to encourage, convince, or influence an individual that your perspective, knowledge, or assumption is correct. This strategy is usually not effective.

Vertical laryngeal height: The height of the larynx in the neck.

Vibrato: The regular and relatively even pattern of oscillation above and below a pitch; a 4 to 6 Hz undulation of frequency and amplitude is considered to be within normal limits. A healthy vibrato adds richness and depth to the tone of the singing voice.

Vicarious experience: Bandura (1986) proposed that self-efficacy improves when we observe others perform a task.

Virilization: In voice, virilization describes an unwanted lowering of the female pitch.

Vital capacity: The quantity of air that can be exhaled after a maximum inhalation.

Vocal athlete: The elite singer and actor whose voice is capable of negotiating extreme pitch and loudness ranges without effort and with great artistic beauty.

Vocal fry (pulse register): A manner of vocal fold vibration by which the fundamental frequency is low enough to hear the individual pulse (vibration). Produced with flaccid vocal folds and low airflow.

Vocal longevity: The stamina and endurance necessary to produce a voice that will last and meet one's needs throughout a lifetime (Titze & Verdolini Abbott, 2012).

Vocal tract: The airway between the glottis and the lips.

Vocalise: A vocal exercise.

Voice Evaluation Form: A form that structures the voice evaluation process.

Voice problem: A voice disturbance that is associated with an inappropriate manner of phonation. The voice no longer meets the individual's professional, social, and emotional needs.

Voice rehabilitation: The process by which an appropriate manner of phonation is developed and generalized to the individual's activities of daily living.

Voice rest: A period of silence following laryngeal surgery when an individual does not speak or sing.

Whisper: Sound produced without vocal fold vibration.

Xerostomia: Dryness in the mouth that may be associated with medication, Sjögren's syndrome, radiation therapy, or idiopathic origins.

Y-Buzz: A physiological training to increase kinesthetic awareness and facilitate resonance and vocal intensity with efficiency of vocal fold vibration; the development of the voice and the body in a holistic way that results in greater power and flexibility (Lessac, 1997).

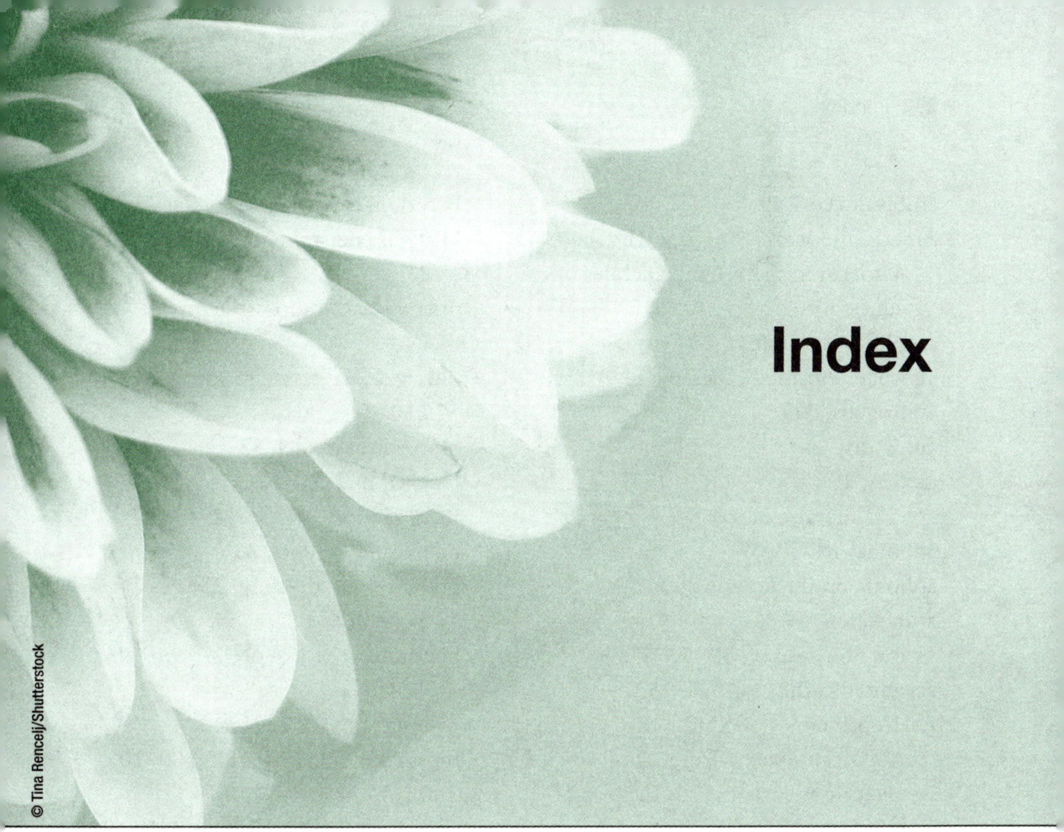

Index

Note: Page numbers followed by b, f, or t indicate materials in boxes, figures, or tables respectively.

A

H

I

J

K

L

M

Q

R

W

X

Y

Z